Sedation and Anesthesia of Zoological Companion Animals

Editors

MIRANDA J. SADAR
JOÃO BRANDÃO

VETERINARY CLINICS OF NORTH AMERICA: EXOTIC ANIMAL PRACTICE

www.vetexotic.theclinics.com

Consulting Editor
JÖRG MAYER

January 2022 • Volume 25 • Number 1

ELSEVIER

1600 John F. Kennedy Boulevard • Suite 1800 • Philadelphia, Pennsylvania, 19103-2899
http://www.vetexotic.theclinics.com

VETERINARY CLINICS OF NORTH AMERICA: EXOTIC ANIMAL PRACTICE Volume 25, Number 1
January 2022 ISSN 1094-9194, ISBN-13: 978-0-323-89676-4

Editor: Stacy Eastman
Developmental Editor: Axell Ivan Jade M. Purificacion

Veterinary Clinics of North America: Exotic Animal Practice (ISSN 1094-9194) is published in January, May, and September by Elsevier, Inc., 360 Park Avenue South, New York, NY 10010-1710. Subscription prices are $296.00 per year for US individuals, $697.00 per year for US institutions, $100.00 per year for US students and residents, $345.00 per year for Canadian individuals, $707.00 per year for Canadian institutions, $359.00 per year for international individuals, $707.00 per year for international institutions, $100.00 per year Canadian students/residents, and $165.00 per year for international students/residents. To receive student/resident rate, orders must be accompanied by name of affiliated institution, date of term, and the *signature* of program/residency coordinator on institution letterhead. Orders will be billed at individual rate until proof of status is received. Foreign air speed delivery is included in all *Clinics* subscription prices. All prices are subject to change without notice. **POSTMASTER:** Send address changes to *Veterinary Clinics of North America: Exotic Animal Practice*, Elsevier Health Sciences Division, Subscription Customer Service, 3251 Riverport Lane, Maryland Heights, MO 63043. **Customer Service: Telephone: 1-800-654-2452** (U.S. and Canada); **1-314-447-8871** (outside U.S. and Canada). **Fax: 1-314-447-8029. E-mail: journalscustomerservice-usa@ elsevier.com (for print support); journalsonlinesupport-usa@elsevier.com (for online support).**

Reprints. For copies of 100 or more of articles in this publication, please contact the Commercial Reprints Department, Elsevier Inc., 360 Park Avenue South, New York, New York 10010-1710. Tel.: 212-633-3874; Fax: 212-633-3820; E-mail: reprints@elsevier.com.

Veterinary Clinics of North America: Exotic Animal Practice is covered in *MEDLINE/PubMed (Index Medicus)*.

Contributors

CONSULTING EDITOR

JÖRG MAYER, Dr med vet, MSc
Diplomate, American Board of Veterinary Practitioners (Exotic Companion Mammals); Diplomate, European College of Zoological Medicine (Small Mammals); Diplomate, American College of Zoological Medicine; Associate Professor of Zoological Medicine, Department of Small Animal Medicine and Surgery, University of Georgia College of Veterinary Medicine, Athens, Georgia, USA

EDITORS

MIRANDA J. SADAR, DVM
Diplomate, American College of Zoological Medicine; Assistant Professor, Avian, Exotic, and Zoological Medicine, College of Veterinary Medicine and Biomedical Sciences, Colorado State University, Fort Collins, Colorado, USA

JOÃO BRANDÃO, LMV, MS
Diplomate, European College of Zoological Medicine (Avian), EBVS® European Veterinary Specialist in Avian Medicine and Surgery, Associate Professor, Zoological Medicine, Debbie and Wayne Bell Professorship in Veterinary Clinical Sciences, College of Veterinary Medicine, Oklahoma State University, Stillwater, Oklahoma, USA

AUTHORS

CHIARA ADAMI, DMV, PhD, MRCVS
Diplomate, American College of Veterinary Anesthesia and Analgesia; Diplomate, European College of Veterinary Anesthesia and Analgesia; School of Veterinary Medicine, Louisiana State University, Baton Rouge, Louisiana, USA

DANIEL ALMEIDA, MV, MS
Diplomate, American College of Veterinary Anesthesia and Analgesia; Associate Professor, Veterinary Clinical Sciences, College of Veterinary Medicine, University of Minnesota, Saint Paul, Minnesota, USA

JULIE A. BALKO, VMD
Diplomate, American College of Veterinary Anesthesia and Analgesia; College of Veterinary Medicine, North Carolina State University, Raleigh, North Carolina, USA

KATARINA BENNETT, DVM
Diplomate, American Board of Veterinary Practitioners (ECM); Avian & Exotics Service, Bluepearl Emergency and Specialty Hospital, Sarasota, Florida, USA

SATHYA K. CHINNADURAI, DVM, MS
Diplomate, American College of Zoological Medicine; Diplomate, American College of Veterinary Anesthesia and Analgesia; Diplomate, American College of Animal Welfare;

Director of Animal Health, Department of Animal Health, Saint Louis Zoo, St Louis, Missouri, USA

INGA-CATALINA CRUZ BENEDETTI, DVM, MSc
Diplomate, European College of Veterinary Anesthesia and Analgesia; Assistant Professor of Anesthesiology and Pain Management, Department of Clinical Sciences, Faculty of Veterinary Medicine, Université de Montréal, Saint-Hyacinthe, Québec, Canada

ANDERSON F. DA CUNHA, DVM, MS
Diplomate, American College of Veterinary Anesthesia and Analgesia; College of Veterinary Medicine, Midwestern University, Glendale, Arizona, USA

CRISTINA DE MIGUEL GARCIA, DVM, MSc, MRCVS
Diplomate, European College of Veterinary Anesthesia and Analgesia; Clinical Fellow, Section of Anesthesiology and Pain Medicine, Department of Clinical Sciences, Cornell University College of Veterinary Medicine, Ithaca, New York, USA

NICOLA DI GIROLAMO, DVM, MSc(EBHC), PhD
Diplomate, European College of Zoological Medicine (Herp); Diplomate, American College of Zoological Medicine; Department of Veterinary Clinical Sciences, College of Veterinary Medicine, Oklahoma State University, Stillwater, Oklahoma, USA

PETER M. DIGERONIMO, VMD, MSc
Diplomate, American College of Zoological Medicine, Adventure Aquarium, Camden, New Jersey, USA; Animal & Bird Health Care Center, Cherry Hill, New Jersey, USA

GRAYSON DOSS, DVM
Diplomate, American College of Zoological Medicine; Clinical Assistant Professor, Zoological Medicine, Department of Surgical Sciences, School of Veterinary Medicine, University of Wisconsin-Madison, Madison, Wisconsin, USA

ANDRÉ ESCOBAR, DVM, MS, PhD
Diplomate, Brazilian College of Veterinary Anesthesia (Anesthesiology); Department of Clinical Sciences, Ross University School of Veterinary Medicine, Basseterre, St Kitts, West Indies

DAVID ESHAR, DVM
Diplomate, American Board of Veterinary Practitioners (ECM), Diplomate, European College of Zoological Medicine (SM & ZHM); Department of Clinical Sciences, Veterinary Health Center, Kansas State University College of Veterinary Medicine, Manhattan, Kansas, USA

TATIANA H. FERREIRA, DVM, MSc, PhD
Diplomate, American College of Veterinary Anesthesia and Analgesia; Department of Surgical Sciences, School of Veterinary Medicine, University of Wisconsin-Madison, Madison, Wisconsin, USA

SARA GARDHOUSE, DVM
Diplomate, American Board of Veterinary Practitioners (ECM); Diplomate, American College of Zoological Medicine; Department of Clinical Sciences, Kansas State University, Manhattan, Kansas, USA

MIKEL SABATER GONZÁLEZ, LV, CertZooMed, MRCVS
Diplomate, European College of Zoological Medicine (Avian); Uplands Way Vets Ltd, Norfolk, United Kingdom; Cambridge Veterinary Group, Cambridge, Cambridgeshire, United Kingdom

GREGG M. GRIFFENHAGEN, DVM, MS
Diplomate, American College of Veterinary Anesthesia and Analgesia; Department of Clinical Sciences, Colorado State University, Veterinary Teaching Hospital, Fort Collins, California, USA

MICHELLE G. HAWKINS, VMD
Diplomate, American Board of Veterinary Practitioners (Avian); Department of Medicine and Epidemiology and One Health Institute, School of Veterinary Medicine, University of California, Davis, California, USA

JAMES G. JOHNSON III, DVM, MS, CertAqV
Diplomate, American College of Zoological Medicine; Staff Veterinarian, Department of Animal Health, Saint Louis Zoo, St Louis, Missouri, USA; Adjunct Assistant Professor, Department of Veterinary Preventative Medicine, College of Veterinary Medicine, The Ohio State University, Columbus, Ohio, USA

NATHANIEL KAPALDO, DVM, MPH
Diplomate, American College of Veterinary Anesthesia and Analgesia; Department of Clinical Sciences, Veterinary Health Center, Kansas State University College of Veterinary Medicine, Manhattan, Kansas, USA

MARTIN KENNEDY, DVM
Diplomate, American College of Veterinary Anesthesia and Analgesia; Associate Professor, Veterinary Clinical Sciences, College of Veterinary Medicine, University of Minnesota, Saint Paul, Minnesota, USA

KERRIE LEWIS, DVM
Diplomate, American College of Veterinary Anesthesia and Analgesia; Pebble Creek Animal Hospital, Tampa, Florida, USA

CHRISTOPH MANS, Dr med vet
Diplomate, American College of Zoological Medicine; Department of Surgical Sciences, School of Veterinary Medicine, University of Wisconsin-Madison, Madison, Wisconsin, USA

CHRISTINE MOLTER, DVM
Diplomate, American College of Zoological Medicine; Animal Health Department, Houston Zoo, Inc., Houston, Texas, USA

ANDREA SANCHEZ, DVM, DVSc
Diplomate, American College of Veterinary Anesthesia and Analgesia; Department of Clinical Studies, Ontario Veterinary College, Ontario, Canada

STEFANIA SCARABELLI, DVM, MRCVS, Cert AVP (VA)
Diplomate, European College of Veterinary Anesthesia and Analgesia; Diplomate, American College of Veterinary Anesthesia and Analgesia; Clinica Veterinaria Malpensa-Anicura, Samarate, Varese, Italy

CARRIE SCHROEDER, DVM
Diplomate, American College of Veterinary Anesthesia and Analgesia; Department of Surgical Sciences, University of Wisconsin-Madison School of Veterinary Medicine, Madison, Wisconsin, USA

REZA SEDDIGHI, DVM, MS, PhD
Diplomate, American College of Veterinary Anesthesia and Analgesia; Professor, Large Animal Clinical Sciences, College of Veterinary Medicine, University of Tennessee, Knoxville, Tennessee, USA

JOE S. SMITH, DVM, MPS, PhD
Diplomate, American College of Veterinary Internal Medicine (Large Animal Internal Medicine); Diplomate, American College of Veterinary Clinical Pharmacology; Assistant Professor, Large Animal Clinical Sciences, College of Veterinary Medicine, University of Tennessee, Knoxville, Tennessee, USA

CLAIRE VERGNEAU-GROSSET, Dr méd vét, IPSAV, CES
Diplomate, American College of Zoological Medicine; Assistant Professor, Service de Médecine Zoologique, Clinical Sciences Department, Université de Montréal, Saint-Hyacinthe, Québec, Canada

ERIN WEND-HORNICKLE, DVM
Diplomate, American College of Veterinary Anesthesia and Analgesia; Associate Professor, Veterinary Clinical Sciences, College of Veterinary Medicine, University of Minnesota, Saint Paul, Minnesota, USA

Contents

Anesthetic drugs must be delivered at the appropriate dose and route of administration to produce the expected anesthetic effects. This is important for patient safety because anesthetic drugs function by depressing the central nervous and cardiovascular systems, which if improperly dosed or administered could cause potentially life-threatening effects. Several routes of administration and different drug delivery methods are available to safely and reliably anesthetize zoologic companion animal patients. Because of the nature of zoologic companion animal practice, anesthetic procedures pose risks that the anesthetist should understand to carefully plan procedures that are as safe and efficient as possible.

Veterinarians often need to sedate or anesthetize fish to perform physical examinations or other diagnostic procedures. Sedation may also be required to transport fish. Painful procedures require complete anesthesia with appropriate antinociceptive agents. Regulations and withdrawal times apply to food animal species in many countries. Specific protocols are therefore warranted in commercial fish versus ornamentals. Tonic immobility of elasmobranchs and electric anesthesia should never be used to perform painful procedures. Anesthetic monitoring in fish remains challenging. This review summarizes ornamental fish anesthesia and discusses techniques used in the commercial fish industry and in field conditions.

Amphibians commonly are managed under human care for research, education, conservation, and companionship and frequently are in need of sedation, anesthesia, or end-of-life care involving euthanasia. Objective investigation of sedative and anesthetic protocols in these taxa still is in its infancy, but knowledge of current best practices is paramount to appropriate care. Tricaine methanesulfonate delivered via immersion (bath) is the most common anesthetic agent in amphibians, but several other effective techniques have been identified. This summary provides a comprehensive review of the current evidence-based literature regarding amphibian sedative, anesthetic, and euthanasia techniques.

developed based on preexisting conditions, size, species, age, and estimated risk. Other key factors to improve safety, quality of perioperative
care, and client satisfaction are anticipation of complications, extension
of close monitoring to the recovery phase, multimodal analgesic approach,
stress prevention/reduction, and transparent communication with the
owner.

Despite anecdotal reports to the contrary, zoologic companion animals are unlikely to be more susceptible to the cardiotoxic effects of local anesthetics than domestic small animals. Local anesthetics can be clinically useful for analgesia and anesthesia in zoologic companion animal practice.

VETERINARY CLINICS OF NORTH AMERICA: EXOTIC ANIMAL PRACTICE

SERIES OF RELATED INTEREST

Veterinary Clinics of North America: Small Animal Practice
Available at: https://www.vetsmall.theclinics.com/

THE CLINICS ARE NOW AVAILABLE ONLINE!
Access your subscription at:
www.theclinics.com

Preface

Sedation and Anesthesia of Zoological Companion Animals

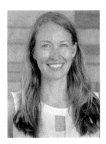
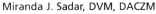
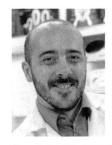

Miranda J. Sadar, DVM, DACZM   João Brandão, LMV, MS, DECZM (Avian)
Editors

Zoological companion animal (ZCA) medicine and surgery have made great strides in recent decades. The evolution of this specialty is a consequence of increased interest by the veterinary community and society to care for nontraditional species. Although still in its infancy in comparison to other areas of veterinary medicine, there is a great wealth of knowledge published in the scientific literature about ZCA species.

Two of the most common procedures performed by a clinician seeing ZCA species in practice are sedation and anesthesia. The use of sedation and anesthesia allows the clinician to perform other procedures in a safe manner, for the patient as well as for the veterinary staff involved. Although sedation and anesthesia are commonly performed, and essential to provide a high standard-of-care for these patients, the last *Veterinary Clinics of North America: Exotic Animal Practice* issue dedicated to anesthesia is now over 20 years old. Due to the vast amount of literature published since then and our special interests in decreasing stress for ZCA species, we were elated when presented with the opportunity to cover this important topic. We were thrilled to be able to bring so many of our highly esteemed colleagues together to assemble this issue. The issue contains a wealth of information that has been gathered and summarized by the authors to present clinically useful information for the veterinary community.

The Sedation and Anesthesia issue provides an up-to-date overview of sedation and anesthesia in ZCA species. The *Veterinary Clinics of North America: Exotic Animal Practice* issue is mostly organized by animal group. A great deal of attention was given to commonly and popular kept species, such as ferrets, rabbits, rodents, and reptiles, but we also wanted to include some of the more underrepresented groups and those that are gaining in popularity, such as fish, amphibians, backyard poultry, and miniature companion pigs. Each article focuses on specifics for the group or species that it covers, as well as refreshers on some of the basics of sedation and anesthesia. We wanted this issue to not only focus on safety for patients but also to cover considerations for veterinary personnel. To address this, an article dedicated to drug delivery and safety considerations was also included. In addition, as part of a multi-modal approach to anesthesia, we wanted to provide a summary on local and regional anesthetic options and techniques across taxonomic groups. We hope the readers will find these articles useful and will allow clinicians worldwide to provide the most current and highest quality of care possible.

We are so thankful to all the authors who contributed to this issue. When we set out to organize this issue, we sought the contribution of renowned veterinarians with expertise in both ZCA and sedation/anesthesia techniques. We are grateful to them for their time and for sharing their expertise in this area. We would also like to express our appreciation to Dr Jörg Mayer and all the staff at Elsevier for their support.

Miranda J. Sadar, DVM, DACZM
Avian, Exotic, and Zoological Medicine
College of Veterinary Medicine and
Biomedical Sciences
Colorado State University
300 West Drake Road
Fort Collins, CO 80523, USA

João Brandão, LMV, MS, DECZM (Avian)
Zoological Medicine
Bell Professorship in Veterinary Clinical Sciences
College of Veterinary Medicine
Oklahoma State University
2065 West Farm Road
Stillwater, OK 74078, USA

E-mail addresses:
miranda.sadar@colostate.edu (M.J. Sadar)
jbrandao@okstate.edu (J. Brandão)

Drug Delivery and Safety Considerations

James G. Johnson III, DVM, MS, CertAqV, DACZM[a,b,]*,
Sathya K. Chinnadurai, DVM, MS, DACZM, DACVAA, DACAW[a]

KEYWORDS

• Anesthesia • Drug delivery • Equipment • Monitoring • Safety • Sedation

KEY POINTS

- Appropriate anesthetic drug delivery is essential to produce expected anesthetic depth and physiologic effects, and provide for safer and more efficient procedures in zoologic companion animal patients.
- It is important to understand anesthetic drug delivery methods available and how to adapt anesthetic plans to the variety of patient species that may be encountered in zoologic companion animal practice.
- Different routes of administration for sedative and anesthetic drugs include oral, transmucosal, inhalational, topical/immersion, intramuscular injection, intravascular injection, or intraosseous injection.
- Reliable patient monitoring should be a part of any anesthetic plan, closely measuring the patient's physiologic and biochemical parameters, and being prepared to intervene to correct any discrepancies.
- Because zoologic companion animal patients may be anesthetized in a clinic or field setting, safety considerations should be carefully planned for, including any hazards associated with the patient based on species, anesthetic drugs, equipment, and environment where the procedure is to be performed.

INTRODUCTION

Sedation and anesthesia are routinely used in zoologic companion animal medicine to induce a temporary state of reduced or complete loss of awareness or sensation, allowing for comprehensive medical evaluation, diagnostic testing, and surgical or other therapeutic procedures. Many zoologic companion animal species, by nature, are predisposed to physiologic stress associated with handling for medical

[a] Department of Animal Health, Saint Louis Zoo, One Government Drive, St Louis, MO 63110, USA; [b] Department of Veterinary Preventative Medicine, College of Veterinary Medicine, The Ohio State University, Columbus, OH 43210, USA
* Corresponding author. Department of Animal Health, Saint Louis Zoo, One Government Drive, St Louis, MO 63110.
E-mail address: johnson.4013@gmail.com

Vet Clin Exot Anim 25 (2022) 1–11
https://doi.org/10.1016/j.cvex.2021.08.014   vetexotic.theclinics.com
1094-9194/22/© 2021 Elsevier Inc. All rights reserved.

procedures, making the use of sedative and anesthetic drugs particularly useful to reduce this stress. As such, sedatives and anesthetic drugs may allow for safer and more efficient procedures and eliminate the sensation of pain or discomfort, especially during painful procedures or surgery. Similar to the pharmacology of other drug classes, anesthetic drugs must be delivered at the appropriate dose, and by the proper route of administration, based on the drug's pharmacokinetics and pharmacodynamics to produce the expected sedative or anesthetic effects. Sedative and anesthetic drugs inherently function by depressing the cardiovascular and central nervous systems, resulting in more narrow safety margins than other pharmacotherapeutics, so reliable drug delivery is critical to the safety and success of any sedation or anesthesia in veterinary practice. Improper handling or delivery of sedative or anesthetic drugs can result in life-threatening complications for the patient or safety risks for the practitioner. In addition to the use of anesthetic drugs, it is important to understand drug delivery methods, and equipment and safety considerations, especially given the often variable nature of zoologic companion animal practice, either because of the patient species or nature of the specific anesthetized procedure.

DRUG DELIVERY METHODS
Oral and Transmucosal

Oral or transmucosal administration of anesthetic premedications or sedatives have been used in a variety of species and may be beneficial in stressed or fractious patients when injection may pose high risk to the patient or anesthetist.[1] Oral delivery is recommended only for premedication where small amounts of drug or drug combined with food are used because oral ingestion immediately before anesthesia can pose a risk for regurgitation and aspiration. Oral delivery of sedative drugs can result in more variable pharmacokinetics compared with intramuscular (IM) or intravenous (IV) delivery, possibly resulting in prolonged induction and recovery times.[1] This is especially true in poikilothermic animals, where metabolism is slower. Some drugs are delivered orally via transmucosal administration. Detomidine is an α_2-adrenergic agonist available in a transmucosal gel form and was recently shown to be effective for sedation of ferrets (*Mustela putorius furo*) for examination and venipuncture but with some side effects including piloerection in the tail, second-degree atrioventricular block in one animal, and hyperglycemia.[2] These side effects were successfully treated with administration of atipamezole, the antagonist agent for detomidine.[2] However, detomidine transmucosal gel was not found to be effective as a sedative in New Zealand white rabbits (*Oryctolagus cuniculus*) because of variable and unpredictable levels and duration of sedation.[3] Beyond transmucosal drug administration, oral benzodiazepines, phenothiazines, and α_2-adrenergic agonists have been used in a variety of species for sedation, including birds, miniature pigs, small carnivores, and nonhuman primates.[1]

Intranasal and Inhalational

The respiratory and olfactory mucosa of the nasal cavity have high vascularity and permeability, making the intranasal route of drug administration an effective and less invasive means of administering anesthetic drugs.[4] Patient factors affecting intranasal drug administration in zoologic companion animals include the size of the nares, thickness of the tissue membrane, nasal blood flow, nasal mucus production inhibiting vascular membrane contact, and mucociliary clearance.[4] Drug factors that may affect intranasal administration include lipophilicity of the compound, size of the molecule, and dissociation constant (pKa) of the drug. Sedative and anesthetic drugs that are effective in smaller volumes are best for intranasal administration to maximize mucosal contact and not overload the mucosal surface area in the nasal cavity. Administration of intranasal drugs is most effective using instruments, such as micropipettes, catheter tip syringes, syringes attached to a soft IV catheter, or atomizers to successfully introduce the drug through varying sized nares. The nasal cavity is generally lipophilic, so lipophilic drugs are ideal because they are best absorbed following intranasal administration.[4] A variety of sedative drugs, including midazolam, diazepam, butorphanol, morphine, ketamine, dexmedetomidine, and xylazine, have been used with varying success in a variety of avian, reptilian, and small mammal patients.[1,5–10] Intranasal administration of atipamezole has also been shown to effectively antagonize intranasally administered dexmedetomidine in several species.[5,6,9,11] In one study, intranasal administration of ketamine in rabbits in dorsal recumbency resulted in two fatalities with intranasal hemorrhage.[10] Chitosan, a polysaccharide compound derived from chitin that is nontoxic to the nasal mucosa, was shown to enhance absorption of xylazine and diazepam in budgerigars in one study.[12]

Inhalational anesthesia is frequently used for induction and maintenance of anesthesia. Isoflurane and sevoflurane are the most commonly used volatile inhalant gases and their use requires an anesthesia machine with a vaporizer, rebreathing or nonrebreathing circuit, and gas flow supplied by an oxygen tank. Inhalant anesthesia is administered via chamber induction, manual restraint with facemask, or via laryngeal mask or endotracheal intubation following induction. Induction chambers are purchased commercially, constructed, or created by placing a plastic bag around a crate containing the patient. Maintenance anesthesia is administered with inhalant gases by face mask, laryngeal mask, or endotracheal intubation (**Fig. 1**). It is important to ensure adequate seals around the facemask, laryngeal mask, or endotracheal tube to avoid exposure of personnel involved with the procedure to inhalant gases. Patients induced with gas in a chamber should be removed from the chamber quickly and the chamber should immediately be removed from the room and left open in a well-ventilated space, preferably outdoors. It is important to consider that anesthetic gas exposure is a significant occupational health hazard, especially when using anesthetic gases in patients via facemask or induction chamber.[13]

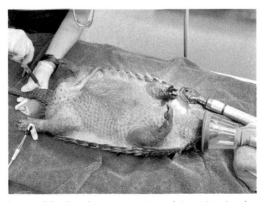

Fig. 1. A six-banded armadillo (*Euphractus sexcinctus*) is maintained under inhalant anesthesia using a tight-fitting facemask. Inhalant anesthesia administered via facemask is useful, especially in species that are challenging to intubate. (*Courtesy of* J. Johnson/Saint Louis Zoo)

Immersion or Topical

Immersion anesthesia is effectively inhalant anesthesia for fish and amphibian species, and is useful in species prone to stress or those difficult to manually restrain because of thick, slippery mucus on the skin.[1,14] Immersion anesthetics are typically dissolved in solution (eg, tank water) and buffered to a physiologic pH before exposure to the patient. When a fish is placed in the water containing the dissolved anesthetic, the anesthetic is ventilated, enters the circulation through the gills that are rich in capillary beds, and then the passes into the central nervous system.[14] This process of drug absorption is similar in amphibians, with absorption either through gills in some gilled species, such as axolotls (*Ambystoma mexicanum*), or through the capillary-rich skin of most others. Depth of sedation or anesthesia using immersion anesthetics is typically controlled by adjusting the drug concentration in the water either through additional buffered anesthetic drug to the water or diluting the anesthetic induction water with unmedicated water. When an animal is returned to unmedicated water for recovery, the circulating anesthetic drug is typically excreted through the skin or gills, although some elimination may occur through the kidneys.[14] It is important to maintain water chemistry parameters within optimal ranges for the species being anesthetized, including temperature, pH, and dissolved oxygen, and to ensure ammonia levels are minimized, especially during longer procedures.[14] Ammonia is more toxic in alkaline water and declining water quality during anesthetic procedures is mitigated using partial water changes during the procedure.[14] For procedures, such as surgery or wound care, which must be performed out of water, medicated water is continuously flushed over gills using a syringe or a water pump device and tubing for maintenance anesthesia (**Fig. 2**). Common agents for fish and amphibian immersion anesthesia include tricaine methanesulfonate (MS-222), metomidate, eugenol, clove oil, alfaxalone, and benzocaine.[14–16] When using immersion anesthetics, it is good practice to wear impervious examination gloves to protect the patient from any oils or compounds from the examiner's hands, and protect personnel from unnecessary exposure to anesthetic chemicals.

Anesthetic drugs can also be administered topically to the skin of amphibians. Terrestrial amphibians that may be at risk of drowning if completely immersed in

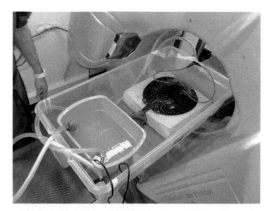

Fig. 2. Anesthetic maintenance and ventilation in an ocellate river stingray (*Potamotrygon motoro*) using a water pump and tubing to pass anesthetic water from the tub over the animal's gills. This stingray was undergoing a computed tomography scan and had to be maintained under anesthesia out of water for the procedure. (*Courtesy of J. Johnson/Zoo Miami*)

anesthetic water are placed in a shallow bath to contact the semipermeable skin on the ventrum. Completely aquatic amphibians are induced in a bath and maintained with topical anesthetic water applied to the skin, especially for a procedure that must occur out of water. For example, aquatic salamanders, such as hellbenders (*Cryptobranchus alleganiensis*), are safely and effectively maintained under anesthesia with MS-222 by applying medicated water over the skin using a syringe.[17] Concentrated liquid isoflurane is administered topically as an anesthetic. However, because of the volatile nature of the gas, it is usually mixed with gel, water, or an absorbent pad with plastic backing to increase contact time with the skin before the isoflurane evaporates.[15] Liquid isoflurane evaporates rapidly at room temperature and because anesthetic gases can pose occupational health hazards to anesthetists, use of liquid isoflurane should be performed in well-ventilated areas, such as a hood, or with proper personal protective equipment, such as a respirator. A recent study in American green tree frogs (*Hyla cinerea*) found that sevoflurane in jelly may be preferable compared with isoflurane jelly, because isoflurane jelly resulted in longer anesthetic recovery times and skin erythema.[18] Benzocaine has also been used for amphibian anesthesia; however, the powder form is poorly soluble in water and must be reconstituted with ethanol.[15] Alternatively, benzocaine is available in a commercial form of benzocaine (Orajel, Church and Dwight, Inc, Ewing Township, NJ) and is used in its original form or in solution.[15] Benzocaine has a narrow safety margin and may be more suitable for euthanasia rather than recovery anesthesia.[19] Caution should also be taken when using lidocaine-prilocaine topical cream (EMLA cream), because high mortality has been documented in anurans with its use.[19] Regardless of the method of topical anesthesia, it is important to keep the skin of amphibians moist at all times with either medicated or unmedicated water, depending on the depth of the patient.

Intramuscular Injection

IM anesthetic drug administration results in a slower onset of action than the IV route, but more predictable effects than orally administered sedatives. In general, drugs that are water-soluble are more completely and predictably absorbed after IM injection because the content of muscle tissue is generally water. Because many muscle bellies are in proximity to fat deposits, especially in overconditioned patients, care must be taken not to inject anesthetic drugs into fat because this may result in either no effects at all or blunted and prolonged effects and metabolism of drugs.

IM administration may be accomplished by a variety of methods. Hand-held injection using a needle and syringe is the most direct method to accurately administer IM drugs.[20] Hand-held injection requires cooperation or safe manual restraint of the patient.[1] When performing hand-held injections, it is helpful to use Luer-Lok syringes to avoid needle detachment.[20] Larger needles are useful to prevent the needle from breaking and more rapid administration of drugs; however, patient size should be considered when choosing the appropriate length and gauge to prevent injury to the patient.[1,20] With this method, there are risks of self-injection or drug aerosolization from broken syringes if the patient suddenly moves, so hand-held administration of ultrapotent anesthetic drugs is not recommended.[1,20]

Although not commonly performed for most "traditional" zoologic companion animals, IM administration of drugs can also be accomplished using pole syringes, which are similar to hand-held injections but with the added safety and convenience of a long pole, especially in uncooperative or dangerous patients.[1,20] Pole syringes are useful if an animal is contained in a squeeze cage or crate, and have the added benefit of administering the injection from a safer distance. Pole syringes are available as manual pressure models where the pole is an extension of the plunger, a modified manual pressure model where the extension pole is attached to the syringe and an internal extension depresses the plunger, or a model with a spring- or gas-loaded plunger that is triggered when the needle pierces the skin.[1,20] Similar to hand-held injections, pole syringes rely on rapid drug delivery through a large-gauge needle, either with committed manual pressure or with the assistance of mechanical pressure in the spring- or gas-loaded models, which are also helpful in larger animals with thicker tissue to penetrate.[20] It is important to also consider that there is risk with using a pole syringe in animals that could grab it and take it away, or animals that could bite the pole syringe.

Although uncommon, in unrestrained zoologic companion animals where pole syringing may be unsafe or unfeasible, the use of a dart and projector is a useful and practical method to administer anesthetic drugs (**Fig. 3**).[20] Multiple types of dart systems are available and specific descriptions are beyond the scope of this article. However, in general, dart types most commonly used include two-chambered compressed (pressurized) gas darts and gunpowder explosive darts, with chemical-powered and spring-powered darts used less commonly.[20] Dart projectors include blow pipes where the dart is propelled by forceful expulsion of the user's breath, compressed gas projectors, air and carbon dioxide rifles and pistols, and gunpowder cartridge-powered rifles.[20] When using dart and projector to administer anesthetic drugs, the biggest patient safety risks include severe tissue injury; hematoma formation; necrosis; bone fractures; and injury to other unintended sites, such as the face, eyes, thorax, or genitalia.[20] These risks are mitigated by using the appropriate type of dart and projector to appropriately control the velocity and minimize excessive kinetic energy of the dart on impact with the animal.[20] Explosive injection of drug from the dart through a large bore needle can also cause tissue injury, so darts that use gunpowder explosive mechanisms to inject drug should be avoided in smaller or thin animals.[20] The use of any projectile device, such as a dart and projector should also raise awareness for human/user safety, so similar precautions to those used for firearms should be taken to avoid accidental firing of the dart toward an unintended target.[20] Given the nature of anesthetic drugs, measures should also be taken to avoid accidental discharge of drug from the dart resulting in exposure of the user or other personnel to potentially dangerous substances.[20] These include preparing darts away from other people, using appropriate personal protective equipment when preparing and firing the darts, and ensuring a dart is fully discharged before removing it from the animal.

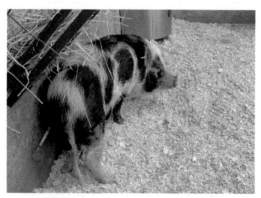

Fig. 3. Anesthetic induction by intramuscular injection using a dart in a miniature companion pig (*Sus scrofa domesticus*). (*Courtesy of* J. Johnson/Saint Louis Zoo)

Intravenous Injection

IV administration of anesthetic drugs results in the shortest onset of action and most predictable effects because the drug is being deposited directly into the bloodstream. Access requires a cooperative, confidently restrained, or sedated patient. IV anesthetics are administered through a needle by direct phlebotomy or through cannulation with an intravascular catheter. IV catheters are more reliably placed in the vein with less risk for extravasation compared with a needle and are placed peripherally or centrally. Peripheral IV catheters are more routinely used for anesthetic events, whereas central catheters that terminate within the thorax are typically used in intensive care cases.[21]

IV catheters are also helpful to ensure venous placement, because there is risk that a needle can inadvertently be advanced into an artery. There is an especially high risk of intra-arterial drug administration when the intended vein lies in close juxtaposition to an associated artery, such as the jugular vein and carotid artery or the femoral vein and femoral artery. Arterial administration of many drugs, including a variety of anesthetics, can result in local irritation, paresthesias, altered motor function, vascular compromise, or tissue necrosis.[22] These complications are thought to be caused by vasospasm after arterial puncture, arterial hemolysis and thrombosis, possible crystallization of drugs blocking the vasculature, endothelial inflammation and cytotoxicity, highly lipid-soluble medications or vehicles, or high osmolarity medications that may result in tissue damage.[22] Additionally, accidental administration of anesthetic drugs specifically into the carotid artery may result in cerebral disturbances that manifest as seizure activity in addition to the severe sequela of local tissue damage in the brain. Overall, intra-arterial administration of anesthetic drugs is discouraged and necessary efforts should be made for prevention.[23]

IV anesthetic inductions are typically performed in sedated patients with a catheter placed. A variety of IV sedatives and anesthetic agents are available including propofol, alfaxalone, dissociatives, benzodiazepines, α_2-adrenergic agonists, and opioids.[1] If IV access is available in an anesthetized patient, total IV anesthesia is administered in situations where inhalant anesthesia with vaporizer is not available. The IV route is also excellent for supplemental anesthetic doses where rapid adjustment of the patient's plane of anesthesia is desired. This may also include administration of euthanasia agents, such as pentobarbital or potassium chloride, in anesthetized patients during end-of-life cases.

Intraosseous Injection

If venous access is difficult or impossible based on the size or clinical condition of the patient, such as small patient size, urgent need for vascular access, hypovolemia, or obesity, intraosseous (IO) catheterization is a suitable alternative and comparable with IV administration.[24] A benefit of the IO route of administration is the rigid venous space in bone does not collapse in cases of systemic circulatory system compromise and even cancellous bone in small zoologic companion animal patients is palpable and accessible.[24,25] Depending on the size of the patient, different methods are used for IO catheterization, including spinal or hypodermic needles that are manually advanced through the bone cortex and left in place as a catheter, spinal needles, various specific IO access kits, or with the assistance of a medical drill to penetrate the bone cortex.[24,25] Care should be taken to avoid bone fracture, especially in smaller species or those with metabolic bone diseases. If IO catheter placement is not an emergency, it is recommended to locally anesthetize the tissue and periosteum surrounding the catheter placement site to decrease pain and discomfort from the procedure. Before administration of any drug via the IO route, it is important to carefully evaluate the safety of that drug in the medullary cavity of bone. In general, anesthetic drugs, such as lidocaine, propofol, alfaxalone, dissociatives, benzodiazepines, opioids, and barbiturates, have been administered via the IO route.[24,26–29]

PATIENT MONITORING AND PHYSIOLOGIC SUPPORT

Induction of anesthesia results in alteration of a patient's physiologic state and, as such, requires reliable anesthetic monitoring to ensure patient safety during the procedure and a smooth, uneventful anesthetic recovery.[1] Although specific patient monitoring plans and parameters are beyond the scope of this article, it is important to consider the variation in anatomy and physiology when using anesthetic monitors because different species present varying challenges for instrument placement on the patient and interpretation. Basic forms of anesthetic monitoring consist of measuring heart rate, peripheral pulse quality as a cursory indirect assessment of blood pressure, respiratory rate, and body temperature, all of which require minimal monitoring equipment. The use of a stethoscope, thermometer, visual evaluation, and palpation of the patient provide for basic anesthetic monitoring.[1] However, the standard of care in a clinical setting should use pulse oximeters, capnography units, electrocardiograph, and Doppler or oscillometric blood pressure monitors for comprehensive anesthetic monitoring of oxygenation, ventilation, and blood pressure.[1] In addition, point-of-care blood analyzers are useful for monitoring a patient's biochemical status during a procedure. Equipment adaptations for monitoring equipment may need to be made, such as avoiding alligator electrocardiograph clamps in small patients or those with thin skin, choosing appropriately sized blood pressure cuffs and placement, location and skin thickness or pigment for placement of pulse oximeter probes, appropriate skin contact for Doppler probes, and appropriate size and type of capnograph based on the ventilatory volume of the patient.

Physiologic support of a patient under anesthesia is the responsibility of the anesthetist and should be based on physiologic and biochemical monitoring values.[1] It is recommended and useful to obtain control of a patient's airway and secure venous access when possible. Airway control is managed through endotracheal intubation or application of a laryngeal mask, and through these methods supplemental ventilation is provided manually or mechanically if a patient is not breathing well spontaneously.[1] Even if intubation is challenging or not feasible based on patient size or anatomy, tight-fitting masks can occasionally be used in an emergency situation to provide supplementary ventilation; however, the patient should be closely monitored for gastric distention in case ventilatory efforts result in aerophagia. Vascular access, usually in the form of placing an IV catheter, is important not only for the administration of anesthetic drugs, as described previously, but also to provide rapid, reliable physiologic support. Physiologic support of the anesthetized patient typically includes IV fluid and electrolyte therapy; vasoactive and cardiac contractility drugs for control of blood pressure; antiarrhythmic therapy for compromising arrhythmias; and emergency drugs, such as epinephrine and atropine in the case of severe bradycardia or cardiac arrest. Methods for venous access are described previously, but it is also important to consider if vascular access is challenging in a patient, catheter placement is time consuming and adds to the overall anesthetic time. In these situations, the type of anesthetic procedure and intended length of the overall procedure should be assessed to determine the priority of gaining vascular or IO access. Often, vascular access attempts are continued while the primary procedure moves forward.

Procedure Risks and Safety

Anesthetic procedures should be performed with patient and personnel safety in mind. The scope of practice in zoologic companion animal medicine covers a wide variety of species posing potential risks to the patient, but also risk to the anesthetist and procedure personnel, especially with larger more dangerous animals. For any anesthetic procedure, hazards should be identified based on the nature of the specific procedure, such as any dangers based on the patient species, method of drug delivery, risk based on drugs used and unintended exposure, and procedures needing to be performed.[30] Patient species that are large, pose a bite or scratch risk, including life-threatening venomous or traumatic bites, or may be carriers of zoonotic disease pose risks to the anesthetist that may not be as frequently encountered in domestic animal practice. Because the anesthetist has the thorough understanding of drug pharmacology and expected physiologic responses, they should guide the assessment of patient anesthetic depth and handling of the anesthetized patient. Also, equipment used, such as darts and projectors, pose unique risks for trauma or drug exposure than what is typically encountered in domestic animal practice. Although more common in zoo or wildlife practice than with zoologic companion animals, ultrapotent narcotics and α_2-adrenergic agonists are life-threatening with unintended exposure. Proper safety considerations and protocols should be in place when using ultrapotent drugs, including accidental exposure protocols and notification of local emergency personnel when ultrapotent drugs are used.[1]

Even use of common medical equipment can pose risks to patient and anesthetist because of the nature of zoologic companion animal practice. For example, fire ignition by surgical cautery in the presence of combustible material is a significant life-threatening complication of surgery in rodents anesthetized with volatile anesthesia delivered via facemask because of high oxygen concentrations and narrow surgical field.[31] Even minor fire ignition that is quickly extinguished is life-threatening in a small zoologic companion animal patient, such as a mouse or a hamster.[31] Additional safety considerations that are commonplace in general veterinary practice but worth reiterating include minimizing exposure to leaked inhalant anesthetics and maintaining radiation safety measures during diagnostic imaging or radiation therapy.

In addition to safety considerations in a clinical setting, environmental risks are also important for anesthetic procedures on zoologic companion animal patients that may need to be performed in the field and outside of the more controlled hospital environment.[30] Considerations include weather conditions, especially temperature extremes or conditions, such as rain, ice, or fog that may cause slippery surfaces or poor visibility, and the physical environment where the procedure is to be performed. Procedures performed on irregular, uneven surfaces or in areas with limited space that require stepping over equipment may pose more of a trip hazard to personnel involved.[30] The procedure environment, whether in a clinic setting or in the field, is more conducive to safely and efficiently accomplishing the procedure goals with organized and ergonomic arrangement of equipment, including examination table or surface, cognizance of and responsible use of extension cords, and proper disposal of sharps or biologic materials, especially when working with species that pose zoonotic disease risks.

SUMMARY

Because anesthetic drugs by nature cause central nervous system and cardiovascular depression, and an altered physiologic state in the patient, safe and reliable drug delivery is essential to the successful execution of any anesthetic procedure. Improper handling or delivery of sedative or anesthetic drugs can result in life-threatening complications for the patient or safety risks for the practitioner. It is important for the anesthetist to be aware of the drug delivery methods available and procedure hazards. These considerations are especially important; because of the diversity of species that are considered zoologic companion animals, procedures are often unconventional and must be adapted based on the species and the nature of the procedure to be performed. With careful planning and understanding of drug delivery and safety considerations, zoologic companion animal patients are safely anesthetized for comprehensive medical evaluation, diagnostic testing, and surgical or other therapeutic procedures.

DISCLOSURE

The authors have nothing to disclose.

REFERENCES

1. Strahl-Heldreth D, Chinnadurai SK. Ambulatory anesthesia for the exotic veterinary practitioner. Vet Clin Exot Anim Pract 2018;21(3):593–608.
2. Phillips BE, Harms CA, Messenger KM. Oral transmucosal detomidine gel for the sedation of the domestic ferret (*Mustela putorius furo*). J Exot Pet Med 2015; 24(4):446–54.
3. Williams MD, Long CT, Durrant JR, et al. Oral transmucosal detomidine gel in New Zealand white rabbits (*Oryctolagus cuniculus*). J Am Assoc Lab Anim Sci 2017; 56(4):436–42.
4. Pires A, Fortuna A, Alves G, et al. Intranasal drug delivery: how, why and what for? J Pharm Durant Sci 2009;12(3):288–311.
5. Canpolat İ, Karabulut E, Cakir S. The efficacy of intranasal administration of dexmedetomidine, ketamine and morphine combination to rabbit. Int J Dev Res 2016;6(7):8634–6.
6. Cermakova E, Ceplecha V, Knotek Z. Efficacy of two methods of intranasal administration of anaesthetic drugs in red-eared terrapins (*Trachemys scripta elegans*). Veterinární medicína 2018;63(2):87–93.
7. Divers SJ. Anaesthesia of zoological species (exotic pets, zoo, aquatic, and wild animals). Veterinary Anaesthesia. Elsevier; 2014:535-569.
8. Sadegh AB. Comparison of intranasal administration of xylazine, diazepam, and midazolam in budgerigars (*Melopsittacus undulatus*): clinical evaluation. J Zoo Wildl Med 2013;44(2):241–4.
9. Schnellbacher RW, Hernandez SM, Tuberville TD, et al. The efficacy of intranasal administration of dexmedetomidine and ketamine to yellow-bellied sliders (*Trachemys scripta scripta*). J Herpetological Med Surg 2012;22(3–4):91–8.
10. Weiland LC, Kluge K, Kutter AP, et al. Clinical evaluation of intranasal medetomidine–ketamine and medetomidine–S (+)-ketamine for induction of anaesthesia in rabbits in two centres with two different administration techniques. Vet Anaesth Analg 2017;44(1):98–105.
11. Emery L, Parsons G, Gerhardt L, et al. Sedative effects of intranasal midazolam and dexmedetomidine in 2 species of tortoises (*Chelonoidis carbonaria* and *Geochelone platynota*). J Exot Pet Med 2014;23(4):380–3.
12. Al-Shebani W. The sedative effect of intranasal administration of some sedative agents in budgerigar (*Melopsittacus undulatus*). Al-anbar J Vet Sci 2011;4(2): 171–7.

13. Pokhrel LR, Grady KD. Risk assessment of occupational exposure to anesthesia isoflurane in the hospital and veterinary settings. Sci Total Environ 2021;783: 146894.
14. Mylniczenko ND, Neiffer DL, Clauss TM. Bony fish (Lungfish, Sturgeon, and Teleosts). In: West G, Heard D, Caulkett N, editors. Zoo animal and wildlife immobilization and anesthesia. 2nd edition. Ames, IA: Wiley Blackwell; 2014. p. 209–60.
15. Baitchman E, Stetter M. Amphibians. In: West G, Heard D, Caulkett N, editors. Zoo animal and wildlife immobilization and anesthesia. 2nd edition. Ames, IA: Wiley Blackwell; 2014. p. 303–11.
16. Minter LJ, Bailey KM, Harms CA, et al. The efficacy of alfaxalone for immersion anesthesia in koi carp (*Cyprinus carpio*). Vet Anaesth Analg 2014;41(4):398–405.
17. Junge RE. Hellbender medicine. In: Miller RE, Fowler M, editors. Fowler's zoo and wild animal medicine: current therapy. St. Louis, MO: Elsevier Saunders; 2012. p. 260–5.
18. Zec S, Clark-Price SC, Coleman DA, et al. Loss and return of righting reflex in American green tree frogs (Hyla cinerea) after topical application of compounded sevoflurane or isoflurane jelly: a pilot study. J Herpetological Med Surg 2014; 24(3–4):72–6.
19. Llewelyn V, Berger L, Glass B. Percutaneous absorption of chemicals: developing an understanding for the treatment of disease in frogs. J Vet Pharmacol Ther 2016;39(2):109–21.
20. Isaza R. Remote drug delivery. In: West G, Heard D, Caulkett N, editors. Zoo animal and wildlife immobilization and anesthesia. 2nd edition. Ames, IA: Wiley Blackwell; 2014. p. 155–69.
21. Cheung E, Baerlocher MO, Asch M, et al. Venous access: a practical review for 2009. Can Fam Physician 2009;55(5):494–6.
22. Sen S, Chini EN, Brown MJ. Complications after unintentional intra-arterial injection of drugs: risks, outcomes, and management strategies. Mayo Clin Proc 2005;783–95.
23. Fikkers BG, Wuis EW, Wijnen MH, et al. Intraarterial injection of anesthetic drugs. Anesth Analg 2006;103(3):792–4.
24. Aliman AC, Piccioni MdA, Piccioni JL, et al. Intraosseous anesthesia in hemodynamic studies in children with cardiopathy. Rev Bras Anestesiol 2011;61(1):45–9.
25. Mayer J. Small mammals: intraosseous catheters. In: Mayer J, editor. Clinical veterinary advisor: birds and exotic pets. St. Louis, MO: Elsevier Saunders; 2012. p. 561–2.
26. Buck ML, Wiggins BS, Sesler JM. Intraosseous drug administration in children and adults during cardiopulmonary resuscitation. Ann Pharmacother 2007; 41(10):1679–86.
27. Kamiloglu A, Atalan G, Kamiloglu N. Comparison of intraosseous and intramuscular drug administration for induction of anaesthesia in domestic pigeons. Res Vet Sci 2008;85(1):171–5.
28. Kleber CH. Intraosseous anesthesia: implications, instrumentation and techniques. J Am Dental Assoc 2003;134(4):487–91.
29. Mazaheri-Khameneh R, Sarrafzadeh-Rezaei F, Asri-Rezaei S, et al. Evaluation of clinical and paraclinical effects of intraosseous vs intravenous administration of propofol on general anesthesia in rabbits. Urmia, Iran: Faculty of Veterinary Medicine, Urmia University; 2012. p. 103.
30. Caulkett N, Shury T. Human safety during wildlife capture. In: West G, Heard D, Caulkett N, editors. Zoo animal and wildlife immobilization and anesthesia. 2nd edition. Ames, IA: Wiley Blackwell; 2014. p. 181–7.
31. Collarile T, Di Girolamo N, Nardini G, et al. Fire ignition during laser surgery in pet rodents. BMC Vet Res 2012;8(1):1–6.

Fish Sedation and Anesthesia

Claire Vergneau-Grosset, Dr méd vét, IPSAV, CES, Dipl ACZM[a,b],
Inga-Catalina Cruz Benedetti, DVM, MSc, Dipl ECVAA[c,*]

KEYWORDS

• Teleosts • Elasmobranchs • Nociception • Immobilization • Sedation • Anesthesia

KEY POINTS

• Fish anesthesia can involve various anesthetic drugs, although few are approved for food animal species.
• Monitoring of fish anesthesia is particularly challenging, because many monitoring techniques used in mammals do not apply to fish.
• Preoperative and postoperative steps follow the same general rules as in small animal medicine, including assessing the health of the patient prior to anesthesia, preemptive antinociception, and thorough postoperative monitoring.

As the popularity of fish as companion animals, conservation efforts in public aquaria, and the fish industry for food production have markedly increased over the past decades, veterinarians in zoologic companion animal practice are exposed more frequently to fish patients in their daily practice. Diagnostic and curative procedures often require sedation or anesthesia, both of which require specific knowledge and abilities. This article summarizes available anesthetic protocols and shares methods and tips to overcome the challenges of fish anesthesia.

Veterinarians anesthetizing fish need to be aware of their unique anatomy and physiology and also should be aware of the hazards associated with the water-borne chemicals that commonly are used for fish anesthesia. When handling tricaine methanesulfonate (MS-222) powder or 2-phenoxyethanol (2-PE), for example, gloves should be worn, because these drugs have a transcutaneous absorption and have been associated, respectively, with retinal lesions[1] and hemolytic anemia and hepatotoxicity.[2]

---

[a] Service de Médecine Zoologique, Department of Clinical Sciences, Université de Montréal, 3200 rue Sicotte, Saint-Hyacinthe, Québec J2S 2M2, Canada; [b] Aquarium du Québec, 1675 Av. des Hôtels, Québec, QC G1W 4S3, Canada; [c] Department of Clinical Sciences, Faculty of Veterinary Medicine, Université de Montréal, 3200 rue Sicotte, Saint-Hyacinthe, Québec J2S 2M2, Canada
* Corresponding author.
E-mail address: inga-catalina.cruz.benedetti@umontreal.ca

Vet Clin Exot Anim 25 (2022) 13–29
https://doi.org/10.1016/j.cvex.2021.08.001
1094-9194/22/© 2021 Elsevier Inc. All rights reserved.

PREANESTHETIC EVALUATION AND PREMEDICATION

Fish patient preanesthetic evaluation includes water quality testing, because this can have a direct impact on both the fish health and quality of the anesthesia. Key water quality parameters include dissolved oxygen level, pH, temperature, hardness, ammonia, and nitrites. Fish also may be evaluated from a distance for any sign of weakness or abnormal buoyancy and for body condition score assessment. Any abnormal clinical signs appreciated may be associated with a higher American Society of Anesthesiologists score. Some clinical signs also may be indicative of discomfort, including anorexia,[3] reduced activity, a lower position in the water column,[4] a rocking behavior from side to side while the fish is static, or rubbing of body parts on the aquarium decor.[5]

Premedication should include preemptive multimodal antinociception whenever a potentially painful procedure is to be performed. This includes the use of local anesthetics and opioids. Lidocaine has been demonstrated to be efficient and safe in rainbow trout (*Salmo gairdneri*), at a dose of 6 mg/kg intramuscularly (IM).[6,7] Topical proparacaine (Alcaine [Alcon Laboratories, Inc, Fort Worth, Texas], 0.5%) also is used commonly for intraocular surgeries, such as lensectomy.[8] Due to the delay of action of local anesthetic drugs, it is good practice to perform these injections prior to gowning and drape placement. Preoperative morphine, at 5 mg/kg IM, has been demonstrated to improve koi (*Cyprinus carpio*) recovery after a gonadectomy.[3] Intraoperative butorphanol, at 0.4 mg/kg IM, also has been demonstrated to improve fish postoperative comfort based on behavior assessment.[4] Although butorphanol, at 10 mg/kg IM, caused temporary buoyancy problems in koi in another study,[3] this potentially was due to the high dose employed. This adverse effect has not been observed in more than 30 fish patients having undergone surgery with preemptive butorphanol, administered at 0.4 mg/kg IM, in the experience of one of the authors (CVG).

INDUCTION

Induction may be performed via injection or immersion. Techniques using electro-immobilization gloves to induce immobility during capture have been demonstrated to increase fish stress compared with chemical anesthesia.[9] Thus, these techniques are not recommended in situations where other anesthetic methods can be used.

IM injections, for example, ketamine (12–88 mg/kg) alone or in combinations with α_2-agonists (medetomidine–ketamine [0.05–0.1 mg/kg and 1–4 mg/kg, respectively][10] and/or benzodiazepines [dexmedetomidine–ketamine–midazolam (0.025–0.1 mg/kg, 1–4 mg/kg, and 0.2 mg/kg, respectively)])[11] can be performed in the epaxial muscles near or just caudal to the dorsal fin, and pectoral fins are used in skates and rays. For large sharks and rays, injection via an automatic pole syringe (Dist-Inject, Animal Care Equipment and Services, Broomfield, Colorado) or darts may be necessary. High doses of atipamezole may be used for reversal of α_2-agonists in sharks, up to 30 times the dose of dexmedetomidine. Portal systems affecting blood flow are present in many fish species, and these should be considered when selecting an injection site. Eight anatomic patterns of blood flow have been defined in the caudal region of fish, which can be classified further into 4 clinically relevant categories.[12] In most fish, the renal portal system receives blood from the caudal part of the body and also from the segmental veins from the flanks. In Cyprinidae, only some of the blood returning from the caudal part of the body is directed toward the renal portal system and the remainder of the blood is shunted toward the hepatic portal system.[12] In the group, including Salmonidae, lumpfish (*Cyclopterus lumpus*), and tuna, the blood originating from the tail does not go through the portal system whereas the blood coming from the segmental veins is directed toward the portal system. The last vascular pattern resembles that of Cyprinidae except the blood diverted from the portal system returns directly to the heart.[12]

The great diversity of fish vasculature makes generalizations about effects of the portal system challenging in the absence of pharmacokinetic studies comparing injection sites. Fish also have white and red muscles, and these may affect pharmacokinetic profiles.[13] Additionally, the volume of drug that can be injected into fish muscle without leakage is relatively small compared with mammals and birds of similar size. Methods to limit drug leakage include minimizing drug volume, using longer needles, and injecting at an oblique angle.[14]

Intravenous (IV) injection of propofol (2.5 mg/kg) also may be used in shark to hasten induction and prevent capture myopathy.[15] The ventral coccygeal vein, which is located on the midline just ventral to the vertebral column, and the posterior cardinal veins, which are located caudolateral to the dorsal fin, are used most frequently for IV injections.[16]

Immersion, for example, with MS-222 (50–400 mg/L, depending on the species), benzocaine (25–150 mg/L), isoeugenol (3.6–120 mg/L), metomidate (0.06–10 mg/L), 2-PE (0.25–600 mg/L), quinaldine (5-20 mg/L),[17] sodium bicarbonate (10–1000 g/L), and alfaxalone (0.5–10 mg/L), should be performed in water from the original tank. It is important to consider that doses can differ significantly between species as well as age and body weight within a species. The water should be well aerated using air stones, and the fish should be captured gently with a net or sling. Whenever possible, positive reinforcement should be used to habituate the fish to enter the net before anesthesia is to be performed. This can be accomplished by target-feeding the fish or feeding in a container used for capture. If anesthetizing fish that tend to jump, such as arowanas or northern pike (*Esox lucius*), a lid should be placed on the tank at all times until an appropriate depth of anesthesia is reached. In these cases, a transparent tank is preferable because it allows for monitoring without opening the top cover. Animal size and water temperature affect the induction and recovery times in several species.[18–23]

MAINTENANCE

Following induction, placement of an IV catheter can be accomplished in the ventral coccygeal vein in fish larger than 500 g. A 24-gauge to 22-gauge catheter can be placed with a lateral or ventral approach with a technique similar to reptiles. Briefly, the catheter is introduced between scales, aiming for the ventral part of the vertebrae, similar to a blood sample; the stylet is removed; and the catheter is sutured in place. This may be useful to administer fluids and avoid hypovolemic shock when excising large, vascularized, or cystic masses. In teleosts, balanced crystalloid fluids may be used, including lactated Ringer solution (Lactated Ringer's Injection, Fresenius Kabi, Lake Zurich, Illinois), Normosol (Normosol® -R, Hospira, Inc., Lake Forest, Illinois), or PlasmaLyte (Plasma-Lyte A, Baxter Healthcare Corporation, Deerfield, Illinois). In elasmobranchs, a customized elasmobranch Ringer solution should be used because of the high osmolarity, which ranges from 900 mOsm/L to 1500 mOsm/L, due to the high urea, trimethylamine N-oxide, sodium chloride, and calcium present in this group. Elasmobranch Ringer solution can be made by mixing lactated Ringer solution with additional sodium chloride (10 g/L), urea (26 g/L), and sodium bicarbonate (0.1 g/L).[24] For blood pressure (BP) monitoring, the dorsal aorta may be used for arterial catheterization in fish larger than 300 g[25] Briefly, a 24-gauge to 22-gauge catheter is introduced on midline, in the most caudal part of the dorsal palate where the first branchial arches join, with the fish positioned in dorsal recumbency. Once a flush is obtained, the catheter can be sutured in place. Because of the intraoral position of this catheter, it should be removed prior to recovery because food prehension with the presence of this type of catheter has not been evaluated and skin erosions have been observed. Catheterization technique of the sinus venosus also has been described in striped bass (*Morone saxatilis*), but this technique requires specific external fixation to maintain the catheter in place.[26]

During maintenance of anesthesia, the position of the fish is key to prevent iatrogenic lesions to the skin and fins and to allow for appropriate water renewal. A custom-made anesthetic table may be used (**Fig. 1**). Care should be taken to avoid tilting large shark species during anesthesia, because some sharks are prone to developing liver fractures with the action of gravity. If access to the oral cavity is needed, the gills may be irrigated through the opercular slit (**Fig. 2**).

Water quality should be evaluated regularly, ensuring that the temperature, nitrogenous wastes, and pH remain adequate. Ideally, duration of anesthesia and anesthetic depth should be minimized for each case. Other anesthetic parameters may be monitored during anesthesia.

ANESTHETIC MONITORING IN FISH

Many indicators of anesthetic depth in mammals cannot be extrapolated to fish. For instance, palpebral reflex is absent in teleost fish given the absence of eyelids. Pulse oximetry is not used due to the aquatic environment and presence of dermal scales. Capnography measures carbon dioxide in its gaseous state in mammals. It, therefore, cannot be used in fish, because their expulsed carbon dioxide is dissolved in water as it moves through the gills.

Visual assessment of the respiratory rate is a crude, but reliable, technique to assess anesthetic depth in fish. This is assessed by measuring the opercular movements to get an opercular rate (OpR). Depending on the species, opercular movements may be more difficult to visualize; for instance, eels, and suckermouth catfish (*Plecostomus* spp) have very small opercular openings. In these species, oral movements may be more easily monitored. Evaluating the effect of a painful (eg, surgical)

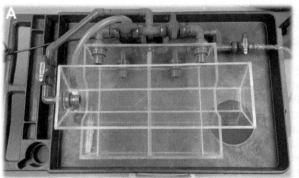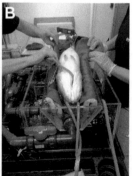

Fig. 1. Anesthesia table designed for fish at the Aquarium du Québec: (*A*) table prior to fish installation and (*B*) set up for a striped bass gonadectomy. Water placed in the lower compartments irrigates the gills through rubber tubing and returns to the table via the large gray pipe in the front. The table compartment toward the fish head contains water with an immersion anesthetic agent whereas the compartment toward the caudal fin contains water without anesthesia. Valves can be opened or closed to adjust anesthetic depth based on a patient's status.

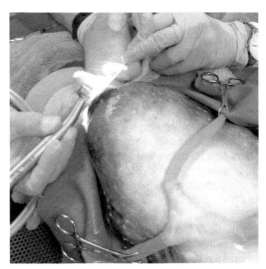

Fig. 2. Gill irrigation from the caudal part of the body during a dental procedure in a puffer-fish. The head of the fish is toward the top of the picture and rubber tubes are positioned in the opercular slits. Water is divided bilaterally with Y-shaped plastic piece.

stimulus on respiratory rate is also a common method to monitor anesthetic depth. Typically, if the OpR increases following surgical stimulation, it is good practice to review the antinociceptive protocol and increase anesthetic depth as needed.

A startle response following fin pinching also is a crude, but effective, technique to assess anesthetic depth. Pinching of the fin, if the fish is insufficiently anesthetized, results in activation of the Mauthner cells, a pair of large neurons in the hindbrain, which elicits a C-start (ie, bending response of half of the body of the fish).[27] This method may be used prior to creating a surgical incision to confirm a surgical depth of anesthesia has been obtained. It should be avoided, however, in fish displaying venomous spines in their fins, such as rockfishes, and in Tetraodontidae (some puffer-fish), which are at risk of inflating suddenly by aspirating air into the esophagus if startled.[28]

Anesthetic monitoring is particularly challenging in fish. Dead fish may display cardiac contractions after brain death, due to the resistance of their tissue to hypoxia. For instance, a heartbeat remained present in goldfish (*Carassius auratus*) up to 4 hours after decapitation.[29] Thus, cardiac contractions do not guarantee life, although cardio-respiratory resuscitation may be performed in cases of confirmed cardiac arrest.

Fish heart rate (HR) may be assessed using a Doppler.[29] Care should be taken to cover the Doppler probe with a glove filled with ultrasonographic transmission gel to protect the probe from water contact, especially in saltwater. The probe may be directed ventrally and medially in the opercular chamber or placed ventral to the gills on the ventral midline. Alternatively, an ultrasound probe may be used to visualize the cardiac contractions.

Electrocardiogram references have been published in zebrafish (*Danio rerio*).[30] Typically, 3 electrodes are placed on the fish; the positive electrode is placed just cranial to the heart to the right of midline, the negative electrode is placed caudal to the heart toward the left, and the reference is placed caudally on the fish midline. When the positive and negative electrodes are parallel to the main heart axis, the R and T waves amplitudes are maximized.

BLOOD GAS ANALYSIS

As in other species, blood gas values can provide useful information during anesthesia. Previous studies have described reference ranges and reference values for blood gas parameters in fish, including rockfish (Sebastes spp),[31] walleye pike (Sander vitreus), koi, yellow perch (Perca flavescens),[32] sandbar sharks (Carcharhinus plumbeus), smooth dogfish (Mustelus canis), gummy sharks (Mustelus antarcticus),[33] and other elasmobranchs.[34] Venipuncture site can influence blood gas values, so the reference corresponding to the sampling site should be selected.[34]

In elasmobranchs, blood lactate, ionized calcium, and glucose concentrations are considered key parameters to determine whether anesthesia should be carried out or terminated. This is true especially for ram ventilators that easily can become acidotic if ventilation is suboptimal under anesthesia. Ideally, lactate concentration should remain below 27 mg/dL (3 mmol/L), glucose should remain between 10 mg/dL and 40 mg/dL (0.56 mmol/L and 2.22 mmol/L) for benthic species and between 50 mg/dL and 70 mg/dL (2.78 mmol/L and 3.89 mmol/L) for pelagic species, ionized calcium should remain higher than 2.5 mmol/L, and base excess should range between -15 mmol/L and 18 mmol/L.[34,35] If these parameters are outside of the normal range, the ventilation should be corrected, or fluids supplemented with calcium may be administered in cases of hypocalcemia.[35]

ELECTROENCEPHALOGRAPHY

Given that heart monitoring is an insensitive way to assess life in a fish patient, electroencephalography (EEG) may be a valid alternative. Pediatric electrodes used for mice also can be implanted in fish to assess cerebral activity. References for EEG parameters have been published in goldfish.[36] Veterinarians should be aware, however, that many anesthetic agents result in a flatline EEG while the fish is still alive, as described in amphibians anesthetized with MS-222.[37] Thus, EEG is a nonspecific parameter to assess patient survival and is used more commonly in laboratory settings.

RECOVERY

During recovery, postoperative antinociceptive agents may be administered if postoperative discomfort is anticipated. Robenacoxib, at 2 mg/kg IM, is a good option for Salmonidae in 12°C water because its duration of action is more than 3 days, which decreases stress associated with repeated captures.[38] For nociceptive stimuli of short duration, meloxicam may be used, at 1 mg/kg to 5 mg/kg IM,[39] due to its high reported margin of safety.[39]

AVAILABLE ANESTHETIC AGENTS IN FISH

Local anesthetics block voltage-gated sodium channels, thereby inhibiting the propagation of action potentials.[40,41] MS-222 and benzocaine, both ester-type local anesthetics, are widely used for anesthesia in fish.

MS-222 is the most commonly used immersion anesthetic in fish. It is approved for use in fish for human consumption in North America and Europe with a withdrawal period of 21 days.[42,43] It is a white, odorless, crystalline powder that is highly soluble in water and needs to be stored in dark, dry, and cool areas. Preparation of immersion solutions is recommended immediately before anesthesia to ensure their potency.[44] Because MS-222 is acidic, the solution needs to be buffered with sodium bicarbonate.[44] MS-222 is metabolized quickly in the liver and excreted via the gills and kidney.[45] Recommended doses to produce anesthesia vary widely depending on the species (**Table 1**).

Minimum anesthetic concentration depression models have shown morphine and ketoprofen to be able to reduce MS-222 requirements in goldfish and indicates these drugs may provide antinociception in this species.[46] Drug effects include transient tachycardia, increased OpR, and hyperglycemia followed by a decrease in HR and OpR.[17] Adverse effects include hypoxemia, hypoglycemia, hyperlactemia, and stress response.[17,44] Although retinal lesions are described in humans, no retinal changes were noted in goldfish anesthetized for 20 minutes daily for 13 days, either by electro-retinography or histopathology.[47] Habituation to MS-222 has been described in gold-fish, requiring progressively higher doses over time. The reason for this observation, however, was not determined and unbuffered MS-222 was used in this study.[48]

Although benzocaine is not an approved anesthetic agent in North America, it is used widely and approved in Norway for fish used for human consumption, with a withdrawal period of 21 days.[43] Recommended immersion dosages are 30 mg/L to 40 mg/L in Salmonidae,[49] whereas no safe dosage has been described in Atlantic cod (*Gadus morhua*) at a temperature of 8°C.[19] This agent is lipid-soluble and may accumulate in cell membranes at low temperature, causing species-specific depression of the central nervous system and immunodepressant effects.[49]

Sodium bicarbonate, or baking soda, releases carbon dioxide when dissolved in water, thereby producing its anesthetic effect. It provided safe dose-dependent anesthesia in greenhead tilapia (*Oreochromis macrochir*) broodstock (10–30 g/L),[50] juvenile Nile tilapia (*Oreochromis niloticus*) (15–50 g/l),[21] juvenile African catfish (*Clarias gariepinus*) (15–50 g/L),[22] and juvenile common carp (1000 g/L at pH 6.5; 600–2000g/L at pH 7.7)[51] in their physiologic temperature range. Associated with hypothermia, sodium bicarbonate caused sedation in rainbow trout, brook trout (*Salvelinus fontinalis*), and common carp (642 mg/L at pH 6.5).[52] A transient excitatory phase prior to anesthesia was noted in common carp.[51] Because it is easily accessible and inexpensive, it may be an interesting alternative to conventional fish anesthetics as an off-label drug use, because sodium bicarbonate is of low regulatory priority in the United States.[53]

Isoeugenol (2-methoxy-4-prop-1-enyl-phenol), like eugenol, is a component of clove oil that exerts its anesthetic and analgesic effects via multiple mechanisms, notably blockage of voltage-gated sodium,[54] potassium,[55] and calcium channels[56]; N-methyl D aspartate (NMDA) receptor antagonism[57]; γ–aminobutyric acid type A (-GABA$_A$) receptor agonism[58]; and by blockage of nicotine$_2$ receptors at the motor end-plate in muscle.[59] It is the active ingredient of AQUI-S (AQUI-S New Zealand, Lower Hutt, New Zealand), which is a commercially available anesthetic solution. In the United States, it currently is under an Investigational New Animal Drug exemption and it is approved for fish used for human consumption in Australia, Chile, New Zealand, and Vietnam without a withdrawal period. Contrary to clove oil, isoeugenol has no carcinogenic potential. Its adverse effects include depression of the respiratory and cardiovascular system, notably by decreasing HR, systemic vascular resistance, cardiac output, and BP.[60–63]

The aromatic ether and phenol derivate, 2-PE, is an anti-infectant with central nervous system depressant effects, partially explained by its antagonistic action at NMDA receptors and neuronal cell membrane expansion.[45,64] It is relatively inexpensive but poses a health risk to users.[65] Described adverse effects include decreased OpR, HR, BP causing hypoxemia, hypercapnia, and acidemia.[66–70] It induces species and dose-dependent modifications in the stress response, and hematological and biochemical parameters.[71–75]

Table 1
Doses of tricaine methanesulfonate used at the Aquarium du Québec to induce anesthesia in healthy fish of various species

Species	Latin Name	Recommended Dose of Tricaine Methanesulfonate (mg/L)	Comment
Clownfish	Amphiprion spp	50	
Bowfin	Amia calva	60	
Pollock	Pollachius virens	60	Prepare to give assisted ventilation (frequent apnea)
Lumpsucker	Cyclopterus lumpus	60	Pectoral fins form a ventouse cup (can stick to bucket)
Red-bellied piranha	Pygocentrus nattereri	70	Difficult reintroduction into a group (cannibalism)
White perch	Morone americana	75	
Shorthead redhorse	Moxostoma macrolepidotum	75	
Lake sturgeon	Acipenser fulvescens	75	
Lake whitefish	Coregonus clupeaformis	75	Very fragile scales
Cownose ray	Rhinoptera bonasus	75	Venomous sting
Largemouth bass	Micropterus salmoides	80	
Leopard shark	Triakis semifasciata	80	
Koi	Cyprinus carpio	90	
Striped bass	Morone saxatilis	90	
Arowana	Osteoglossum spp	90	Jumps
Atlantic halibut	Hippoglossus hippoglossus	90	
Atlantic wolffish	Anarhichas lupus	90	
Rockfish	Sebastes spp	90	Venimous lepidotrichs
Brook trout	Salvelinus frontinalis	100	
Southern stingray	Hypanus americanus	100	Venomous sting
American eel	Anguila rostrata	200	Close the bucket tightly

Metomidate hydrochloride (methyl 3-[1-phenylethyl] imidazole-4-carboxylate hydrochloride) is an imidazole-based nonbarbiturate hypnotic agent exerting its anesthetic action via its agonistic action at $GABA_A$ receptors, the presence of which have been confirmed in the brain and spinal cord of teleost fish.[76–78] Its adverse effects include respiratory, circulatory, and adrenal depression.[60,61,66,79–81]

Ketamine (2-[o-chlorophenol]-2-[methylamino]-cyclohexanone) hydrochloride, a dissociative anesthetic, is a noncompetitive antagonist at the NMDA receptors. Ketamine additionally interacts with opioid, monoaminergic, cholinergic, muscarinic, and nicotinic receptors in mammals.[82] Ketamine usually is available as a racemic mixture in an aqueous solution. In most species, it is metabolized by the liver and excreted by the kidney. Ketamine alone or in combination with α_2-agonists, magnesium oxide, or benzodiazepines have been used for immersion and IM anesthesia in fish.[20,83] Doses required for immersion anesthesia in Persian sturgeon (Acipenser persicus) were very high compared with clove oil, propofol, and 2-PE; doses of 5000 mg/L exceeded 5 minutes to induce anesthesia.[20] Xylazine-ketamine immersion induced smooth anesthesia in common carp that was approximately twice as long as anesthetic duration induced by each of the agents alone, but onset of action was longer.[84] IM ketamine combined with medetomidine, dexmedetomidine, or xylazine has been used successfully to anesthetize sharks, mackerels (Scomber japonica), bonitos (Sarda chiliensis), and Gulf of Mexico sturgeon (Acipenser oxyrinchus desotoi).[10,24,83] Noted adverse effects included bradycardia and respiratory depression of less importance than that induced by propofol.[85] IM ketamine-dexmedetomidine-midazolam combinations provided safe sedation for black sea bass (Centropristis striata) but led to severe and often fatal lactic acidosis in red porgy (Pagrus pagrus).[11] Reversal of α_2-agonists in these studies was obtained with 5 times and 10 times the dose of medetomidine or dexmedetomidine, respectively.

Quinaldine has been described as an anesthetic agent for Salmonidae, Esocidae, and elasmobranchs[86] in combination with MS-222 or benzodiazepines or alone, at concentrations ranging from 1-7.5 mg/L for up to 4 minutes.[87] Its mechanism of action remains unknown. Adverse effects include apnea and hyperglycemia secondary to increased cortisol secretion, compared with metomidate.[79] It is rarely used in public aquaria because its use is not legally approved in fish.

Propofol (2,6-diisopropylphenol) is a highly lipophilic phenolic derivate that induces dose-dependent sedation and anesthesia through its agonistic action at $GABA_A$ receptorsmight not be necessary because already mentioned at the top of the page - citation would have to be removed as well.[78] Propofol commonly is formulated as a white oil in water emulsion containing 1% propofol, 10% soybean oil, 2.25% glycerol, and 1.2% phosphate of purified eggs. Readily available in general practice, it is an interesting alternative to traditional fish anesthetics. Propofol metabolic pathways in fish remains unassessed, although indications for hepatic metabolism exist.[88] It causes rapid anesthetic induction in fish and is commonly used in large sharks for this reason.[20,83,89–96] It is generally used as an immersion anesthetic but has also been used IV successfully in bamboo shark (Chylloscyllium plagiosum), at 2.5 mg/kg.[15] It has been used in combination with butorphanol, dexmedetomidine, ketoprofen, and morphine in goldfish.[89] Dose recommendations are presented in **Table 2**. Adverse effects include bradycardia and respiratory depression that sometimes requires ventilatory assistance and prolonged recoveries.[83,89,90,92,97,98] A transient stress response, as well as isolated elevation in liver enzymes, has also been observed in Siberian sturgeon (Acipenser baerii), Russian sturgeon (Acipenser gueldenstaedtii), and European whitefish (Coregonus lavaretus).[95,97,99] Other hematological changes varied among species.[88,92,97,99] In addition to its anesthetic properties, propofol has

Table 2
Doses of propofol described to induce anesthesia in healthy fish of various species

Species	Latin Name	Described Dosage of Propofol (mg/L)	Comments
Goldfish	Carassius auratus	5–10	
Gulf of Mexico sturgeon	Acipenser oxyrinchus desotoi	3.5–7.5	
Koi	Cyprinus carpio	2.5–10	Prolonged recoveries observed
Levantine scraper	Capoeta damascina	12.5	
Nile tilapia	Oreochromis niloticus	1.5–6	
Tambaqui fish	Colossoma macropomum	0.004	Short anesthesia
Persian sturgeon	Acipenser persicus	1–5	Mortality at highest dosage
Rainbow trout	Oncorhynchus mykiss	10	

also been useful for transport sedation in silver catfish (*Rhamdia quelen*) and Jack Dempsey (*Rocio octofasciata*).[88,91] In an experimental setting, the administration of propofol alone or in combination with α_2-agonists has led to mortality in Persian sturgeons,[20] goldfish[89] and Benni fish (*Barbus sharpeyi*).[100] In goldfish, the 96-hour lethal concentration for 50% of the studied population (6.353 mg/L) was determined, but more studies on therapeutic windows for propofol may be warranted.[101]

Alfaxalone (3α-hydroxy-5α-pregnane-11, 20-dione) in 2-hydroxypropyl-β cyclodextrin is a synthetic neurosteroid anesthetic, which exerts its action through its agonistic action at the GABA$_A$ and glycine receptors, thereby causing hyperpolarization of the postsynaptic cell membrane and consequently inhibition of the propagation of action potentials.[102] The clinical effects are dose-dependent unconsciousness, myorelaxation, and respiratory depression.[103] Alfaxan (Jurox, Kansas City, Missouri) is a clear, aqueous, isomolar sterile solution presented in 10-mL vials at a concentration of 10 mg/mL. To date, its use has been studied in only a few fish species. In immersion, it provides reliable anesthesia in oscar (*Astronotus ocellatus*), 5 mg/L[104]; koi, 10 mg/L[105]; blackspot barbs (*Dawkinsia filamentosa*), 5 mg/L; peacock cichlids (*Aulonocara* sp), 5 mg/L[106]; and goldfish, 0.5 mg/L–2 mg/L for sedation or a light plane of anesthesia, 2–10 mg/L, to reach a surgical plane of anesthesia,[107–110] but response after IM administration, 5 mg/kg–10 mg/kg, has varied largely, with high mortality observed in koi.[111] In oscar, it led to an increase in HR, which persisted after the end of anesthesia and was considered reflex tachycardia resulting from vasodilation and hypotension induced by alfaxalone.[104] Significant respiratory depression was noted in oscar and koi but not in goldfish.[104,105,108] A significant increase in lactate was noted in koi and oscar and was thought to be a consequence of hypoventilation and/or decreased cardiac output and resultant tissue hypoxia as well as the stress of capture, removal from water, and repeated venipuncture.[104,105] Readily available in general practitioners, it is an interesting alternative to traditional fish anesthetics.

Several other drugs used more frequently in the past are available for fish anesthesia. A full resume of all drugs and dosages is beyond the scope of this article and readers are directed toward specialized reviews.[10,17,44,49,112] Additionally, current research on plant-derived anesthetics for fish is gaining popularity. Studies include catnip, citronella, tobacco, rosewood, and avishan-e-shirazi.

In conclusion, many advances in the field of fish anesthesia have been made over the past 2 decades in regard to management, monitoring, and anesthetic drugs. A larger variety of drugs have become available allowing for adaptation of anesthetic protocols to the different species and procedural demands, thereby improving animal safety and well-being. Nonetheless, it is of utmost importance to consider species differences as well as the differences in developmental stages of the fish prior to anesthesia and the authors emphasize the importance of consulting specialized veterinary literature and/or expert reports before treating fish species they are not familiar with. Additionally, the importance of water quality parameters remains essential for optimal patient care and outcome.

DISCLOSURE

No conflict of interest to disclose.

REFERENCES

1. Bernstein PS, Digre KB, Creel DJ. Retinal toxicity associated with occupational exposure to the fish anesthetic MS-222. Am J Ophthalmol 1997;124(6):843–4.
2. Dreno B, Zuberbier T, Gelmetti C, et al. Safety review of phenoxyethanol when used as a preservative in cosmetics. J Eur Acad Dermatol Venereol 2019; 33(Suppl 7):15–24.
3. Baker TR, Baker BB, Johnson SM, et al. Comparative analgesic efficacy of morphine sulfate and butorphanol tartrate in koi (Cyprinus carpio) undergoing unilateral gonadectomy. J Am Vet Med Assoc 2013;243(6):882–90.
4. Harms CA, Lewbart GA, Swanson CR, et al. Behavioral and clinical pathology changes in koi carp (Cyprinus carpio) subjected to anesthesia and surgery with and without intra-operative analgesics. Comp Med 2005;55(3):221–6.
5. Sneddon LU, Braithwaite VA, Gentle MJ. Novel object test: examining nociception and fear in the rainbow trout. J Pain 2003;4(8):431–40.
6. Mettam JJ, Oulton LJ, McCrohan CR, et al. The efficacy of three types of analgesic drugs in reducing pain in the rainbow trout, Oncorhynchus mykiss. Appl Anim Behav Sci 2011;133(3–4):265–74.
7. Chatigny F, Creighton CM, Stevens ED. Intramuscular infiltration of a local anesthetic, lidocaine, does not result in adverse behavioural side effects in rainbow trout. Sci Rep 2018;8(1):10250.
8. Vergneau-Grosset C, Weber ESI. Chapter 5 : Fish Surgery. In: Bennett RA, Pye G, eds Surgery of Exotic Animals: Wiley Blackwell. Available at: https://www.amazon.com/Surgery-Exotic-Animals-Avery-Bennett/dp/1119139589.
9. Lamglait B, Lair S. Ethical considerations for electro-immobilization in adult brook trout (Salvelinus frontinalis). Proceedings of the joint conference of the AAZV and EAZWV (American Association of Zoo Veterinarians and European Association of Zoo and Wildlife Veterinarians). Prague, Czech Republic, 2018.
10. Neiffer DL, Stamper MA. Fish sedation, analgesia, anesthesia, and euthanasia: considerations, methods, and types of drugs. Ilar J 2009;50(4):343–60.
11. Christiansen EF, Mitchell JM, Harms CA, et al. Sedation of red porgy (Pagrus pagrus) and black sea bass (Centropristis striata) using ketamine (K), dexmedetomidine (D) and midazolam (M) delivered via intramuscular injection. J Zoo Aquarium Res 2014;2(3):62–8.
12. Stoskopf M. Anatomy. Fish medicine, vol. 1. 2. Baltimore (MD): ART Sciences LLC; 1992. p. 2–30.

13. Bosch AC, O'Neill B, Sigge GO, et al. Mercury accumulation in Yellowfin tuna (*Thunnus albacares*) with regards to muscle type, muscle position and fish size. Food Chem 2016;190:351–6.
14. Fredholm DV, Mylniczenko ND, KuKanich B. Pharmacokinetic evaluation of meloxicam after intravenous and intramuscular administration in Nile Tilapia (*Oreochromis niloticus*). J Zoo Wildl Med 2016;47(3):736–42.
15. Miller SM, Mitchell MA, Heatley JJ, et al. Clinical and cardiorespiratory effects of propofol in the spotted bamboo shark (*Chylloscyllium plagiosum*). J Zoo Wildl Med 2005;36(4):673–6.
16. Murray MJ. Avoiding the bitey end: restraint, sedation, and anesthesia of sharks. Gainesville: The North American Veterinary Conference; 2009. p. 1657–9.
17. Sneddon LU. Clinical anesthesia and analgesia in fish. J Exot Pet Med 2012; 21(1):32–43.
18. Zahl IH, Kiessling A, Samuelsen OB, et al. Anaesthesia of Atlantic halibut (*Hippoglossus hippoglossus*) Effect of pre-anaesthetic sedation, and importance of body weight and water temperature. Aquacult Res 2011;42(9):1235–45.
19. Zahl IH, Kiessling A, Samuelsen OB, et al. Anaesthesia of Atlantic cod (*Gadus morhua*)—effect of pre-anaesthetic sedation, and importance of body weight, temperature and stress. Aquacult 2009;295(1–2):52–9.
20. Adel M, Sadegh AB, Yeganeh S, et al. Anesthetic efficacy of clove oil, propofol, 2-phenoxyethanol, and ketamine hydrochloride on Persian Sturgeon, *Acipenser persicus*, juveniles. J World Aquacult Soc 2016;47(6):812–9.
21. Opiyo MA, Ogello EO, Charo-Karisa HJIJoAS. Effectiveness of sodium bicarbonate as an anaesthetic for different sizes of Nile tilapia (*Oreochromis niloticus* L., 1758) juveniles. Intern J Aquat Sc 2013;4(2):14–22.
22. Githukia C, Kembenya E, Opiyo M. Anaesthetic effects of sodium bicarbonate at different concentrations on african catfish (*Clarias gariepinus*) juveniles. J Aquacult Engineer Fish. Res 2016;2(3):151–8.
23. Park IS. The anesthetic effects of clove oil and MS-222 on far eastern catfish, *Silurus asotus*. Dev Reprod 2019;23(2):183–91.
24. Andrews AJC, Jones RT. A method for the transport of sharks for captivity. J Aquaricult Aquat Sc 1990;5:70–2.
25. Smith LS, Bell GR. A technique for prolonged blood sampling in free-swimming salmon. J Fish Res Board Can 1964;21(4):711–&.
26. Bakal RS, Harms CA, Khoo LH, et al. Sinus venosus catheterization for repeated vascular access in the hybrid striped bass. J Aquat Anim Health 1999;11(2): 187–91.
27. Greenwood AK, Peichel CL, Zottoli SJ. Distinct startle responses are associated with neuroanatomical differences in pufferfishes. J Exp Biol 2010;213(4):613–20.
28. Zhao S, Song JK, Wang XJ. [Functional morphology of puffing behavior in pufferfish (*Takifugu obscurus*)]. Dongwuxue Yanjiu 2010;31(5):539–49.
29. Balko JA, Oda A, Posner LP. Use of tricaine methanesulfonate or propofol for immersion euthanasia of goldfish (*Carassius auratus*). J Am Vet Med Assoc 2018; 252(12):1555–61.
30. Zhao Y, Yun M, Nguyen SA, et al. In vivo surface electrocardiography for adult zebrafish. J Vis Exp 2019;150. https://doi.org/10.3791/60011.
31. Harrenstien LA, Tornquist SJ, Miller-Morgan TJ, et al. Evaluation of a point-of-care blood analyzer and determination of reference ranges for blood parameters in rockfish. J Am Vet Med Assoc 2005;226(2):255–65.
32. Hanley CS, Clyde VL, Wallace RS, et al. Effects of anesthesia and surgery on serial blood gas values and lactate concentrations in yellow perch (*Perca*

flavescens), walleye pike (*Sander vitreus*), and koi (*Cyprinus carpio*). J Am Vet Med Assoc 2010;236(10):1104–8.

33. Gallagher AJ, Frick LH, Bushnell PG, et al. Blood gas, oxygen saturation, pH, and lactate values in elasmobranch blood measured with a commercially available portable clinical analyzer and standard laboratory instruments. J Aquat Anim Health 2010;22(4):229–34.

34. Naples LM, Mylniczenko ND, Zachariah TT, et al. Evaluation of critical care blood analytes assessed with a point-of-care portable blood analyzer in wild and aquarium-housed elasmobranchs and the influence of phlebotomy site on results. J Am Vet Med Assoc 2012;241(1):117–25.

35. Mylniczenko ND. Monitoring stress in sharks and rays. Paper presented at: Shark Reef Aquarium Seminar. Las Vegas, Nevada, March 1-3, 2019.

36. Laming PR. Electroencephalographic studies on arousal in the goldfish (*Carassius auratus*). J Comp Physiol Psychol 1980;94(2):238–54.

37. Lalonde-Robert V, Desgent S, Duss S, et al. Electroencephalographic and physiologic changes after tricaine methanesulfonate immersion of African clawed frogs (*Xenopus laevis*). J Am Assoc Lab Anim Sci 2012;51:622–7.

38. Raulic J, Beaudry F, Beauchamp G, et al. Pharmacokinetic, pharmacodynamic and toxicology study of robenacoxib in rainbow trout (*Oncorhynchus mykiss*). J Zoo Wild Med 2021;52(2):529–37.

39. Larouche CB, Limoges MJ, Lair S. Absence of acute toxicity of a single intramuscular injection of meloxicam in goldfish (*Carassius auratus auratus*): a randomized controlled trial. J Zoo Wildl Med 2018;49(3):617–22.

40. Frazier DT, Narahashi T. Tricaine (MS-222): effects on ionic conductances of squid axon membranes. Eur J Pharmacol 1975;33(2):313–7.

41. Neumcke B, Schwarz W, Stämpfli RJPA. Block of Na channels in the membrane of myelinated nerve by benzocaine. Pflugers Arch 1981;390(3):230–6.

42. Approved Aquaculture Drugs. Available at: https://www.fda.gov/animal-veterinary/aquaculture/approved-aquaculture-drugs. Accessed February 10, 2021.

43. Anon. Pharmaceutical use in Norwegian fish farming in 2001–2007, Wholesale-based drug statistics. Norwegian Institute of Public Health; 2007.

44. Carter KM, Woodley CM, Brown RS, et al. A review of tricaine methanesulfonate for anesthesia of fish. Rev Fish Biol Fisheries 2011;21(1):51–59.

45. Burka JF, Hammell KL, Horsberg TE, et al. Drugs in salmonid aquaculture - A review. J Vet Pharmacol Ther 1997;20(5):333–49.

46. Ward JL, McCartney SP, Chinnadurai SK, et al. Development of a minimum-anesthetic-concentration depression model to study the effects of various analgesics in goldfish (*Carassius auratus*). J Zoo Wildl Med 2012;43(2):214–22.

47. Bailey KM, Hempstead JE, Tobias JR, et al. Evaluation of the effects of tricaine methanesulfonate on retinal structure and function in koi carp (*Cyprinus carpio*). J Am Vet Med Assoc 2013;242(11):1578–82.

48. Posner LP, Scott GN, Law JM. Repeated exposure of goldfish (*Carassius auratus*) to tricaine methanesulfonate (MS-222). J Zoo Wildl Med 2013;44(2):340–7.

49. Zahl IH, Samuelsen O, Kiessling A. Anaesthesia of farmed fish: implications for welfare. Fish Physiol Biochem 2012;38(1):201–18.

50. Hasimuna OJ, Monde C, Mweemba M, et al. The anaesthetic effects of sodium bicarbonate (baking soda) on greenhead tilapia (*Oreochromis macrochir*, Boulenger 1912) broodstock. Egypt J Aquat Res 2020;46(2):195–9.

51. Altun T, Bilgin R, Danabaş DJT, et al. Effects of sodium bicarbonate on anaesthesia of common carp (*Cyprinus carpio* L., 1758) juveniles. Turkish J Fish Aquat Sci 2009;9(1):29–31.

52. Booke HE, Hollender B, Lutterbie GJTPFC. Sodium bicarbonate, an inexpensive fish anesthetic for field use. Progressive Fish-Culturist 1978;40(1):11–3.

53. Noga EJ. Chapter 16: General concepts in therapy. In: Noga EJ, editor. Fish disease diagnosis and treatment. 2nd edition. Ames (IO): Wiley-Blackwell; 2010. p. 347–73.

54. Park C-K, Li H, Yeon K-Y, et al. Eugenol inhibits sodium currents in dental afferent neurons. J Dent Res 2006;85(10):900–4.

55. Li H, Park C-K, Jung S, et al. Eugenol inhibits K$^+$ currents in trigeminal ganglion neurons. J Dent Res 2007;86(9):898–902.

56. Lee M, Yeon K-Y, Park C-K, et al. Eugenol inhibits calcium currents in dental afferent neurons. J Dent Res 2005;84(9):848–51.

57. Wie M-B, Won M-H, Lee K-H, et al. Eugenol protects neuronal cells from excitotoxic and oxidative injury in primary cortical cultures. Neurosci Lett 1997; 225(2):93–6.

58. Aoshima H, Hamamoto KJB. Potentiation of GABAA receptors expressed in *Xenopus* oocytes by perfume and phytoncid. Biosci Biotechnol Biochem 1999;63(4):743–8.

59. Ingvast-Larsson JC, Axén VC, Kiessling AKJA. Effects of isoeugenol on in vitro neuromuscular blockade of rat phrenic nerve-diaphragm preparations. Am J Vet Res 2003;64(6):690–3.

60. Hill J, Davison W, Forster MJFP, et al. The effects of fish anaesthetics (MS222, metomidate and AQUI-S) on heart ventricle, the cardiac vagus and branchial vessels from Chinook salmon (*Oncorhynchus tshawytscha*). Fish Physiol Biochem 2002;27(1):19–28.

61. Hill JV, Forster ME. Cardiovascular responses of Chinook salmon (*Oncorhynchus tshawytscha*) during rapid anaesthetic induction and recovery. Comp Biochem Physiol C Toxicol Pharmacol 2004;137(2):167–77.

62. Rothwell S, Forster MJFP, Biochemistry. Anaesthetic effects on the hepatic portal vein and on the vascular resistance of the tail of the Chinook salmon (*Oncorhynchus tshawytscha*). Fish Physiol Biochem 2005;31(1):11–21.

63. Putland R, Rogers L, Giuffrida B, et al. Anesthetic effects of AQUI-S 20E® (eugenol) on the afferent neural activity of the oyster toadfish (*Opsanus tau*). Fish Physiol Biochem 2020;46(6):2213–26.

64. Mußhoff U, Madeja M, Binding N, et al. Effects of 2-phenoxyethanol on N-methyl-D-aspartate (NMDA) receptor-mediated ion currents. Arch Toxicol 1999;73(1):55–9.

65. Morton WE. Occupational phenoxyethanol neurotoxicity: a report of three cases. J Occup Med 1990;32(1):42–5.

66. Iwama GK, McGeer JC, Pawluk MP. The effects of five fish anaesthetics on acid–base balance, hematocrit, blood gases, cortisol, and adrenaline in rainbow trout. Can J Zool 1989;67(8):2065–73.

67. Ortuño J, Esteban MA, Meseguer J. Effects of four anaesthetics on the innate immune response of gilthead seabream (*Sparus aurata* L.). Fish Shellfish Immunol 2002;12(1):49–59.

68. Cuesta A, Meseguer J, Esteban MJVI, et al. Total serum immunoglobulin M levels are affected by immunomodulators in seabream (*Sparus aurata* L.). Vet Immunol Immunopathol 2004;101(3–4):203–10.

69. Fredricks K, Gingerich W, Fater DJCB, et al. Comparative cardiovascular effects of four fishery anesthetics in spinally transected rainbow trout, *Oncorhynchus mykiss*. Compar Biochem Physiol Part C: Comp Pharmacol 1993;104(3): 477–83.

70. Lambooij B, Pilarczyk M, Bialowas H, et al. Anaesthetic properties of Propiscin (Etomidaat) and 2-phenoxyethanol in the common carp (*Cyprinus carpio* L.), neural and behavioural measures. Aquaculture 2009;40(11):1328–33.

71. Adámek Z, Fašaić K, Paul A, et al. The effect of 2-phenoxyethanol (Quinaldine-Eastman Kodak) narcosis on blood parameters of young carp (*Cyprinus carpio* L.). Veterinarski Arhiv 1993;63(5):245–50.

72. Javadi Moosavi M, Salahi Ardekani MM, Pirbeigi A, et al. The effects of exposure duration to optimal concentration of 2-phenoxyethanol on primary and secondary stress responses in kutum (*Rutilus frisii kutum*). J Anim Physiol Anim Nutr (Berl) 2015;99(4):661–7.

73. Witeska M, Dudyk J, Jarkiewicz N. Haematological effects of 2-phenoxyethanol and etomidate in carp (*Cyprinus carpio* L.). Vet Anaesth Analg 2015;42(5): 537–46.

74. Toni C, Martos-Sitcha JA, Baldisserotto B, et al. Sedative effect of 2-phenoxyethanol and essential oil of Lippia alba on stress response in gilthead sea bream (*Sparus aurata*). Res Vet Sci 2015;103:20–7.

75. Shaluei F, Hedayati A, Jahanbakhshi A, et al. Physiological responses of great sturgeon (*Huso huso*) to different concentrations of 2-phenoxyethanol as an anesthetic. Fish Physiol Biochem 2012;38(6):1627–34.

76. Delgado L, Schmachtenberg OJTC. Immunohistochemical localization of GABA, GAD65, and the receptor subunits GABA Aα1 and GABA B1 in the zebrafish cerebellum. Cerebellum 2008;7(3):444–50.

77. Uematsu K, Shirasaki M, Storm-Mathisen JJJ. GABA-and glycine-immunoreactive neurons in the spinal cord of the carp. *Cyprinus carpio* 1993;332(1):59–68.

78. Ying S-W, Goldstein PAJMP. Propofol suppresses synaptic responsiveness of somatosensory relay neurons to excitatory input by potentiating GABAA receptor chloride channels. Mol Pain 2005;1:2.

79. Davis KB, Griffin BR. Physiological responses of hybrid striped bass under sedation by several anesthetics. Aquaculture 2004;233(1/4):531–48.

80. Olsen YA, Einarsdottir IE, Nilssen KJJA. Metomidate anaesthesia in Atlantic salmon, *Salmo salar*, prevents plasma cortisol increase during stress. Aquaculture 1995;134(1-2):155–68.

81. Karlsson A, Rosseland BO, Massabuau JC, et al. Pre-anaesthetic metomidate sedation delays the stress response after caudal artery cannulation in Atlantic cod (*Gadus morhua*). Fish Physiol Biochem 2012;38(2):401–11.

82. Mion G, Villevieille T. Ketamine pharmacology: an update (pharmacodynamics and molecular aspects, recent findings). CNS Neurosci Ther 2013;19(6): 370–80.

83. Fleming GJ, Heard DJ, Floyd RF, et al. Evaluation of propofol and medetomidine-ketamine for short-term immobilization of Gulf of Mexico sturgeon (*Acipenser oxyrinchus* de soti). J Zoo Wild Med 2003;34(2):153–8.

84. Al-Hamdani AH, Ebrahim SK, Mohammad FK. Experimental xylazine-ketamine anesthesia in the common carp (*Cyprinus carpio*). J Wildl Dis 2010;46(2):596–8.

85. Williams TD, Rollins M, Block BA. Intramuscular anesthesia of bonito and Pacific mackerel with ketamine and medetomidine and reversal of anesthesia with atipamezole. J Am Vet Med Assoc 2004;225(3):417–21.

86. Brown EA, Franklin JE, Pratt E, et al. Contributions to the pharmacology of quinaldine (uptake and distribution in the shark and comparative studies). Comp Biochem Physiol A Comp Physiol 1972;42(1):223–31.

87. Mylniczenko ND, Neiffer DL, Clauss TM, Chapter 15: Bony fish (lungfish, sturgeon and teleosts), In: West G, Heard D, Caulkett N. (editors) Zoo Animal and Wildlife Immobilization and Anesthesia, 2nd edition. Ames (IO): Wiley Blackwell; 2014. p. 209–60.

88. Gressler LT, Sutili FJ, da Costa ST, et al. Hematological, morphological, biochemical and hydromineral responses in *Rhamdia quelen* sedated with propofol. Fish Physiol Biochem 2015;41(2):463–72.

89. Balko JA, Wilson SK, Lewbart GA, et al. Propofol as an immersion anesthetic and in a minimum anesthetic concentration (MAC) reduction model in goldfish (*Carassius auratus*). J Zoo Wildl Med 2017;48(1):48–54.

90. Oda A, Messenger KM, Carbajal L, et al. Pharmacokinetics and pharmacodynamic effects in koi carp (*Cyprinus carpio*) following immersion in propofol. Vet Anaesth Analg 2018;45(4):529–38.

91. Yaşar TÖ, Yağcılar Ç, Yardımcı M. Comparative efficacy of propofol and clove oil as sedatives in transportation of Jack Dempsey fish (*Rocio octofasciata*). Eurasian J Vet Sc 2020;36(1):8–15.

92. Oda A, Bailey KM, Lewbart GA, et al. Physiologic and biochemical assessments of koi (*Cyprinus carpio*) following immersion in propofol. J Am Vet Med Assoc 2014;245(11):1286–91.

93. Adel M, Cholicheh HR, Gholamhosseini A, et al. A comparison between sedation using propofol and clove oil in Levantine scraper (*Capoeta damascina*). Iranian J Fish Sci 2020;19(6):2893–900.

94. Valenca-Silva G, Braz MG, Barreto RE, et al. Low dose of the anesthetic propofol does not induce genotoxic or mutagenic effects in nile tilapia. Trans Am Fish Soc 2014;143(2):414–9.

95. Gomulka P, Czerniak E, Dągowski J, et al. Effects of propofol and carbon dioxide on acid-base balance in Siberian sturgeon. Pol J Vet Sci 2015;18(2):267–72.

96. Gomulka P, Fornal E, Berecka B, et al. Pharmacokinetics of propofol in rainbow trout following bath exposure. Pol J Vet Sci 2015;18(1):147–52.

97. Gomulka P, Dagowski J, Wlasow T, et al. Haematological and biochemical blood profile in russian sturgeon following propofol and eugenol anaesthesia. Turkish J Fish Aquat Sc 2015;15(1):13–7.

98. Lobao de Souza AdS, Peret AC, Hamoy M, et al. Propofol and essential oil of Nepeta cataria induce anaesthesia and marked myorelaxation in tambaqui *Colossoma macropomum*: implications on cardiorespiratory responses. Aquacult 2019;500:160–9.

99. Gomulka P, Wlasow T, Szczepkowski M, et al. The effect of propofol anaesthesia on haematological and biochemical blood profile of european whitefish. Turkish J Fish. Aquat Sc 2014;14(2):331–7.

100. Mortazevi Zadeh S, Peyghan R, Yooneszadeh Feshalami M, et al. Determine of appropriate concentration of propofol anesthetic drug in Benni (*Barbus sharpeyi*). Iran J Fish Sci 2012;21(2):133–42.

101. Gholipourkanani H, Ahadizadeh S. Use of propofol as an anesthetic and its efficacy on some hematological values of ornamental fish *Carassius auratus*. Springerplus 2013;2(1):76.

102. Cottrell GA, Lambert JJ, Peters JA. Modulation of GABAA receptor activity by alphaxalone. Br J Pharmacol 1987;90(3):491–500.

103. Lambert JJ, Belelli D, Peden DR, et al. Neurosteroid modulation of GABAA receptors. Prog Neurobiol 2003;71(1):67–80.
104. Bugman AM, Langer PT, Hadzima E, et al. Evaluation of the anesthetic efficacy of alfaxalone in oscar fish (*Astronotus ocellatus*). Am J Vet Res 2016;77(3): 239–44.
105. Minter LJ, Bailey KM, Harms CA, et al. The efficacy of alfaxalone for immersion anesthesia in koi carp (*Cyprinus carpio*). Vet Anaesth Analg 2014;41(4): 398–405.
106. Zellar AK, Olea-Popelka FJ, Campbell TW. A comparison of alfaxalone and tricaine methanesulphonate (MS-222) in two fish species. J Exot Pet Med 2018; 27(4):82–8.
107. Leonardi F, Costa GL, Interlandi CD, et al. Immersion anaesthesia in goldfish (*Carassius auratus*) with three concentrations of alfaxalone. Vet Anaesth Analg 2019;46(1):79–83.
108. Bauquier SH, Greenwood J, Whittem T. Evaluation of the sedative and anaesthetic effects of five different concentrations of alfaxalone in goldfish, *Carassius auratus*. Aquaculture 2013;396-399:119–23.
109. Fernández-Parra R, Donnelly TM, Pignon C, et al. Immersion anesthesia with alfaxalone in a goldfish (*Carassius auratus*). J Exot Pet Med 2017;26(4):276–82.
110. O'Hagan BJ, Raidal SR. Surgical removal of retrobulbar hemangioma in a goldfish *(Carassius auratus)*. Vet Clin North Am Exot Anim Pract 2006;9(3):729–33.
111. Bailey KM, Minter LJ, Lewbart GA, et al. Alfaxalone as an intramuscular injectable anesthetic in koi carp (*Cyprinus carpio*) J Zoo Wildl Med 2014;45(4): 852–8.
112. Javahery S, Nekoubin H, Moradlu AH. Effect of anaesthesia with clove oil in fish (review). Fish Physiol Biochem 2012;38(6):1545–52.

Sedation and Anesthesia of Amphibians

Peter M. DiGeronimo, VMD, MSc, DACZM[a,b,]*, Julie A. Balko, VMD, DACVAA[c]

KEYWORDS

- Amphibian • Anesthesia • Euthanasia • Sedation • Tricaine methanesulfonate

KEY POINTS

- Objective investigation of sedative and anesthetic protocols in these taxa still is in its infancy, but knowledge of current best practices is paramount to appropriate care.
- Tricaine methanesulfonate delivered via immersion (bath) is the most common anesthetic drug used in amphibians.
- Close monitoring of anesthetic depth, cardiorespiratory status, and patient status (eg, skin moisture and positioning) is an important consideration in the perianesthetic period.
- Due to the large interspecies variability within these taxa, extrapolation of pharmacokinetic and pharmacodynamic data between amphibian species should be practiced with caution.

TAXONOMY

Amphibians are a class of tetrapod vertebrates that includes the orders Anura, Urodela, and Gymnophiona and commonly are managed under human care for research, education, conservation, and companionship. Anurans include 55 families of frogs and toads. Aquatic larval forms (tadpoles) and adults have striking anatomic differences, translating to different anesthetic requirements and responses between these 2 stages, even in animals of the same species. Urodeles (caudates) have tails as adults and include 10 families of newts and salamanders. Some (eg, axolotls [*Ambystoma mexicanum*], sirens [Sirenidae], and mud puppies [Proteidae]), exhibit neoteny, retaining anatomic features of juveniles, such as external gills, even after reaching sexual maturity.[1] Gymnophiona includes 10 families of legless caecilians and, although gills are present in larvae, they are shed prior to or shortly after hatching or birth.

The authors do not have any commercial or financial conflicts of interest, or any funding sources to disclose.
[a] Adventure Aquarium, 1 Riverside Drive, Camden, NJ 08103, USA; [b] Animal & Bird Health Care Center, 1785 Springdale Road, Cherry Hill, NJ 08003, USA; [c] College of Veterinary Medicine, North Carolina State University, 1060 William Moore Drive, Raleigh, NC 27607, USA
* Corresponding author. Adventure Aquarium, 1 Riverside Drive, Camden, NJ 08103.
E-mail address: pmdigeronimo@gmail.com

INDICATIONS FOR SEDATION AND ANESTHESIA

Sedation and anesthesia are indicated to facilitate diagnostics and treatment, and/or to mitigate pain or distress associated with veterinary intervention and physical restraint. Despite lacking a cerebral neocortex, amphibian neuroanatomy is analogous to mammalian structures responsible for the experience and perception of pain.[2] Analgesia is not the focus of this article, and literature regarding the recognition and management of pain in amphibians if referenced in other texts.

ANATOMY AND PHYSIOLOGY

Amphibians are a diverse taxon with unique anatomic and physiologic characteristics. Most species have little subcutaneous (SC) tissue and a highly developed lymphatic system; thus, injections intended to be SC inadvertently may be administered intralymphatically.[3] The amphibian heart is 3-chambered and found on ventral midline just caudal to the thoracic limbs. The clinical significance of the amphibian renal portal venous system is unknown.[3] Regurgitation and/or emesis with subsequent aspiration is rare in amphibians undergoing anesthesia. Preanesthetic fasting for 24 hours to 48 hours is recommended only for large specimens or those undergoing intracoelomic surgery to reduce the size of the gastrointestinal tract.[3,4] Gastric eversion can occur spontaneously in anurans and is not necessarily a sign of illness but has been reported secondary to anesthesia. Amphibians are heterothermic and should be maintained within their preferred optimal temperature zones (POTZs) during the perianesthetic period.[3] Although the POTZ is species-specific, room temperature (15°C–23°C; 59°F–73°F) falls within the POTZs of most species.[4] Clinicians should review the natural history, husbandry, and anatomy of the target species to guide sedative or anesthetic choices.

The amphibian integument is highly permeable and has several important functions, including fluid uptake and gas and electrolyte exchange. If gular movements weaken or cease, cutaneous oxygen uptake can minimize the development of hypoxemia. Amphibian skin also permits transcutaneous administration of anesthetic agents. Furthermore, many terrestrial anurans have a patch of highly permeable skin on their ventrum.[3] Immersion of the ventrum (not to exceed the level of the shoulders) may be used for fluid therapy or administration of anesthetics.[5] The degree of absorption can be influenced by drug lipophilicity, with lipophilic agents equally absorbed from any skin surface of adult terrestrial amphibians and hydrophilic agents more preferentially absorbed via the ventral pelvic skin.[6] The permeability of the skin renders amphibians susceptible to integumentary trauma and accidental intoxication.

Physical restraint for preanesthetic evaluation or induction can be achieved with properly washed and rinsed, clear plastic containers. When manual restraint is indicated, moistened, powder-free, nonlatex gloves must be worn to mitigate the risks of trauma to the skin, exposure of the patient to commensal flora of human skin, and/or transfer of residues that may be present on human hands.[5] Handling without moistened gloves is not recommended because it may disrupt mucus or waxy layers on the outer surface of amphibian skin that serve as barriers to potential pathogens and, in terrestrial species, prevent excessive water loss. The mucus layer of many aquatic amphibians makes them difficult to restrain manually, especially with moistened gloves, so a wet cloth towel may facilitate handling.[7]

Amphibians utilize 4 modes of respiration, depending on species and life stage. Tadpoles and neotenic adults use gills for branchial respiration. Adult amphibians rely on buccopharyngeal, pulmonary, and cutaneous respiration to varying degrees.

Buccopharyngeal respiration is monitored by observing gular pumping in the ventral cervical region. Pulmonary respiration may be more challenging to accurately assess and pulmonary respiratory rates (RR) can be quite low (eg, 4–7 breaths/hour reported for caecilians).[8] All amphibians, even fully aquatic species, require an air-water interface because even neotenic species with external gills concurrently have lungs. Cutaneous respiration is used by all amphibians to some extent, especially in urodeles,[1] and is the primary mode of respiration for amphibians under a surgical plane of anesthesia. Anurans and caecilians undergo oxygen uptake and carbon dioxide elimination via the lungs and skin, respectively. In contrast, in urodeles, the skin is the primary site of oxygen uptake.[1,8]

In most anurans, the trachea is short or absent, with the lungs opening directly into the buccopharyngeal cavity. Most caecilians have a functional right and a vestigial left lung and some (eg, Rio Cauca caecilians [*Typhlonectes natans*]) also have a tracheal lung.[8] Lungs are absent in lungless salamanders (Plethodontidae) and significantly reduced in torrent salamanders (Rhyacotritonidae).[1] In these species, cutaneous respiration is the primary mode of gas exchange.

MONITORING

During sedation or anesthesia, monitoring is important to assess patient response, titrate drug administration, and allow rapid intervention in case of complications. Monitored responses should include escape response, righting reflex, superficial and deep pain responses, and palpebral and corneal reflexes and are recorded as present, absent, or delayed.[5] Knowledge of a baseline, or conscious, response for a particular species is crucial to interpretation of a result subsequently obtained under the influence of anesthetic drugs. A loss of the righting reflex often is the first indication of successful sedation or induction of anesthesia.[3,4] In most species, light anesthesia is indicated by loss of withdrawal reflex, cessation of gular respiration,[4] and loss of the corneal reflex.[9] Under a surgical plane of anesthesia, all reflexes, including response to deep pain and abdominal respirations, are absent.[3–5] Deep pain can be assessed by firmly pinching a digit,[4] being careful to not damage tissue.

Gular pumping and abdominal breathing are monitored to assess the respiratory system.[5] Amphibians under a surgical plane of anesthesia are apneic and rely on cutaneous respiration. Maintaining moist skin promotes gas exchange and prevents dehydration due to insensible losses. This is accomplished using well-oxygenated, anesthetic-free water either via partial immersion or intermittent application.[4] As long as the skin is kept moist, even fully aquatic species can be kept out of water during anesthesia.[4] Oxygen can be bubbled into the water using a standard anesthesia circuit to maintain adequate dissolved oxygen concentrations.[9]

Heart rate (HR) is monitored by visual observation, ultrasonography, or Doppler ultrasound (**Fig. 1**).[5,9] A significant decrease in HR from baseline (>20%)[10] may suggest the patient is in a deep plane of anesthesia[4,9,11] and decrease/cessation of drug delivery and/or transfer to anesthetic-free water may be considered.[9] Amphibian hearts may continue to beat after death, so myocardial arrest may not equate to brain death.[5] Electrocardiogram leads acquisition generally is not recommended because leads may be traumatic and the use of alcohol can be deleterious.[3] A pulse oximetry device may be used to collect HR and rhythm and can be applied on an extremity or directly over the heart.[9] Because commercially available pulse oximeters calculate oxygen saturation based on mammalian hemoglobin saturation curves, this tool is unreliable for oxygen assessment in amphibians.[5]

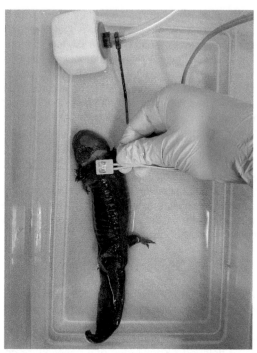

Fig. 1. HR is monitored by placing a Doppler probe over the thoracic girdle of an axolotl (*Ambystoma mexicanum*) under general anesthesia with buffered MS-222 administered by bath. Gills are submerged fully and an air stone is used to keep the water well aerated.

ANESTHETIC AGENTS

The most commonly used drugs to sedate and/or anesthetize amphibians are water-soluble agents administered via partial immersion (bath), although the use of volatile inhalants anesthetics and injectable drugs also has been described.

Tricaine Methanesulfonate

Tricaine methanesulfonate (MS-222) is an isomer of benzocaine commercially available as a white, water-soluble powder.[11] It is an effective anesthetic among species and life stages in which it has been previously tested[4] and is considered by some the anesthetic agent of choice for amphibians.[3] MS-222 is an amide anesthetic that blocks sodium-gated ion channels impeding the conduction of action potentials. Its mechanism of central nervous system depression is not fully understood, but likely involves crossing the blood-brain barrier to exert its effects.[12] In an in vitro African clawed frog (*Xenopus laevis*) tadpole model, MS-222 caused a dose-dependent, reversible blockade of motor and sensory nerve activity and, thus, acted closer to a true anesthetic agent rather than a paralytic agent[13]; however, this has not yet been demonstrated in vivo.

MS-222 is acidic (pH 3)[12] and poorly absorbed in its unionized form.[11] Therefore, MS-222 solutions should be buffered to a neutral pH (7.0–7.4) prior to administration using twice the weight of sodium bicarbonate (ie, baking soda).[9] Unbuffered MS-222 likely induces significant stress in amphibians and should not be used. In *X laevis*, plasma corticosterone concentrations were significantly higher in frogs exposed to unbuffered (pH 3) compared with buffered (pH 7) MS-222.[14]

MS-222 can be reconstituted with bottled or distilled water at room temperature.[4] Alternatively, the animal's tank water can be used if it is of good quality with negligible concentrations of ammonia and nitrites. Amphibians never should be exposed to water that has been chlorinated or treated with chloramines. Chlorine can be removed by leaving tap water out overnight in an open container exposing it to air. Chlorine and chloramines can be removed from water by carbon filters or by sodium thiosulfate or sodium hydroxymethanesulfonate, the active ingredients in commercially available water conditioning products. Lactated Ringer solution,[15] amphibian Ringer solution (ARS),[16] reverse osmosis water,[17] and carbon filtered tap water[18] also have been successfully used to dissolve MS-222. If routine use is expected, stock solutions of MS-222 can be made, but the agent is not stable long term once reconstituted, especially if exposed to light.[4] Stored solutions should be discarded if a brown discoloration is noted because this may indicate the presence of toxic byproducts.

Prior to MS-222 administration, keep patients in a quiet, dimly lit environment to reduce stress.[5] Anesthesia may be induced by immersion in a lidded aquarium or sealed plastic container or bag.[4] Many animals exhibit an excitement phase on initial exposure to MS-222[11]; thus, using a closed container and lining the interior with a soft material (eg, plastic bubble wrap) can reduce the risk of escape and trauma, respectively, during induction.[11] Fully aquatic amphibians may be induced by complete immersion with access to air (**Fig. 2**), but partial immersion is recommended for all other

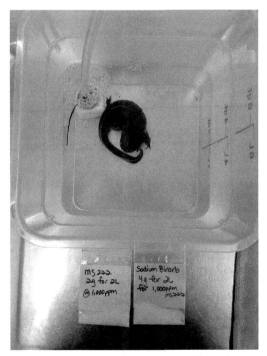

Fig. 2. An axolotl (*Ambystoma mexicanum*) is maintained in well-aerated water in a deep plastic container prior to induction of anesthesia with 1 g/L MS-222 buffered with 2 g/L sodium bicarbonate.

species because drowning can occur with accidental submersion of the head.[5] Animals should be observed carefully upon induction and recovery.[5,9]

MS-222 induction times usually are less than 30 minutes,[9] but initial effects may not be appreciable until 15 minutes, with peak effects requiring up to 30 minutes in some instances.[4,12] Higher MS-222 concentrations can produce shorter induction times.[10] As a result, induction time can be highly variable, so careful monitoring of reflexes throughout the induction period is warranted. Once the desired anesthetic plane is achieved, or at 30 minutes, the patient may be removed from the MS-222 induction solution and rinsed with anesthetic-free water to prevent excessive anesthetic depth.[9] If a patient's anesthetic plane subsequently lightens prior to conclusion of the procedure, immersion in a bath at half the induction concentration can be used to increase anesthetic depth.[4,9]

Species-specific variations in the response to MS-222 exist (**Table 1**). Hellbenders (*Cryptobranchus alleganiensis*) typically require lower MS-222 concentrations for anesthetic induction (250 mg/L) compared with other amphibians.[7] Similarly, larval amphibians generally require a fraction of the concentration used to anesthetize adults of the same species.[9,10] In White's tree frogs (*Litoria caerulea*), tadpoles may be anesthetized with 0.2-g/L MS-222,[9] whereas 0.5 g/L resulted in only mild sedation in postmetamorphic individuals after 25 minutes of exposure.[19]

Higher concentrations of MS-222 also can result in a longer duration of anesthesia. In African clawed frogs, a 20-minute bath of buffered (pH 7) MS-222 at 1-g/L induced surgical anesthesia for up to 30 minutes, whereas, 2-g/L induced surgical anesthesia for up to 60 minutes. As expected, these protocols caused pronounced respiratory depression, but no significant effects on HR, oxygen saturation, or histopathology (heart, lungs, liver, kidneys, and skin) 24 hours following exposure.[20] Prolonged immersion in MS-222 can decrease oxygen saturation over time, especially at higher concentrations.[24] A time-dependent decrease in HR also has been reported in White's tree frogs anesthetized with MS-222.[19]

In waxy monkey frogs (*Phyllomedusa sauvagii*) undergoing cystotomy, anesthesia was induced with immersion in buffered 1-g/L to 3.3-g/L MS-222 in reverse osmosis water. Lower concentrations (1–2 g/L) were used to maintain anesthesia.[17] Anesthesia with MS-222 (2 g/L for induction; 0.5–1 g/L for maintenance to effect) sufficiently

Table 1
Published concentrations of tricaine methanesulfonate administered by immersion for induction and maintenance of general anesthesia in select amphibian species

Species	Concentration
Hellbender (*Cryptobranchus alleganiensis*)	250 mg/L[7]
White's tree frog[a] (*Litoria caerulea*)	2 g/L[19]
African clawed frog (*X laevis*)	1–2 g/L[20]
American toad (*Anaxyrus americanus*)	2 g/L for induction 0.5–1 g/L for maintenance[18]
American bullfrog (*Lithobates catesbeianus*)	1.4 g/L[21]
Axolotl[b] (*Ambystoma mexicanum*)	2–4 g/L[22]
Rio Cauca caecilian (*Typhlonectes natans*)	1 g/L for induction 0.5 g/L for maintenance[16]

[a] Surgical anesthesia induced in 5 min to 20 min and full recovery achieved 10 min to 43 min after rinsing with fresh water.[19]
[b] Lower concentrations (0.5 g/L) may be efficacious in smaller individuals.[23]

immobilized an American toad (*Anaxyrus americanus*) for phacoemulsification without the use of topical ophthalmic neuromuscular blocking agents. Despite the use of standard MS-222 concentrations, the animal failed to recover and subsequently died postoperatively following 6 hours in an anesthetic-free water bath.[18] A concentration of 1-g/L MS-222 failed to induce surgical anesthesia in an American bullfrog (*Lithobates catesbeianus*), and the concentration had to be increased to 1.4 g/L for performance of digit amputation.[21]

Immersion in 2 g/L MS-222 for 20 minutes successfully induced surgical anesthesia in adult axolotls (118–187g) for 15 minutes to 30 minutes, with lower concentrations (1 g/L) having no appreciable effects. HR and blood oxygen saturation were not affected significantly, and all animals recovered by 75 minutes postexposure. Concentrations of up to 4 g/L resulted in a prolonged anesthetic duration (>90 minutes), but no other adverse effects.[22] A single case report describes successful endoscopic removal of a gastrointestinal foreign body in an axolotl using much lower concentrations of MS-222 (0.5 g/L).[23] The lower effective dose in this case may be attributed to the small size of the animal (36 g) and subsequent higher body surface area to volume ratio. A similar effect has been observed in Chinese giant salamanders (*Andrias davidianus*) for which longer induction times were observed in individuals with higher body mass compared with smaller conspecifics at equivalent MS-222 concentrations.[25]

Buffered MS-222 (1 g/L) dissolved in ARS-induced surgical anesthesia in a relatively short time (5–6 minutes) in Rio Cauca caecilians undergoing cesarean section. Following induction, animals were exposed to either oxygenated anesthetic-free ARS or 0.5-g/L MS-222 reconstituted in ARS in order to maintain appropriate depth of anesthesia. In that cohort, the authors reported an approximately 30% decrease in HR compared with baseline and prolonged recovery times.[16]

MS-222 is excreted by the kidneys and/or skin; therefore, keeping the skin moistened with anesthetic-free water can hasten anesthetic recovery.[11] Water also may be changed periodically during recovery to promote excretion and prevent potential accumulation of waste products.[23] For aquatic amphibians, gently rocking the animal may facilitate recovery by encouraging gas exchange.[7] For many species, withdrawal reflex and gular respirations return to baseline prior to return of the righting reflex during the recovery period.[4] Delayed adverse events following anesthesia with MS-222 have not been reported. Anesthesia with MS-222, or its parent compound benzocaine, did not alter circulating leukocyte concentrations nor resistance to larval trematode infection in Cuban treefrogs (*Osteopilus septentrionalis*) compared with negative controls.[26] In another study, chemical restraint of White's tree frogs with MS-222 did not cause significant changes in intraocular pressure as measured by rebound tonometry.[27]

Techniques to create sterile solutions of MS-222 for injection have been described but offer no advantage over topical administration by bath and generally are not recommended.[11] MS-222 has been administered intracoelomically and SC in the dorsal lymph sacs, but the potential to cause tissue damage or toxicity by these routes is unknown.[12]

Benzocaine

Benzocaine, the parent compound of MS-222, is commercially available the an over-the-counter topical anesthetic Orajel (Church & Dwight, Ewing, New Jersey). Because of its efficacy, safety, and availability, benzocaine has been used in clinical practice and field studies of free-ranging amphibians. Similar to MS-222, the mechanism of action of benzocaine is unclear and it is unknown whether it actually depresses the central nervous system or has a paralytic effect at higher doses.[12] The variable anesthetic times reported for topical application of benzocaine gel (15–60 minutes)[12] likely are due to variation in the applied volume and duration of exposure. Stock solutions made with the commercial product are reported to be stable for up to 2 weeks at room temperature.[11]

In African clawed frogs, benzocaine (1 g/L) induced surgical anesthesia within approximately 3 minutes and had a duration of action of about 40 minutes.[28] Marine toads (Bufo marinus) have been anesthetized successfully within 5 minutes in a 1-g/L (0.1%) benzocaine bath with a loss of corneal reflex and an anesthetic plane that allowed femoral artery catheterization.[29]

In small (≤1-g) red-spotted newts (Notophthalmus viridescens dorsalis), a 20% benzocaine solution, made by adding 1g of 10% benzocaine to 500-mL distilled water, induced anesthesia within 4 minutes and lasted for 20 minutes with no reported adverse effects.[30] In other species, benzocaine concentrations as low as 0.02% to 0.3% may effectively anesthetize adults, and even lower concentrations, 0.005% to 0.01%, can be used for tadpoles.[11] Topical application of approximately 9 mg of 10% benzocaine gel (regular-strength Orajel) to the shoulder or pelvic region of red-spotted newts caused immediate local limb paralysis and decreased activity within 3 minutes and surgical anesthesia within 15 minutes. Animals recovered within 15 minutes following a rinse in freshwater.[30]

Baths of benzocaine (0.02%) were compared with MS-222 (0.02% [0.2 g/L]) in metamorphic (terrestrial) and paedomorphic (aquatic) adult tiger salamanders. Benzocaine exhibited shorter and less variable induction times (21.5 minutes ± 14.1 minutes) compared with MS-222 (106.6 minutes ± 18.1 minutes) but longer and more variable recovery times (73.8 minutes ± 4.5 minutes for benzocaine and 9.7 minutes ± 1.6 minutes for MS-222).[31] The prolonged induction time associated with MS-222 in this study may be due to the relatively low exposure concentration compared with standard concentrations of MS-222 used for adult amphibians.

Essential Oils

Essential oils have been used successfully to anesthetize amphibians. Clove oil contains several related compounds that have various biologic effects; clinically, the most important of these compounds is isoeugenol. Higher concentrations of isoeugenol (10 µL/L, 20 µL/L, and 50 µL/L) were associated with short induction times, prolonged recovery, and deeper anesthetic planes in larval brown tree frogs (Litoria ewingii), with no adverse effects during or following recovery.[32] In general, exposure of adult amphibians to 350 mL/L of eugenol for 15 minutes induces a surgical plane of anesthesia for up to 30 minutes with little or no effect on HR or oxygen saturation; however, the efficacy and safety of this technique are inconsistent. Recovery usually occurs within 1 hours to 2 hours.[33]

African clawed frogs exposed to 350 µL/L eugenol reached a surgical plane of anesthesia for 15 minutes to 30 minutes. Frogs exhibited loss of the withdrawal reflex, righting reflex, and response to noxious stimuli for 30 minutes to 60 minutes, with longer duration of effects in smaller frogs. Despite lower HR, oxygen saturation was not affected and no side effects were observed in the 24-hour postanesthetic period.[34] In a related study by the same investigators, renal tubular apoptosis, massive hepatic necrosis, pulmonary lesions, and/or hemorrhage in adipose tissue were observed histologically following exposure to anesthetic concentrations of eugenol.[35]

Surgical anesthesia was achieved in only 67% of tiger salamanders (Ambystoma tigrinum) exposed to 450-mg/L clove oil in water. After 30 minutes of exposure, HR was decreased but RR remained unchanged.[5] In leopard frogs (Rana pipiens) anesthetized with clove oil, up to 50% of subjects prolapsed their stomachs following exposure with spontaneous resolution in all animals.[36] When used as a direct topical application to the skin (compared with bath immersion), eugenol was not effective at inducing anesthesia and caused cutaneous necrosis at the application site within 24 hours of exposure.[37] Thus, topical application of essential oils to amphibians is not recommended.

The use of other essential oils (*Aniba rosaeodora*, *Lippia origanoides*, *L alba* chemotype *citral*, and *L alba* chemotype *linalool*) diluted in ethanol and administered at concentrations of 25 μL/L to 200 μL/L to tadpoles of map treefrogs (*Hypsiboas geographicus*) has been investigated. Results revealed prolonged induction at lower concentrations and prolonged recovery at higher concentrations with no mortalities observed.[38]

Inhalant Halogens (Isoflurane and Sevoflurane)

Halogenated ethers, such as isoflurane and sevoflurane, are commonly available in clinical practice. In amphibians, they have been administered topically, via immersion (bath), injection, and inhalation.[12,39]

Administration of 2% to 5% isoflurane in oxygen into an airtight chamber has been reported to induce surgical anesthesia within 5 minutes to 20 minutes in amphibians.[11,12] Isoflurane administered via an airtight container in northern leopard frogs (*R pipiens*) effectively induced anesthesia and, although potency was similar to mammals, time to equilibration was prolonged.[40] With administration by inhalation, time to induction and resultant plane of anesthesia were highly variable, and animals often resumed spontaneous movement as soon as they were removed from the induction chamber, limiting the clinical usefulness of these protocols.[4,11,12] In experimental models, 1.15% isoflurane administered by chamber effectively anesthetized 50% of leopard frogs; however, it required up to 80 minutes to achieve a surgical plane of anesthesia.[41] Because pulmonary ventilation often ceases within the first 20 minutes of exposure, subsequent isoflurane uptake is presumed to be via transcutaneous absorption, which may account for prolonged induction times.[41] Placing cotton or gauze-soaked inhalant on the animal may be more effective. Although animals often exhibit excitement initially when exposed to isoflurane-soaked gauze, induction of anesthesia can be rapid (approximately 2 minutes in some cases). Duration of anesthesia may be up to 40 minutes and recovery time may be prolonged.[11]

For delivery of inhalant via the lungs, amphibians can be intubated using short uncuffed endotracheal tubes or red rubber, intravenous (IV), or tomcat urinary catheters.[11] Intubation is complicated by the narrow glottis,[12] a short or absent trachea, and difficulty adequately securing the tube to prevent inadvertent extubation.[11] When inserted, the device should be introduced just past the larynx.[4] Inhalant anesthetics delivered via this route do not contact the buccopharynx or skin for additional uptake.[11]

Anesthesia was successfully induced in mountain chicken frogs (*Leptodactylus fallax*) by placing each animal in a sealed clear plastic bag containing 5% isoflurane in oxygen. The righting reflex was lost in 2.4 minutes ± 2.3 minutes and gular respirations were absent by 7.6 minutes ± 2.7 minutes. Although this species lacks a trachea, the frogs were intubated successfully using a modified cuffed tube 2.5 mm to 3.5 mm in diameter and maintained on 2% isoflurane with manual intermittent positive pressure ventilation every 5 seconds to 10 seconds. A surgical plane of anesthesia was achieved within a few minutes of intubation. No complications were observed and following approximately 21 minutes of anesthesia; the frogs were ventilated using room air and recovered the righting reflex in 40.4 seconds ± 10.1 minutes.[42]

Various techniques to administer isoflurane by immersion have been described. These include using a syringe and 25-gauge needle to spray liquid isoflurane into a water bath (2–3 mL isoflurane per liter of water)[4] or bubbling 5% isoflurane in pure oxygen through a water column,[12] the latter of which did not successfully anesthetize African clawed frogs.[39] The use of volatile inhalants necessitates proper scavenging systems (eg, hood) to limit excessive ambient contamination and personnel exposure.[9,11] A mixture of 3-mL isoflurane, 1.5-mL water, and 3.5-mL water soluble lubricant can be made and administered topically at 0.025 mL/g to 0.035 mL/g of body weight to achieve 45 minutes to 80 minutes of anesthesia time.[4,11,12] Lower doses are recommended for aquatic species and higher doses for terrestrial species.[4] An isoflurane-soaked pad applied to the dorsum and covered with an impermeable barrier to prevent evaporation rapidly induced anesthesia in 7 of 11 exposed African clawed frogs with no reported side effects and uneventful recoveries.[39] Topical application of sevoflurane mixed with a water-soluble lubricant to American bullfrogs resulted in sufficient transdermal absorption to produce anesthesia.[43] Topical isoflurane is not considered as reliable for anesthesia in urodeles as it is in anurans.[1]

Isoflurane administered by injection (intracoelomic, SC, or IM) carries high mortality rates and low margins of safety and efficacy. Following isoflurane administered intracoelomically, most African clawed frogs died whereas others experienced variable recovery times (38 minutes to 15 hours). SC administration failed to induce anesthesia in 3 frogs and resulted in prolonged (>1 hour) induction times in 3 others and a single death. Anesthesia was not achieved in any frog following intramuscular (IM) administration of isoflurane.[39] Until efficacy and safety are demonstrated, injection of volatile anesthetics is contraindicated.

Propofol

Propofol may be administered to amphibians IV, intracoelomically, or by immersion, but results generally are inconsistent. IV administration is challenging because placement of an IV catheter may require sedation and may be possible only in larger individuals. Intraosseous administration may be more feasible in smaller species. Although not recommended in other species due to side effects, intra-arterial injection of propofol was tolerated in bullfrogs.[44]

In a study of 3 individual White's tree frogs, 9.5-mg/kg propofol administered intracoelomically induced sedation, whereas 30-mg/kg propofol induced anesthesia and 53-mg/kg propofol resulted in death.[45] In contrast, 40% and 83% of tiger salamanders achieved anesthesia with 25-mg/kg and 35-mg/kg intracoelomic propofol, respectively. Lower RR and HR were observed 60 minutes to 90 minutes after administration.[46]

Propofol administered via immersion has been poorly studied. A single study in African clawed frogs investigated a 15-minute propofol immersion at 3 doses: 88 mg/L, 175 mg/L, and 330 mg/L. The lowest dose produced less than 30 minutes of anesthesia and many individuals remained responsive to noxious stimuli. All frogs exposed to the higher doses died. This study concluded that propofol baths are neither safe nor effective in this species[47] and further research in other species is warranted.

Alfaxalone

Alfaxalone can be used to sedate amphibians but has not been demonstrated to induce a surgical plane of anesthesia. Studies have investigated its use IM, SC, and by immersion (**Table 2**). As in other species, alfaxalone has no analgesic effects.

The dose range reported for American bullfrogs is 10 mg/kg IM to 17.5 mg/kg IM, with higher doses producing shorter times to recumbency, but similar durations of

Table 2
Published doses of alfaxalone for sedation in select amphibian species

Species	Dosage	Onset and Duration	Notes
American bullfrog (*Lithobates catesbeianus*)	10–17.5 mg/kg IM[48]	Higher doses shortened time to recumbenc, but had similar duration of effect.	No change in HR; remained responsive to noxious stimuli
	2 g/L by bath[48]	No effect	
Spanish ribbed newt (*Pleurodeles waltl*)	15–30 mg/kg IM[49]	Higher doses resulted in shorter times to first effect.	Lost righting and escape reflexes but not corneal reflexes; remained responsive to noxious stimuli
Oriental fire-bellied toad (*Bombina orientalis*)	2 g/L by bath[50]	Exposure for 14 min resulted in sedation for 10–30 min.	No change in HR; remained responsive to noxious stimuli
Australian green tree frog (*Litoria caerulea*)	30 mg/kg IM[51]	First effect observed at 3–10 min and lasted 25–90 min.	No change in HR but decreased gular RR; lower doses (20 mg/kg IM) failed to sedate subjects
Green and golden bell frog (*Litoria aurea*)	20 mg/kg IM[51]	First effect observed at 4–10 min and lasted 40–60 min.	No change in HR but decreased gular RR
Booroolong frog (*Litoria booroolongensis*)	20 mg/kg IM[51]	First effect observed at 3–10 min and lasted 65–100 min.	No change in HR but decreased gular RR

effect. Frogs remained responsive to noxious stimuli throughout and no changes in HR were noted.[48] In a different study in bullfrogs, 10-mg/kg alfaxalone IM produced shorter induction times (approximately 5–10 minutes), and the difference was attributed to higher ambient temperatures (25°C). Both HR and mean arterial pressure increased following administration, the latter transiently, and recovery of muscle tone occurred within 60 minutes.[44] In a single case report, 7-mg/kg alfaxalone IM with a lidocaine ring block provided sufficient sedation to perform a nuptial pad amputation in an American bullfrog; additional 5-mg/kg alfaxalone IM was administered 40 minutes following the initial dose to complete the procedure.[52] Spanish ribbed newts (*Pleurodeles waltl*) were sedated in 4.5 minutes to 8.7 minutes with 15-mg/kg, 20-mg/kg, or 30-mg/kg alfaxalone IM in the forelimb, with faster effects at higher dosages. Newts lost escape response and righting reflex, but many retained corneal reflexes. None lost response to noxious stimuli. Similarly, duration of sedation (30–60 minutes) was dose-dependent. No lesions or complications were observed.[49]

Species-specific variation in response to alfaxalone administration via immersion has been noted. American bullfrogs exhibited no signs of sedation using alfaxalone immersion at concentrations as high as 2 g/L.[48] In contrast, 10 of 11 oriental fire-bellied toads (*Bombina orientalis*) were anesthetized successfully for 10 minutes to 30 minutes when exposed to the same concentration for approximately 14 minutes.

A surgical plane of anesthesia never was achieved, animals never lost nociceptive withdrawal response, and HR did not significantly change compared with baseline.[50]

Other Agents

Local anesthetics have been sparsely investigated in amphibians. Anecdotally, the use of lidocaine and bupivacaine has been reported and recommended doses, up to 5 mg/kg, both undiluted and diluted (3:1 with sodium bicarbonate), are extrapolated empirically from use in mammals.[53] The ultimate effect of local anesthetics in the presence of MS-222 anesthesia is unknown because these drugs share a class and mechanism.[53] Additionally, the efficacy and duration of topically applied local anesthetics are unknown, given likely rapid systemic absorption.[53,54] In American bullfrogs, topical lidocaine caused dose-dependent sedation without evidence of local antinociception at the site of application.[54]

Injectable anesthetics generally are considered unreliable in amphibians and can be associated with narrow margins of safety.[4,9] Injectable agents ideally are administered according to species-specific dosages that, for the most part, remain unknown.[4]

Ketamine (70–100 mg/kg IM) has been used to anesthetize amphibians and was associated with muscle contractions and rigidity and prolonged recovery times (up to 12–18 hours).[9,11] Additionally, individuals may remain responsive to painful stimuli.[12] Other sources have recommended ketamine, 20 to 40 mg/kg IM, for premedication.[5] The efficacy of tiletamine-zolazepam (Telazol, Zoetis, Parsippany, New Jersey) has received little investigation in amphibians and currently is not considered clinically useful.[11,12] Tiletamine-zolazepam (5 mg/kg, 10 mg/kg, 20 mg/kg, and 50 mg/kg IM) in American bullfrogs and leopard frogs produced significant interspecies variation in depth and duration of anesthesia. Greater effects were noted in leopard frogs, with recovery times of up to 32 hours. Mortality was noted at the highest doses in both groups.[11]

α_2-Agonists may sedate or anesthetize amphibians but are less studied and effectiveness may be species-specific. Medetomidine (0.15 mg/kg IM) did not produce sedation and caused cardiopulmonary depression in leopard frogs.[5] In juvenile blue poison dart frogs (*Dendrobates tinctorius azureus*), dexmedetomidine (5 mg/kg) and midazolam (40 mg/kg) combined with either ketamine (100 mg/kg) (KMD) or alfaxalone (20 mg/kg) (AMD) resulted in a rapid loss of righting reflex (median 5 minutes for both groups). Following partial reversal with atipamezole (50 mg/kg) and flumazenil (0.05 mg/kg), time to recovery was similar in both groups (approximately 90 minutes). Although HR was not significantly different between groups, pulmonary respiration was depressed in AMD and muscle rigidity was observed in KMD, which became more pronounced following reversal. Gastric prolapse was observed in a subset of frogs in both groups and was easily reducible. All frogs ate within 24 hours of chemical restraint.[55] In an experimental model using leopard frogs, intraspinal dexmedetomidine induced analgesia for at least 4 hours without motor or sedative effects.[56] Intraspinal dexmedetomidine as part of a multimodal approach to anesthesia has yet to be investigated clinically. Dexmedetomidine, 40 mg/kg to 120 mg/kg, injected into the dorsal lymph sac has been shown to provide analgesia, but not anesthesia, in leopard frogs.[2]

Opioid research in amphibians suggests potential benefit for clinical practice and the use of opioids in leopard frogs has been reviewed elsewhere.[2] Relative to mammals, extremely high doses are required to achieve analgesia and sedation has not been a reported side effect.[2] In an experimental model using red-spotted newts, administration of 50-mg/kg buprenorphine intracoelomically or 0.5-mg/L butorphanol in tank water seemed to have analgesic but not sedative effects.[57] The role of opioids in balanced anesthetic protocols for amphibians requires further investigation.

Metomidate hydrochloride has shown promise administered via immersion (bath), but more research is indicated. In leopard frogs, a 30-mg/L bath for 60 minutes caused sedation in all exposed subjects, but a surgical plane of anesthesia was achieved in less than a third of frogs. In the latter frogs, loss of the righting reflex and escape response occurred within approximately 18 minutes but lasted only 9 minutes to 20 minutes.[58] Recovery time was prolonged and variable (5 hours->10 hours), limiting the clinical usefulness of this drug.[58] The related drug etomidate induced a surgical plane of anesthesia within approximately 15 minutes when used as a bath (22.5 mg/L) in African clawed frogs and lasted approximately 30 minutes.[28]

Ethanol, ether, diazepam, hexobarbital, and thiopental have been used via immersion to induce loss of righting reflex, and in some cases, loss of response to noxious stimuli, in bullfrog tadpoles, but none of these is recommended for clinical use.[59] Use of 5% ethanol for sedation of amphibians is not recommended unless immediately followed by euthanasia (eg, with prolonged immersion in 20% ethanol).[11] Barbiturates, in general, have a low margin of safety in amphibians and, therefore, should not be used for sedation or anesthesia.[11,60]

The use of hypothermia as a sole or adjunctive method to facilitate restraint or euthanasia of amphibians remains controversial. Arguments in favor of its use[61,62] are based in part on studies demonstrating that high doses of naloxone and naltrexone can reverse the apparent analgesic effects of hypothermia, suggesting hypothermia-induced analgesia is at least partially mediated by opioid receptors.[63] According to the American Veterinary Medical Association Guidelines for the Euthanasia of Animals, however, "Hypothermia is an inappropriate method of restraint or euthanasia for amphibians [...] unless animals are sufficiently small (<4 g) to permit immediate and irreversible death if placed in liquid nitrogen"[64(p94)]; this recommendation is based on the precautionary principle—it is best to avoid its use until there is more evidence that it is humane.[65] The authors agree with this statement and do not recommend the use of hypothermia for amphibian restraint.

Euthanasia

Recent literature has begun to fill the deficit in evidence-based recommendations for amphibian euthanasia. Immersion in 6-g/L MS-222 for 15 minutes successfully euthanized X laevis tadpoles, whereas exposure to eugenol, 800 μL/L, had variable effects depending on the stage of larval development and the batch of stock solution used. Rapid chilling was ineffective for euthanasia.[66] In adult frogs, MS-222 alone may not be appropriate for euthanasia. Although death was achieved in 17 of 18 smoky jungle frogs (Leptodactylus pentadactylus) immersed in 2.5-g/L to 10-g/L MS-222 for 60 minutes to 90 minutes, most frogs had repeated and unpredictable episodes of regained consciousness and a prolonged time to loss of heartbeat, making this technique neither rapid nor distress-free.[67] As clinical signs of a surgical plane of MS-222 anesthesia, including unconsciousness and apnea, overlap significantly with death, asystole must be confirmed to ensure euthanasia has occurred.[24] Barbiturates, specifically intracoelomic sodium pentobarbital, can induce cardiac rapidly arrest[24] and are recommended for euthanasia following induction of general anesthesia.

SUMMARY

Sedation and anesthesia may be indicated for amphibians undergoing examination, sample collection, surgical intervention, or euthanasia. The unique anatomy and physiology of amphibians present unique anesthetic considerations for clinicians. Knowledge of current best practices and clinical investigation allows clinicians to practice evidence-based medicine to appropriate standards.

REFERENCES

1. Baitchman EJ, Herman TA. Caudata (Urodela): tailed amphibians. In: Miller RE, Fowler ME, editors. Fowler's zoo and wild animal medicine, vol. 8. St. Louis, MO: Elsevier Saunders; 2015. p. 13–20.
2. Machin KL. Amphibian pain and analgesia. J Zoo Wildl Med 1999;30:2–10.
3. Chai N. Anurans. In: Miller RE, Fowler ME, editors. Fowler's zoo and wild animal medicine, vol. 8. St. Louis, MO: Elsevier Saunders; 2015. p. 1–13.
4. Stetter M. Amphibians. In: West G, Heard D, Caulkett N, editors. Zoo animal and wildlife immobilization and anesthesia. Ames, IA: Blackwell Publishing; 2007. p. 205–9.
5. Mitchell MA. Anesthetic considerations for amphibians. J Exot Pet Med 2009; 18:40–9.
6. Llewelyn VK, Berger L, Glass BD. Effects of skin region and relative lipophilicity on percutaneous absorption in the toad *Rhinella marina*. Environ Toxicol Chem 2019;38:361–7.
7. Junge RE. Hellbender medicine. In: Miller RE, Fowler ME, editors. Fowler's zoo and wild animal medicine, vol. 7. St. Louis, MO: Elsevier Saunders; 2012. p. 260–5.
8. Clayton LA, Mylniczenko ND. Caecilians. In: Miller RE, Fowler ME, editors. Fowler's zoo and wild animal medicine, vol. 8. St. Louis, MO: Elsevier Saunders; 2015. p. 20–6.
9. Gentz EJ. Medicine and surgery of amphibians. ILAR J 2007;48:255–9.
10. Downes H, Kienle EA, Pederson. Metamorphosis and the steady state anesthetic concentrations of tricaine, benzocaine and ethanol. Comp Biochem Physiol 1994; 107C:95–103.
11. Wright KM. Restraint techniques and euthanasia. In: Wright KM, Whitaker BR, editors. Amphibian medicine and captive husbandry. Malabar, FL: Krieger Publishing Company; 2001. p. 111–22.
12. Guénette SA, Giroux MC, Vachon P. Pain perception and anaesthesia in research frogs. Exp Anim 2013;62:87–92.
13. Ramlochansingh C, Branoner F, Chagnaud BP, et al. Efficacy of tricaine methanesulfonate (MS-222) as an anesthetic agent for blocking sensory-motor responses in *Xenopus laevis* tadpoles. PLoS One 2014;9:e101606.
14. Archard GA, Goldsmith AR. Euthanasia methods, corticosterone and haematocrit levels in Xenopus laevis: evidence for differences in stress? Anim Welfare 2010; 19:85–92.
15. Yaw TJ, Swanson JE, Pierce CL, et al. Placement of intracoelomic radiotransmitters and silicone passive sampling devices in Northern leopard frogs (*Lithobates pipiens*). J Herpetol Med Surg 2017;27:111–5.
16. Barbon AR, Goetz M, Lopez J, et al. Uterine rupture and cesarean surgery in three Rio Cauca caecilians (*Typhlonectes natans*). J Zoo Wildl Med 2017;48: 164–70.
17. Archibald KE, Minter LJ, Dombrowski DS, et al. Cystic urolithiasis in captive waxy monkey frogs (*Phyllomedusa sauvagii*). J Zoo Wildl Med 2015;46:105–12.
18. Kilburn JJ, Bronson E, Shaw GC, et al. Phacoemulsification in an American toad (*Anaxyrus americanus*). J Herpetol Med Surg 2019;29:17–20.

19. Krisp AR, Hausmann JC, Sladky KK, et al. Anesthetic efficacy of MS-222 in White's tree frogs (*Litoria caerulea*). J Herpetol Med Surg 2020;30:38–41.

20. Lalonde-Robert V, Beaudry F, Vachon P. Pharmacologic parameters of MS222 and physiologic changes in frogs (*Xenopus laevis*) after immersion at anesthetic doses. J Am Assoc Lab Anim Sci 2012;51:464–8.

21. Dombrowski DS, Vanderklok C, Van Wettere AJ. Curative surgical excision of a squamous cell carcinoma associated with the digit of an American bullfrog (*Lithobates catesbeianus*). J Herpetol Med Surg 2016;26:42–5.

22. Zullian C, Dodelet-Devillers A, Roy S, et al. Evaluation of the anesthetic effects of MS222 in the adult Mexican axolotl (*Ambystoma mexicanum*). Vet Med Res Rep 2016;7:1–7.

23. Burns PM, Langlois I, Dunn M. Endoscopic removal of a foreign body in a Mexican axolotl (*Ambystoma mexicanum*) with the use of MS222-induced immobilization. J Zoo Wildl Med 2019;50:282–6.

24. Lalonde-Robert V, Desgent S, Duss S, et al. Electroencephalographic and physiologic changes after tricaine methanesulfonate immersion of African clawed frogs (*Xenopus laevis*). J Am Assoc Lab Anim Sci 2012;51:622–7.

25. Marcec R, Kouba A, Zhang L, et al. Surgical implantation of coelomic radiotransmitters and postoperative survival of Chinese giant salamanders (*Andrias davidianus*) following reintroduction. J Zoo Wildl Med 2016;47:187–95.

26. Sears B, Snyder P, Rohr J. No effects of two anesthetic agents on circulating leukocyte counts or resistance to trematode infections in larval amphibians. J Herpetol 2013;47:498–501.

27. Hausmann JC, Krisp A, Sladky K, et al. Measuring intraocular pressure in White's tree frogs (*Litoria caerulea*) by rebound tonometry: comparing device, time of day, and manual versus chemical restraint methods. J Zoo Wildl Med 2017;48: 413–9.

28. Smith BD, Vail KJ, Carroll GL, et al. Comparison of etomidate, benzocaine, and MS222 anesthesia with and without subsequent flunixin meglumine analgesia in African clawed frogs (*Xenopus laevis*). J Am Assoc Lab Anim Sci 2018;57: 202–9.

29. Andersen JB, Wang T. Effects of anaesthesia on blood gases, acid-base status and ions in the toad *Bufo marinus*. Comp Biochem Physiol 2002;131:639–46.

30. Brown HHK, Tyler HK, Mousseau TA. Orajel as an amphibian anesthetic: refining the technique. Herpetol Rev 2004;35:252.

31. Crook AC, Whiteman HH. An evaluation of MS-222 and benzocaine as anesthetics for metamorphic and paedomorphic tiger salamanders (*Ambystoma tigrinum nebulosum*). Am Midl Nat 2006;155:417–21.

32. Speare R, Speare B, Muller R, et al. Anesthesia of tadpoles of the southern brown tree frog (*Litoria ewingii*) with isoeugenol (Aqui-S). J Zoo Wildl Med 2014;45: 492–6.

33. Guénette SA, Hélie P, Beaudry F, et al. Eugenol for anesthesia of African clawed frogs (*Xenopus laevis*). Vet Anaesth Analg 2007;34:164–70.

34. Goulet F, Hélie P, Vachon P. Eugenol anesthesia in African clawed frogs (*Xenopus laevis*) of different body weights. J Am Assoc Lab Anim Sci 2010;49:460–3.

35. Goulet F, Vachon P, Hélie P. Evaluation of the toxicity of eugenol at anesthetic doses in African clawed frogs (*Xenopus laevis*). Toxicol Pathol 2011;39:471–7.

36. Lafortune M, Mitchell MA, Smith JA. Evaluation of medetomidine, clove oil and propofol for anesthesia of leopard frogs. J Herp Med Surg 2001;11:13–8.

37. Ross A, Guénette, Hélie P, et al. Cas de nécrose cutanée chez des grenouilles africaines à une application topique d'eugénol. Can Vet J 2006;47:1115–7.

38. Salbego J, Maia JLS, Toni C, et al. Anesthesia and sedation of map treefrog (*Hypsiboas geographicus*) tadpoles with essential oils. Ciência Rural 2017;47: e20160909.
39. Smith JM, Stump KC. Isoflurane anesthesia in the African clawed frog (*Xenopus laevis*). Contemp Top Am Assoc Lab Anim Sci 2000;39:39–42.
40. Barter LS, Antognini JF. Kinetics and potency of halothane, isoflurane, and desflurane in the Northern leopard frog *Rana pipiens*. Vet Res Commun 2008;32: 357–65.
41. Barter LS, Mark LO, Smith AC, et al. Isoflurane potency in the Northern leopard frog *Rana pipiens* is similar to that in mammalian species and is unaffected by decerebration. Vet Res Comm 2007;31:757–63.
42. Barbon AR, Routh A, Lopez J. Inhalatory isoflurane anesthesia in mountain chicken frogs (*Leptodactylus fallax*). J Zoo Wildl Med 2019;50:453–6.
43. Ardente AJ, Barlow BM, Burns P, et al. Vehicle effects on in vitro transdermal absorption of sevoflurane in the bullfrog, *Rana catesbeiana*. Environ Toxicol Pharmacol 2008;25:373–9.
44. Williams CJA, Alstrup AKO, Bertelsen MF, et al. Cardiovascular effects of alfaxalone and propofol in the bullfrog, *Lithobates catesbeianus*. J Zoo Wildl Med 2018;49:92–8.
45. Von Esse FV, Wright KM. Effect of intracoelomic propofol in White's tree frogs, *Pelodryas caerulea*. Bull Assoc Reptil Amphib Vet 1999;9:7–8.
46. Mitchell MA, Riggs SM, Singleton CB, et al. Evaluating the clinical and cardiopulmonary effects of clove oil and propofol in tiger salamanders (*Ambystoma tigrinum*). J Exot Pet Med 2009;18:50–6.
47. Guénette SA, Beaudry F, Vachon P. Anesthetic properties of propofol in African clawed frogs (*Xenopus laevis*). J Am Assoc Lab Anim Sci 2008;47:35–8.
48. Posner LP, Bailey KM, Richardson EY, et al. Alfaxalone anesthesia in bullfrogs (*Lithobates catesbeiana*) by injection or immersion. J Zoo Wildl Med 2013;44: 965–71.
49. Cermakova E, Oliveri M, Ceplecha V, et al. Anesthesia with intramuscular administration of alfaxalone in Spanish ribbed newt (*Pleurodeles waltl*). J Exot Pet Med 2020;33:23–6.
50. Adami C, Spadavecchia C, Angeli G, et al. Alfaxalone anesthesia by immersion in oriental fire-bellied toads (*Bombina orientalis*). Vet Anaesth Analgesia 2015;42: 547–51.
51. Sladakovic I, Johnson RS, Vogelnest L. Evaluation of intramuscular alfaxalone in three Australian frog species (*Litoria caerulea, Litoria aurea, Litoria booroolongensis*). J Herp Med Surg 2014;24:36–42.
52. Latney LV, Miller E, Pessier AP. Nuptial pad amputation in an American bullfrog (*Lithobates catesbeianus*) with squamous cell carcinoma. J Zoo Wildl Med 2015;46:941–4.
53. Chatigny F, Kamunde C, Creighton CM, et al. Uses and doses of local anesthetics in fish, amphibians, and reptiles. J Am Assoc Lab Anim Sci 2017;56:244–53.
54. Williams CJA, Alstrup AKO, Bertelsen MF, et al. When local anesthesia becomes universal: pronounced systemic effects of subcutaneous lidocaine in bullfrogs (*Lithobates catesbeianus*). Comp Biochem Physiol 2017;209:41–6.
55. Yaw TJ, Mans C, Martinelli L, et al. Comparison of subcutaneous administration of alfaxalone-midazolam-dexmedetomidine with ketamine-midazolam-dexmedetomidine for chemical restraint in juvenile blue poison dart frogs (*Dendrobates tinctorius azureus*). J Zoo Wildl Med 2019;50:868–73.

56. Stevens CW, Brenner GM. Spinal administration of adrenergic agents produces analgesia in amphibians. Europ J Pharmacol 1996;316:205–10.
57. Koeller CA. Comparison of buprenorphine and butorphanol analgesia in the Eastern red-spotted newt (*Notophthalmus viridescens*). J Am Assoc Lab Anim Sci 2009;48:171–5.
58. Doss GA, Nevarez JG, Fowlkes N, et al. Evaluation of metomidate hydrochloride as an anesthetic in leopard frogs (*Rana pipiens*). J Zoo Wildl Med 2014;45:53–9.
59. Downes H, Courogen PM. Contrasting effects of anesthetics in tadpole bioassays. J Pharmacol Exp Ther 1996;278:284–96.
60. Downes H, Koop DR, Klopfenstein B, et al. Retention of nociceptor responses during deep barbiturate anesthesia in frogs. Comp Biochem Physiol 1999;124:203–10.
61. Lillywhite HB, Shine R, Jacobson E, et al. Amphibians and reptiles used in scientific research: should hypothermia and freezing be prohibited? Bio Sci 2016;67:53–61.
62. Medler S. Anesthetic MS-222 eliminates nerve and muscle activity in frogs used for physiology teaching laboratories. Adv Physiol Educ 2019;43:69–75.
63. Suckow MA, Terril LA, Gridgesby CF, et al. Evaluation of hypothermia-induced analgesia and influence of opioid antagonists in leopard frogs (*Rana pipiens*). Pharmacol Biochem Behav 1999;63:39–43.
64. AVMA. Guidelines for the euthanasia of animals 2020. Available at: www.avma.org/sites/default/files/2020-01/2020-Euthanasia-Final-1-17-20.pdf. Accessed December 8, 2020.
65. Warwick C, Bates G, Arena PC, et al. Reevaluating the use of hypothermia for anesthetizing and euthanizing amphibians and reptiles. J Am Vet Med Assoc 2018;253:1536–9.
66. Galex IA, Gallant CM, D'Avignon N, et al. Evaluation of effective and practical euthanasia methods for larval African clawed frogs (*Xenopus laevis*). J Am Assoc Lab Anim Sci 2020;59:269–74.
67. Balko JA, Posner LP, Chinnadurai SK. Immersion in tricaine methanesulfonate (MS-222) is not sufficient for euthanasia of smokey jungle frogs (*Leptodactylus pentadactylus*). J Zoo Wildl Med 2019;50:89–95.

Chelonian Sedation and Anesthesia

Stefania Scarabelli, DVM, MRCVS, Cert AVP (VA), Dipl ECVAA, Dipl ACVAA[a],
Nicola Di Girolamo, DVM, MSc(EBHC), PhD, Dipl ECZM (Herp), Dipl ACZM[b],*

KEYWORDS

- Anesthesia • Sedation • Intrathecal • Turtle • Tortoise • Terrapin

KEY POINTS

- Knowledge of respiratory and cardiac anatomy and physiology is of paramount importance to provide safe anesthesia in chelonians
- Alternatives to general anesthesia, such as sedation and locoregional anesthesia (especially intrathecal), are indicated for specific procedures
- Patient history and preoperative clinical examination should be performed together with patient stabilization, when needed, before general anesthesia
- Induction of general anesthesia with inhalant anesthetics is not warranted in chelonians; instead, hypnotic injectable agents (propofol and alfaxalone) are preferred
- Despite inhalant agents being the most common drugs used for maintenance of general anesthesia, due to chelonians' ability to shunt, total intravenous anesthesia should be considered

 Video content accompanies this article at http://www.vetexotic.theclinics.com.

INTRODUCTION

Anesthetic management of chelonians represents a unique challenge; the order Chelonia includes numerous species that display diverse anatomic features, habitats, body sizes, temperaments, and metabolic rates. Body size and temperament should be considered when determining the approach for an anesthetic procedure. The anesthetist must be familiar with the peculiar anatomy and physiology of the cardiovascular and respiratory system as these heavily influence drug disposition, equipment, and monitoring during the procedure. Besides considerations related to the patient, an anesthetic plan should be related to the procedure, including the setting (hospital,

[a] Clinica Veterinaria Malpensa-Anicura, Via G. Marconi 27, Samarate, VA 21017, Italy;
[b] Department of Veterinary Clinical Sciences, College of Veterinary Medicine, Oklahoma State University, 2065 West Farm Road, Stillwater, OK 74078, USA
* Corresponding author.
E-mail address: nicoladiggi@gmail.com

Vet Clin Exot Anim 25 (2022) 49–72
https://doi.org/10.1016/j.cvex.2021.08.009
1094-9194/22/© 2021 Elsevier Inc. All rights reserved.
vetexotic.theclinics.com

field), available resources, length of the procedure, possible complications, and the expected degree of pain. In addition, the clinician should be familiar with the pharmacology of the drugs used in the perianesthetic period and be aware of differences regarding doses and effects.

CARDIOVASCULAR ANATOMY AND PHYSIOLOGY

The heart in chelonians is located within the pericardial sac and lies on the ventral midline where the humeral, pectoral, and abdominal scutes of the plastron intersect.[1] As for Squamata, the heart is 3-chambered with 2 anatomically separated atria and a single ventricle that is functionally divided by a muscular ridge into 2 main chambers, the *cavum dorsale* and *cavum pulmonale*. The *cavum dorsale* can be functionally compared to the left ventricle of mammals and is further subdivided into a *cavum arteriosus*, into which the left atrium empties, and a *cavum venosum*, which receives blood from the right atrium and from which both the right and left aortic arches originate.[2] The *cavum pulmonale* gives origin to the pulmonary artery and can be functionally compared to the right ventricle of mammals. The *cavum venosum* and the *cavum arteriosum* are connected by an interventricular canal[2] that is responsible for chelonians' ability to shunt blood from systemic to pulmonary circulation, and vice versa. In physiologic conditions of normal ventilation and temperature, the muscular ridge in the ventricle minimizes mixing of well oxygenated and poorly oxygenated blood, but the shunt fraction and direction can be influenced by several factors. The main determinant of blood direction is the balance of pulmonary and systemic vascular resistance (SVR)[2,3]; for example, periods of apnea during diving will lead to an increase in pulmonary vascular resistance (PVR) with shunting of blood "away" from the nonfunctional lung to the systemic circulation. This is a protective mechanism to preserve oxygen when ventilation is absent. The opposite will occur during periods of respiratory activity with a decrease in PVR and a left-to-right (L-R) shunt.[2]

Sympathetic and parasympathetic nervous systems play a pivotal role in shunt direction. The pulmonary vasculature of chelonians exhibits a cholinergic vasoconstrictor innervation; therefore, stimulation of the vagus nerve will result in an increase in PVR and development of a right-to-left (R-L) shunt. In fact, when atropine (5 mg/kg intra-arterial), an antagonist at muscarinic cholinergic receptors, was administered in pond sliders (*Trachemys scripta*), an L-R shunt was elicited.[4] An increase in pulmonary arterial flow after atropine administration (1 mg/kg IV) has also been reported in anesthetized red-footed tortoises (*Chelonoidis carbonaria*).[5] Sympathetic stimulation has been reported to have different effects on the pulmonary vasculature depending on the species considered; however, even if the adrenergic control of intracardiac shunting is not completely understood, a net L-R shunt seems to be the predominant effect of sympathetic activation.[5] For example, epinephrine infusion has been reported to increase blood flow in the pulmonary circulation in pond sliders[6] and an L-R shunt due to sympathetic activation has been suspected in common snapping turtles (*Chelydra serpentina*).[7]

Another factor strictly related to cardiac shunting is thermoregulation. It has been proposed that cardiac shunt patterns can influence the rate of temperature change in chelonians. However, the changes in blood flow pattern may not be the cause of a decrease in SVR, but a consequence, and reflect differences in vascular resistance rather than represent an actual regulation of the shunt pattern.[8] A net L-R shunt has been reported in pond sliders during moments of activity, but the direction and magnitude of shunting was much more variable when turtles were kept at unstable temperatures, supporting the hypothesis that temperature affects shunts.[9]

The ability of chelonians to shunt is particularly relevant for the anesthetist in the perioperative period. An R-L shunt may affect induction, making inhalant anesthetics less effective as induction agents. If R-L shunting develops, the anesthetic gas that reaches the lungs will not achieve a similar concentration in the systemic circulation because of the 2 circulations being independent. An R-L shunt will influence respiratory monitoring. Capnography is one of the most useful tools in mammalian anesthesia, as end-tidal carbon dioxide ($ETCO_2$) is reflective of the partial pressure of carbon dioxide in arterial blood ($Paco_2$). In chelonians, the presence of shunting will make information gathered with capnography difficult to interpret.

An R-L shunt, moving blood away from the pulmonary circulation, can affect depth and stability when using inhalant anesthesia and may be one cause of prolonged recoveries. A study in common snapping turtles[7] reported the administration of epinephrine 0.1 mg/kg intramuscularly (IM) after 90 minutes of isoflurane anesthesia shortened recovery times, and the authors speculated that shunt reduction was a possible explanation. Other authors investigated the influence of shunt fraction and direction on minimum anesthetic concentration (MAC) of isoflurane in red-footed tortoises, and found MAC was decreased after atropine administration and subsequent increase in pulmonary arterial flow when measured with electrocardiogram-gated MRI.[5]

Most of the drugs used in the perioperative period, through their direct or indirect activity on the autonomic nervous system, can potentially influence shunting. Ventilation strategies, pain (and its control), and maintenance of a preferred body temperature are other fundamental factors.

Blood pressure (BP) in chelonians seems to be controlled by mechanisms similar to those described in mammals, and the adrenergic system plays a pivotal role. For example, alpha-1 receptor activation with norepinephrine has been reported to increase systemic BP, whereas a decrease was seen after phentolamine administration and receptor blockade in pond sliders.[3] However, unlike in mammals, BP in chelonians is directly affected by factors such as temperature changes,[10] and, indirectly, by changes in the levels of activity and amount and direction of shunting.

Another important feature of the cardiovascular system of chelonians is the presence of the renal and hepatic portal systems. Briefly, the renal system is believed to be activated during periods of dehydration, where blood in the caudal part of the body will flow directly to the kidneys through the coccygeal and iliac veins, perfuse the renal tubules, and leave the kidneys by the efferent portal vein to join the postcaval vein.[11] When hydration status is normal, this system can be bypassed and blood flows directly into the ventral abdominal vein, to the hepatic portal vein, and enters the liver (hepatic portal system). Flow direction is ruled by valves positioned between the femoral and abdominal veins.[12] Some studies have shown differing effects of drugs with administration into the caudal half of the body compared to the cranial half. Propofol administered in the coccygeal vein of yellow-bellied sliders (Trachemys scripta scripta) had less efficacy compared with the cranial half.[12] A pharmacokinetic study on buprenorphine in red-eared sliders reported plasma concentrations were lower with administration into the pelvic limbs compared with forelimbs,[13] likely due to first pass extraction by the liver. Given this potential difference, drugs with hepatic or renal metabolism in chelonians should be administered in the cranial half of the body.

RESPIRATORY ANATOMY AND PHYSIOLOGY

Chelonians are obligate nasal breathers, with the glottis being located at the base of the tongue and leading directly into the trachea. The trachea has complete cartilaginous rings, necessitating the use of uncuffed endotracheal tubes (ETTs). The trachea runs on the left side of the neck, is relatively short, and bifurcates at the thoracic inlet into a left and right intrapulmonary bronchus. Attention should be paid to avoid endobronchial intubation. The lungs are paired, multichambered, and are located dorsally beneath the carapace and the vertebral column. Chelonians have a larger lung volume but smaller respiratory surface area relative to lung volume[14] compared with mammals. In addition, chelonians also have a higher lung compliance.[15] It is recommended to use low peak inspiratory pressures (PIPs) during mechanical ventilation, not exceeding 10 cm H_2O.[16] Chelonians lack a true diaphragm and rely on thoracic and abdominal musculature for ventilation. A pseudodiaphragm is present, which separates the lungs from the celomic cavity, and limb movements stretch this septum downward resulting in lung expansion. This relationship between breathing and locomotion has been studied by several authors[17,18] and should be considered when immobilization will lead to ventilatory depression. For this reason, positive pressure ventilation (PPV) is generally recommended in anesthetized chelonians.

Respiration in chelonians is controlled by oxygen, carbon dioxide, and environmental temperature, and different responses to changes in these parameters have been reported among species.[19] Hypoxia and hypercapnia induce an increase in ventilation, most commonly achieved with an increase in respiratory rate (RR) rather than an increase in tidal volume (TV), whereas hyperoxia decreases ventilation.[19,20] During diving, hypoxia induces bradypnea and hypercapnia causes tachypnea[21]; the physiologic aim is to preserve oxygen and eliminate carbon dioxide.

Chelonians have low oxygen consumption compared with mammals and can tolerate hypoxic conditions with cardiovascular adaptations, such as shunting, changes in heart rate (HR), reduction in their metabolic rate, and an ability to buffer lactic acid produced from the conversion to anaerobic metabolism.[22]

Chelonians are predisposed to respiratory disease because of their inability to cough and their poorly developed mucociliary apparatus, and inflammatory exudates can accumulate in the dependent portion of the lungs and worsen gas exchange. Clinical signs of respiratory distress may be delayed because of their resistance to hypoxia,[23] but these alterations can become relevant during an anesthetic event.

Some important differences between ventilation in turtles and tortoises, and aquatic and terrestrial species, should be mentioned. In turtles, both inspiration and expiration are active, whereas in tortoises, inspiration can be passive.[24] Respiratory patterns are different between aquatic and terrestrial species. One study,[19] comparing breathing patterns in leopard tortoises (*Testudo pardalis*) and African side-necked turtles (*Pelomedusa subrufa*), found periods of breath-holding and single breaths alternated in leopard tortoises, whereas breathing in side-necked turtles was characterized by episodes of several consecutive breaths separated by periods of breath-holding. In both species, breath-holding was preceded by inspiration and resumption of breathing was initiated by expiration. Several studies have evaluated TV in tortoises[19,25] and turtles[19,26,27] with variable results; however, in general, turtles have higher values per kilogram. This may be due to the lungs serving 2 functions, ventilation and buoyancy, in aquatic species. In mammals, where TV is generally considered around 10 mL/kg for all species, volume-controlled ventilation is often an option when mechanical ventilation is required. In chelonians, differences in TV make pressure-controlled ventilation strategies the favorite choice. Appropriate ventilation may also be relevant for cardiovascular shunting, as PPV will influence PVR which, in turn, will influence shunt direction. In mammals, PVR is increased if too low or too high TV is applied.[28] Lastly, some aquatic species can respire across their skin, pharyngeal mucosa, and/or cloacal bursae; however, the clinical impact of these modes of respiration is unclear.

THERMOREGULATION

Chelonians are ectothermic and the regulation of body temperature depends on the external environment. Some species, such as leatherback sea turtles (*Dermochelys coriacea*), can maintain their body temperature near the optimal zone over a large range of ambient temperatures through different mechanisms.[29] The preferred optimal temperature range (POTR) varies among species; however, 26 to 38°C and 25 to 35°C are considered adequate for terrestrial and aquatic/semiaquatic species, respectively.[30]

Maintenance of adequate temperature is particularly relevant in the perioperative period. As discussed previously, temperature influences cardiac shunting, and shunting influences anesthesia. Temperature is one of the main determinants of metabolic rate. If temperature decreases, metabolism will slow and increase the duration of administered drugs and prolong recovery. The influence of temperature on anesthetic drug effects has been extensively studied in reptiles. In chelonians, 2 studies evaluating the effects of alfaxalone in red-eared sliders (*Trachemys scripta elegans*) at different body temperatures reported that, at lower temperatures, turtles were more sedate, and the drugs' effects lasted longer.[31,32] Temperature influences the onset of sedation as well, with prolonged time to reach maximal effects at lower temperatures.[32]

PREANESTHETIC EVALUATION

Preoperative patient assessment is important to evaluate the anesthetic risks, discuss these with the owner, plan the perioperative management, and to stabilize the animal before the anesthetic event. Identification of the species is important due to anatomic differences, POTR, and drug dosing. A complete history should be collected to gain information about husbandry, diet, and environment, and to evaluate for underlying diseases and their duration. A thorough physical examination is of paramount importance, even if limited in conscious chelonians. An accurate weight is needed for appropriate drug dosing and can be used to estimate overall health. Chelonians are resilient to respiratory diseases and mild signs may indicate severe underlying problems. RR, depth, and patterns should be assessed together with the presence of nasal, oral, and ocular discharge or conjunctivitis. If indicated, diagnostic tests, such as radiographs and bacterial culture, should be performed.[33]

A basic assessment of the cardiovascular system should include HR or pulse rate. A Doppler probe, placed at the level of the carotid or femoral artery, can be used.[15] Hydration status is difficult to evaluate in chelonians but can be estimated from history, skin turgor, presence of sunken eyes, increased hematocrit, and hyperproteinemia. In turtles, total body water is around 75% of body mass and it is nearly equally distributed between the intracellular and extracellular compartments with a total blood volume around 7% of body mass.[34] These values should be considered for fluid therapy planning.

Body temperature should be measured before anesthesia and, if not an emergency, animals should be acclimatized, and temperature maintained within POTR before drug administration.

Hematology and biochemistry are useful before sedation or anesthesia, as in other animals. Hematocrit, total protein, and albumin contribute to the evaluation of hydration status. Glucose levels are lower in reptiles compared with mammals and are variable among chelonian species. Hematocrit and glucose can provide prognostic indications in chelonians that may be helpful when discussing the anesthetic event with the owner.[35] Electrolytes, particularly calcium and phosphorus levels, can be altered during nutritional or renal hyperparathyroidism and chronic renal disease. The usefulness of uric acid, blood urea nitrogen, and ammonia may vary in the evaluation of kidney function depending on the species (aquatic vs semiaquatic/semiterrestrial vs terrestrial).[36]

SEDATION AND ROUTES OF ADMINISTRATION

Sedation may be needed in large, uncooperative chelonians for physical examination, blood sampling, and diagnostic imaging, in addition to being used before general anesthesia. Sedative drugs used in chelonians include alpha-2 agonists and benzodiazepines that may be combined with ketamine and/or opioids to improve sedation and provide further analgesia. Sedation and local anesthesia can be used for certain types of procedures. Several routes of drug administration are available for sedation (Table 1).

The IM route is commonly used for premedication in chelonians. These injections are generally performed in the pectoral, triceps, or caudal aspect of the biceps muscles.[37] The pelvic limb muscles are generally avoided because of potential renal portal system and/or hepatic first-pass effects.

Subcutaneous (SC) injections can be performed by tenting the skin in the axillary or inguinal region.[30]

Intravenous access is critical for induction, maintenance, and recovery of chelonians under general anesthesia. As in other species, IV drug administration will lead to a faster onset of action and decrease the variability in drug uptake; moreover, some drugs can only be administered IV. The jugular vein is the most accessible location for catheterization (Fig. 1). The external jugular vein in chelonians is superficial and located at different levels of the lateral aspect of the neck. To identify the vein, the chelonian is placed in lateral recumbency with the neck extended and the head slightly flexed laterally to increase exposure. In small to medium species (300–500 g and up to 3–5 kg), the jugular vein is visible after compression is applied at the cranial coelomic inlet. If the vein is not readily visible, latero-lateral maneuvering of the head may aid in visualization. If it is not visible externally, in most chelonians, the dorsal edge of the tympanic membrane can be used as an effective landmark for catheterization, as the vein runs caudal to it. Before placing the catheter, the authors modify it by adding 2 small pieces of medical tape to create wings. These custom-made wings adhere better to the neck of the animal than the plastic wings available on specific catheters. The use of silk-like tape (Durapore, 3M, St. Paul, MN, USA) is preferred over plastic tape (Transpore, 3M, St. Paul, MN, USA). Cyanoacrylate glue is effective when applied in small amounts (1 drop per side) to create an adherence between the tape and the skin. The superficial layer of skin with the glue is typically shed in the following days after application, without leaving evident markings or inflammation.

The subcarapacial venous sinus, located on the midline of the cranial aspect of the carapace in the region where the cervical vertebrae join the shell, has been historically used for IV drug administration in chelonians. However, death and transient or permanent paresis and paralysis have been reported after IV administration in this site,[38,39] and as such this site should not be used for clinical purposes.

Intranasal (IN) drug administration for sedation has inconsistent effects in chelonian.[40,41] Intraosseous (IO), intracoelomic, and intracloacal routes are less commonly used in chelonians. The IO route has suboptimal distribution of fluids,[42] but the gular scutes are readily accessible for catheter placement (Fig. 2). The intracoelomic route carries the risk of inadvertent organ puncture, and the intracloacal route has been reported to be poorly reliable for sedative administration.[43]

Table 1
Anesthetic agents used in selected chelonian species

Specie	Drug and Dose (mg/kg)	Route	Comments	Reference
Red-eared sliders	0.1 Mede + 5 Keta	IM	Anesthesia for minor procedures and ETI	Greer et al,[44] 2001
Red-eared sliders	0.2 Mede + 10 Keta	IM	Anesthesia for skin incision and suture	Greer et al,[44] 2001
Green sea turtles	0.05 Mede + 5 Keta + 5 Tramadol	IM	Deep sedation, loss of reflexes (except palpebral), no reaction to flipper pinch and venipuncture, partially maintained jaw tone	Scheelings et al,[45] 2020
Leatherback sea turtles	0.03–0.08 Mede + 3–8 Keta	IV	Sole combination for field anesthesia	Harms et al,[46] 2007
Loggerhead sea turtles	0.05 Mede + 5 Keta	IV	Induction of general anesthesia followed by maintenance with sevoflurane	Chittick et al,[47] 2002
Yellow-bellied sliders	0.2 Dexmed + 10 Keta	IN	Sedation for clinical examination, venipuncture, minor procedures	Schnellbacher et al,[41] 2012
Yellow-bellied sliders	0.2 Dexmed + 10 Keta	IC	Unpredictable results	Morici et al,[43] 2017
Loggerhead sea turtles	5 Propofol	IV	Anesthesia for 30 min laparoscopy, rapid recovery	MacLean et al,[60] 2008
Amazon turtles	5–10 Propofol	IV	Dose-dependent depth of anesthesia and recovery times	Quagliatto Santos et al,[61] 2008
Red-eared sliders	10–20 Propofol	IV	Dose-dependent depth of anesthesia and recovery times	Ziolo et al,[62] 2009
Various chelonians	5 Alfax	IV	Anesthetic plan suitable for ETI and surgical plan for about 27 min	Knotek,[63] 2014
Loggerhead sea turtles	3,5, 10 Alfax	IV	All doses allowed ETI, dose-dependent recovery times. At the highest dose, IPPV was required	Phillips et al,[64] 2017
Macquarie River Turtles	9 Alfax	IV	Anesthetic plan suitable for ETI but not surgical plan was reached; short recovery times.	Scheelings,[65] 2013
Russian tortoises	10–20 Alfax ± 0.1–0.05 Mede	IM	Alfaxalone alone sedation for nonpainful procedures. Adding mede provided deeper	Hansen & Bertelsen,[66] 2013

(continued on next page)

Table 1
(continued)

Specie	Drug and Dose (mg/kg)	Route	Comments	Reference
			sedation but with cardiovascular and respiratory depression	
Red-eared sliders	10–20 Alfax	IM	Effects at two different ambient temperatures were evaluated. Dose-dependent and inconsistent response. At higher temperature, higher doses needed and shorter duration	Shepard et al,[31] 2013
Red-eared sliders	10–20 Alfax	IM	Effects at two different ambient temperatures were evaluated. Dose-dependent response. At higher temperature, higher doses needed and shorter duration	Kischinovsky et al,[32] 2012
Macquarie River Turtles	9 Alfax	IM	No sedation	Scheelings,[65] 2013

Abbreviations: Alfax, alfaxalone; Dexmed, dexmedetomidine; ETI, endotracheal intubation; IPPV, intermittent positive pressure ventilation; Keta, ketamine; Mede, medetomidine; PPV, positive pressure ventilation.

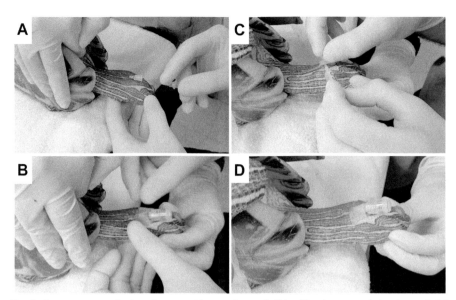

Fig. 1. Intravenous catheter placement in a red-eared slider (*Trachemys scripta elegans*). (*A*) Placement of the catheter. To identify the external jugular vein, the chelonian is placed in lateral recumbency with the neck extended and the head slightly flexed laterally to increase exposure. Notice the small amount of flush in the catheter. (*B*) Two small pieces of medical tape are added to the catheter to create wings. These wings adhere to the neck of the animal better than the plastic wings available on some catheters. The use of silk-like tape (eg, Durapore, 3M) is preferred over plastic (eg, Transpore, 3M). (*C*) Cyanoacrylate glue is applied (1 drop per side) to create an adherence between the tape and the skin. (*D*) Intravenous drugs can be administered through the catheter.

Alpha-2 Agonists and Ketamine

Alpha-2 agonists provide sedation, muscle relaxation, and analgesia. Reported doses are variable depending on route of administration, species of interest, desired level of sedation/anesthesia, and drug combinations.

The IM route is advantageous for ease of administration in uncooperative animals or when IV access is unavailable. Alpha-2 agonists are often combined with ketamine and effects are dose-dependent. For example, in red-eared sliders, 0.1 mg/kg medetomidine and 5 mg/kg ketamine IM provided an anesthesia level adequate for minor procedures and endotracheal intubation (ETI), whereas when 0.2 mg/kg medetomidine and 10 mg/kg ketamine were administered, skin incision and suture could be performed.[44] In green sea turtles (*Chelonia mydas*), medetomidine 0.05 mg/kg combined with ketamine 5 mg/kg and tramadol 5 mg/kg IM provided deep sedation with loss of all reflexes except the palpebral, no reaction to flipper pinch and venipuncture, and only partially maintained jaw tone.[45] In leatherback sea turtles (*D coriacea*), IV medetomidine (0.03–0.08 mg/kg) and ketamine (3–8 mg/kg) have been used for field anesthesia as a sole combination,[46] and lower doses (0.05 mg/kg medetomidine and 5 mg/kg ketamine) have been used in loggerhead sea turtles (*Caretta caretta*) for induction of general anesthesia before maintenance with sevoflurane.[47]

The sedative effects of dexmedetomidine 0.2 mg/kg with ketamine 10 mg/kg have been evaluated IN[41] and intracloacally[43] in yellow-bellied sliders. After IN administration, an adequate level of sedation for clinical examination, venipuncture, or minor

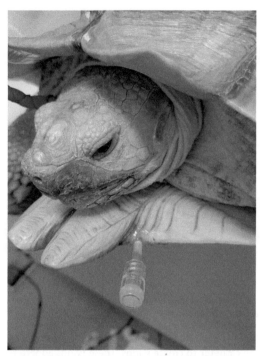

Fig. 2. Intraosseous catheter placed in the gular scute of an African-spurred tortoise (*Centrochelys sulcata*).

procedures was achieved, whereas intracloacal administration produced unpredictable results.

One of the advantages of the use of alpha-2 agonists is they can be antagonized to have faster and more predictable recoveries. Atipamezole using 5 times the dose of administered medetomidine has been used in chelonians.[46,48] Hypotension has been reported in gopher tortoises (*Gopherus polyphemus*) after IV atipamezole administration[48]; therefore, this route should be reserved for emergency situations. The use of IN atipamezole at 2.5 times the dose of IN dexmedetomidine has been reported to be efficacious.[41]

The main side effects of alpha-2 agonists are cardiovascular and respiratory depression. Decrease in HR, BP, and RR have been reported in desert tortoises (*Gopherus agassizii*) after administration of high doses (0.15 mg/kg) of medetomidine IM.[49] Another study evaluating the cardiopulmonary effects of medetomidine 0.1 mg/kg with ketamine 5 mg/kg IV reported a transient increase in BP and mild hypoventilation.[48] Apnea has been reported after medetomidine 0.05 mg/kg combined with ketamine and tramadol IM.[45]

Ketamine is a dissociative anesthetic which provides analgesia at subanesthetic doses. It is commonly used in chelonians as a component of a premedication protocol, and often in combination with sedatives and/or opioids. When high doses are used, induction of general anesthesia can be achieved; however, recovery times can be extremely prolonged. Ketamine is a racemic mixture consisting of the 2 enantiomers R-ketamine and S-ketamine; in some mammalian species, the use of S-ketamine has been reported to induce better analgesia and shorter recovery times.[50,51] No differences were found when effects of ketamine and S-ketamine, in association with medetomidine, were compared in Hermann's (*Testudo hermanni*) and spur-thighed tortoises (*Testudo graeca*).[52] Several doses have been reported in the literature; it is the authors' opinion that doses between 5 and 10 mg/kg should be used for premedication.

Benzodiazepines

Benzodiazepines provide sedation and muscle relaxation, but do not have analgesic effects. Both midazolam and diazepam have been used in chelonians; however, midazolam can be administered IM because of its physicochemical properties and diazepam should only be administered IV because of poor absorption when injected IM. Benzodiazepines are considered safe from a cardiovascular standpoint and are commonly combined with ketamine to decrease its dose, counteract muscle rigidity, and avoid prolonged recoveries. Reported doses vary between 0.25 and 2 mg/kg in association with ketamine, and the duration of sedation is dose-dependent.[53] Midazolam has been evaluated as a sole agent in chelonians; however, sedation was achieved only in some species.[54] Midazolam IN failed to produce sedation in red-footed and Burmese star tortoises (*Geochelone platynota*).[55]

Opioids

Opioids can be added to a premedication protocol to provide analgesia. In particular, morphine, hydromorphone, and tramadol have been proven to have analgesic effects in chelonians. Morphine at 1.5 or 6.5 mg/kg SC[56] and 2 mg/kg SC[57] provided analgesia in turtles, with respiratory depression being the most relevant side effect. Hydromorphone, another full mu-agonist, was efficacious in red-eared slider turtles.[58] In contrast, both butorphanol[56,57] and buprenorphine[58] failed to provide adequate antinociception. Tramadol, administered at 5 and 10 mg/kg PO, provided thermal analgesia in turtles with less respiratory depression than morphine.[59]

INDUCTION OF GENERAL ANESTHESIA

General anesthesia in chelonians is induced with hypnotic agents, such as propofol and alfaxalone (see **Table 1**). Induction with inhalant anesthetics should be avoided because of chelonians' ability to breath-hold, the potential triggering of the dive reflex, and the high doses of inhalants required which may be unsafe for the patient (cardiovascular depressant) and personnel (environmental contamination).

Propofol

Propofol is a common induction agent used in reptiles. It is a propyl phenol derivate that works on γ-aminobutyric acid (GABA) receptors. In mammals, it produces a rapid and smooth induction of anesthesia and can be used for maintenance as a constant rate infusion. It does not provide analgesia and it has partial extrahepatic metabolism. The main disadvantage is it can only be administered IV or IO. In chelonians, it has been used as an induction agent to facilitate ETI or as a sole agent for short procedures.[16] In loggerhead sea turtles, 5 mg/kg IV propofol was sufficient for 30 minutes of laparoscopy and provided rapid recoveries with a safe return to water shortly after the procedure.[60] Doses of 5 to 10 mg/kg IV have been reported in Arrau river turtle (*Podocnemis expansa*),[61] whereas 10 to 20 mg/kg has been successfully used in red-eared sliders via supravertebral sinus injection, with depth of anesthesia and recovery times being dose-dependent.[62] Owing to the reported accidental submeningeal injection of propofol after administration by this route,[38] supravertebral sinus injections should be avoided. As in mammals, hypoventilation and apnea are reported side effects of propofol administration in chelonians, and the anesthetist should be prepared for ETI and PPV when using this drug. Administration of propofol using an IV catheter rather than a direct injection has the advantage of titrating the drug to effect (Video 1). Typically, for premedicated chelonians with an IV catheter, the authors give small boluses (2–4 mg/kg) until the desired effect is reached.

Alfaxalone

Alfaxalone is a synthetic neuroactive steroid and, similar to propofol, it works on GABA receptors producing hypnosis and muscle relaxation without analgesic properties. In mammals, it is metabolized mainly by the liver. The main advantage is it can be administered IM. Several studies have investigated the use of alfaxalone as a single dose administered IV or IM. In several terrapin and tortoise species, 5 mg/kg IV led to an anesthetic plan suitable for ETI and a surgical plane of anesthesia for about 27 minutes.[63] In loggerhead sea turtles, 3 doses (3, 5, and 10 mg/kg) were administered IV and all doses allowed ETI; recovery times were dose-dependent, and at the highest dose, all animals required PPV.[64] With 9 mg/kg IV in Macquarie River Turtles (*Emydura macquarii*), a suitable anesthetic plane for intubation was reached but not a surgical plane of anesthesia.[65] Moreover, recovery time was shorter compared with other species.[65] Studies investigating the use of alfaxalone IM have been performed in Russian tortoises (*Agrionemys horsfieldii*)[66] and in red-eared sliders.[31,32] Doses of 10 to 20 mg/kg IM were used; at higher temperatures, higher doses were needed and the duration of the effect was shorter because of the increased metabolism. When 9 mg/kg IM was given to Macquarie River Turtles, no sedation was obtained.[65]

Dose-dependent respiratory depression is the most frequently reported side effect of alfaxalone; an increase in $Paco_2$ with a decrease in partial pressure of arterial oxygen and pH, confirming hypoventilation, has been reported in loggerhead sea turtles.[64] The effects on the cardiovascular system have been poorly investigated in chelonians. An increase in HR has been reported in loggerhead sea turtles after IV administration,[64] whereas no changes were reported in Macquarie river turtles[65] and in 2 studies in red-eared sliders[31,32] after IM injection; however, in the last 2 studies, different temperatures were evaluated and influenced the animals' HR, possibly masking direct effects. Studies evaluating changes in BP after alfaxalone administration should be performed in chelonians to better understand the impact on hemodynamics.

INTUBATION

ETI is straightforward to perform in most chelonians as the glottis is located at the aboral termination of the tongue and is typically visible (**Fig. 3**). Owing to tracheal anatomy, short and uncuffed ETT should be used. For small chelonians, appropriately sized tubes can be made from IV or feeding catheters connected to an ETT adapter. The length of the ETT from the patient's oral cavity to the anesthetic circuit should be minimal in order to decrease dead space. In order to expose the glottis, gentle pressure in a caudo-rostral direction is applied to the gular area of the animal, between the aboral termination of the mandibles. The tongue of chelonians is extremely friable and should not be pulled or manipulated with hands or forceps (including plastic atraumatic forceps). Once the glottis is visualized, time is allowed for it to open, or the bevel of the ETT can be used gently to open it. Several commercial or custom-made mouth gags can be used to keep the mouth open around the tube and to prevent biting of the ETT in case of a sudden recovery. This is especially important in chelonians with a stronger bite, such as snapping turtles (**Fig. 4**). In small patients, a tongue depressor

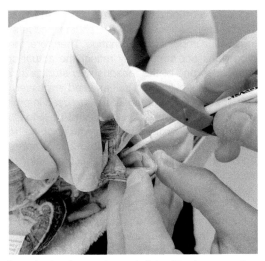

Fig. 3. Endotracheal intubation in a red-eared slider (*Trachemys scripta elegans*).

can be used to attach the animal's head, the ETT, and the circuit end to prevent ETT kinking or extubation.

MAINTENANCE OF ANESTHESIA

There are several options for the maintenance of general anesthesia in chelonians. High doses of injectable drugs used in premedication can directly lead to general anesthesia and be sufficient for procedures of short duration. However, ETI and PPV have been advocated for procedures lasting longer than 15 minutes.[16]

Inhalants

Inhalant agents (sevoflurane and isoflurane) are commonly used for the maintenance of general anesthesia in reptiles; however, in chelonians, inhalant anesthetics can be less reliable. Their abilities to cardiac shunt and breath-hold, especially in aquatic

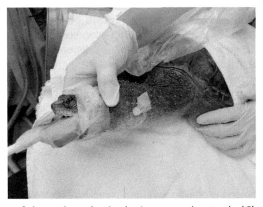

Fig. 4. Arrangement of the endotracheal tube in a snapping turtle (*Chelydra serpentina*).

species, make anesthesia with inhalants unpredictable and susceptible to sudden changes in depth. As discussed earlier, when R-L shunting occurs, there is decreased blood flow to the lungs which impairs gas exchange. Therefore, the monitored expired inhalant concentration does not adequately reflect the actual concentration in the blood and brain. This is also one of the reasons why studies investigating the MAC of inhalants in chelonians are lacking and values used are based on studies in other reptiles and mammals. If sevoflurane or isoflurane are used in premedicated animals, typical concentrations should be around 2% to 3% and 1.5% to 2%, respectively. Isoflurane MAC after elimination of cardiac shunting with atropine has been reported to be 2.2%.[5] In anesthetic events lasting longer than 2 to 3 hours, anesthetic gases can be decreased and even discontinued 20 to 30 minutes before the predicted termination of the procedure to have a smoother recovery.

Propofol and Alfaxalone—total intravenous anesthesia

Another method for maintenance of general anesthesia is to use repeated boluses of injectable drugs; however, this technique will lead to large variations in plasma drug concentrations and a higher risk of drug overdose (increased side effects) and underdose (loss of drug effect). In order to maintain a drug steady therapeutic dose, total intravenous anesthesia (TIVA) is commonly used in humans. The use of TIVA is well recognized in dogs and cats and is gaining popularity in zoologic companion animals. Drugs used for TIVA should have specific pharmacokinetic properties, including a rapid onset of action, rapid metabolism, high clearance, and no cumulative effect. Generally, a hypnotic drug is used in combination with drugs providing analgesia, such as a short-acting opioid. Propofol and alfaxalone can be safely used in TIVA in chelonians.[67] The main disadvantage of TIVA is the need for venous access.

The authors have used propofol and alfaxalone TIVA in a range of species including both terrestrial and aquatic chelonians, and for a range of procedures (**Fig. 5**). For propofol, after premedication with dexmedetomidine, ketamine, and midazolam, an IV catheter is placed in the jugular vein and boluses of propofol 2 to 3 mg/kg are administered until there is loss of jaw tone. ETI is performed and propofol is continued at a variable rate infusion (VRI), starting at 0.2 mg/kg/min and decreasing after the first hour of surgery. If needed, additional propofol boluses are administered IV. For alfaxalone, loading doses of 10 to 20 mg/kg IM are administered, and VRI is performed at 0.2 to 1 mg/kg/min. Both drugs require mechanical ventilation throughout the anesthetic procedure.

PPV should always be performed for chelonians under general anesthesia (**Fig. 6**). As already discussed earlier, pressure-controlled ventilation is preferred with PIP below 10 cm H_2O and RR 2 to 6 breaths/min. Nonrebreathing systems are used for patients less than 10 kg with fresh gas flow (FGF) depending on the breathing system and mechanical ventilator used. For patients weighing greater than 10 kg, a rebreathing system can be used starting with FGF of 100 to 200 mL/kg/min and decreasing to 10 to 20 mL/kg/min when a suitable anesthetic depth has been reached. Pure oxygen or a mix of oxygen and air can be used as carrier gas, considering the chelonian tolerance to hypoxemia. The influence of the inspired gases on recovery times has been studied in other reptile species.[68,69]

MONITORING

Monitoring in chelonians is challenging, and visual and tactile monitoring by a trained and experienced person is of paramount importance.

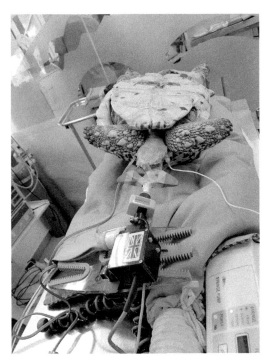

Fig. 5. Leopard tortoise (*Stygmochelis pardalis*) set up for a variable rate infusion of propofol for total intravenous anesthesia. Notice the catheter in the right jugular vein, presence of mainstream capnography, a Doppler pencil probe, and the mechanical ventilator.

Depth of Anesthesia

Depth of anesthesia can be assessed by evaluating the corneal and palpebral reflexes, head withdrawal, muscle tone, movements, and reaction to painful stimuli. Muscle relaxation and loss of response to tactile stimuli in turtles undergoing inhalant anesthesia will appear in the cranial part of the body first and move caudally[70]; tail tone will be lost last. An appropriate surgical plane of anesthesia is usually associated with complete lack of movement, total muscle relaxation, no response to painful stimuli, absent palpebral reflex, and present corneal reflex.

Cardiovascular Monitoring

HR can be measured with ultrasonic Doppler devices (**Fig. 7**). Pencil or flat probes can be placed on either side of the neck, within the thoracic inlet, to detect pulse rate via the carotid artery or to detect HR directly from the heart. In anesthetized chelonians, HR can also be easily evaluated via direct auscultation with an esophageal stethoscope placed into the thoracic esophagus at the level of the heart. Esophageal stethoscopes are inexpensive, easy to use, and should always be available. Respiratory sounds can also be audible using the Doppler or esophageal stethoscope. Electrocardiography (ECG) is useful to detect the electrical activity of the heart, keeping in mind that electrical activity can be present without heart contraction, therefore an ECG signal does not always correspond to adequate stroke volume. A II lead or a base-apex configuration can be used; needles can be placed through the skin to improve signal strength. Chelonian ECG is similar to mammals with P, QRS, and T complexes.

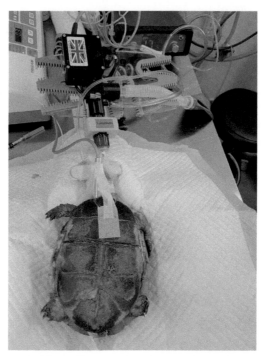

Fig. 6. Chinese box turtle (*Cuora flavomarginata*) set up for mechanical ventilation with a pressure-cycled ventilator (Vetronics, UK) during total intravenous anesthesia.

A wave from the sinus venosus may be seen just before the P wave; in fact, contraction is initiated by the cardiac muscle fibers at this level.[71] There are no definitive reference values for normal HR in chelonians, and because HR is influenced by factors such as body temperature, metabolism, and pain, trends are more useful than single measured values.

Respiratory Monitoring

Chelonians under general anesthesia commonly require PPV. PIP, TV, and compliance can be monitored if a spirometer is available, but the clinical utility of these values still needs to be studied. When breathing spontaneously, RR can be gathered from movements of the skin at the level of the prefemoral fossae or at each side of the thoracic inlet. Pulse oximetry, capnography, and blood gas analysis have limited accuracy in chelonians, but trends can be evaluated (Video 3).

Temperature

Patient temperature should be continuously monitored in the perioperative period. Esophageal or cloacal probes (**Fig. 8**) can be used and temperature should be maintained within the POTR. Hypothermia will lead to decreased metabolism and prolonged recoveries, whereas overheating will increase oxygen consumption and drug metabolism with shortened effects. Several warming devices are available including heating blankets, warm air blankets, and heating mats (see **Fig. 8**); incubators and heat lamps can be used during recovery.

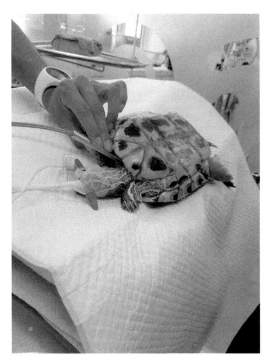

Fig. 7. Placement of a Doppler pencil probe in the left pectoral area of a red-eared slider (*Trachemys scripta elegans*).

FLUID SUPPORT

Fluid therapy should be administered before anesthesia if the animal is considered dehydrated. Fluids can be administered PO, IV, IO, SC, or intracoelomic depending on the degree and duration of dehydration. There is a lack of evidence regarding the most appropriate fluid type to administer in chelonians; species, patient condition, underlying disease, and acid-base status can all influence the type of fluid preferred. One study[72] compared the efficacy of different types of crystalloids in stranded juvenile loggerhead sea turtles in restoring acid-base values and electrolyte imbalances. The highest efficacy was obtained with mixed 0.9% saline-lactated Ringer's solution followed by physiologic saline and lactated Ringer's solution. Reported fluid maintenance for chelonians is 25 to 30 mL/kg/d; fluid volume should not exceed 2% to 3% of total body weight.[15,16] In case of massive blood loss, the use of hetastarch, diluted 1:2 or 1:3 with 0.9% saline administered 0.1 mL/kg every 10 to 15 minutes, has been reported; in case of PCV less than 5%, blood transfusions should be considered.[73] In order to accurately control infusion rate, especially in small chelonians, syringe pumps should be used.

RECOVERY

Recovery from anesthesia with inhalants is generally prolonged in chelonians compared with mammals. For this reason, it is critical to maintain venous and respiratory access during recovery (**Fig. 9**). Inhalant anesthetic concentration should be gradually decreased toward the end of the procedure to fasten recoveries; it is still unclear

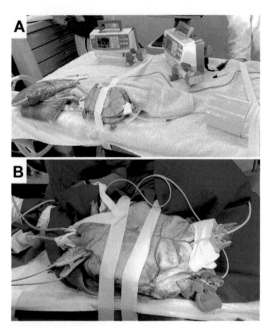

Fig. 8. Examples of devices used to maintain body temperature in chelonians. (A) A three-toed box turtle (*Terrapene carolina triunguis*) is prepared for a prefemoral ovariectomy. Temperature is controlled via a heating mat below the towel and a forced air warming device after covering the patient with the surgical drapes. (B) A Texas tortoise (*Gopherus agassizii*) is prepared for a prefemoral ovariectomy. Temperature is controlled via a forced air warming device.

if switching to lower oxygen concentrations is of any benefit in shortening recovery times. During recovery, chelonians can be ventilated with a bag valve mask (also known as Ambu bag) with room air (Video 2). Hypothermia can further prolong recovery times, therefore maintenance of the POTR is of paramount importance. In snapping turtles, epinephrine (0.1 mg/kg IM) and acupuncture with electrical stimulation at GV-26 were reported to increase HR and decrease recovery time after 90 minutes of isoflurane anesthesia.[7] It is hypothesized that administration of epinephrine reversed the R-L shunt resulting in increased pulmonary blood flow, which allowed inhalant anesthetic removal by the lungs. However, it has been mentioned that the administration of large doses of epinephrine postoperatively in chelonians may also increase SVR and cardiac afterload, thus resulting in compromised perfusion.[74] Considering the effect of postoperative epinephrine has been evaluated in only a limited number of healthy chelonians, further clinical research is required before implementing these treatments.

For the recovery period, the animal should be in a temperature-controlled zone, HR and RR should be monitored, and extubation performed once spontaneous breathing is returned and movements are present. It is not uncommon for chelonians to take a few breaths with the ETT in place and, once extubated, develop apnea again, therefore spontaneous ventilation should be constant and continuous before extubation. Fluid therapy and appropriate analgesia should be continued during the recovery phase. Owing to occasional prolonged recoveries, it is ideal to perform procedures early in the morning when possible so personnel will be available for monitoring.

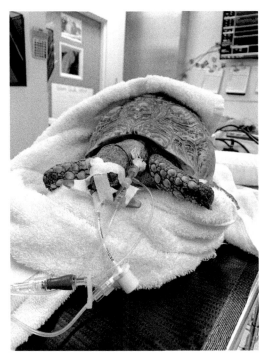

Fig. 9. A leopard tortoise (*Stygmochelis pardalis*) recovering from surgery. The intravenous catheter and endotracheal tube are maintained until the animal has resumed voluntary breathing and is starting to move its head. The endotracheal tube could have been shortened to reduce dead space.

LOCAL ANESTHESIA

Local techniques that can be applied in chelonians include topical application, local infiltration, and intrathecal anesthesia. There are no studies investigating local anesthetic toxicity in chelonians and several toxic doses have been anecdotally reported, mainly based on mammalian studies. The authors consider 4 mg/kg and 1 mg/kg as standard doses for lidocaine and bupivacaine, respectively. In small patients, care must be taken to avoid exceeding these doses; if an adequate volume is not reached, the local anesthetic can be diluted with 0.9% NaCl.

Intrathecal Anesthesia

Intrathecal anesthesia has revolutionized the way certain procedures are performed in chelonians. When performed properly, intrathecal anesthesia can provide desensitization to the tail, cloaca (including phallus and clitoris), and pelvic limbs (Video 3). Several protocols for intrathecal anesthesia in chelonians have been described.[75] Bupivacaine (preservative-free) 1 mg/kg is a safe and effective option. The author typically prepares multiple (2–3) bupivacaine injections in case the injection gets contaminated with blood from the dorsal tail vein. Including a small air bubble between the drug and the syringe plunger helps to determine the typical decrease in resistance encountered when entering the intrathecal space. The tail is pulled firmly and the dorsal vertebral processes are palpated. The needle is inserted on the midline between 2 vertebral processes (**Fig. 10**). The plunger is withdrawn. If blood is sampled, the needle is retracted gently

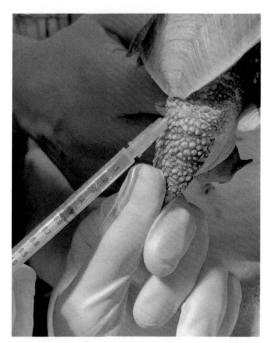

Fig. 10. Administration of intrathecal anesthesia in an African-spurred tortoise (*Centrochelys sulcata*).

and the plunger withdrawn again until no blood is sampled. The injection is given when (1) no blood is sampled and (2) no resistance is perceived. If compression of the air bubble is noticed, the needle should be redirected. On some occasions, a loss of resistance on entrance into the intrathecal space is noted (Video 4).

SUMMARY

Anesthesia in chelonians can be challenging because of their anatomic and physiologic features. Potential differences in drugs' effectiveness because of species, size, body/environment temperature, and administration site should be always be considered. Premedication with sedatives and opioids, induction of general anesthesia with injectable agents, and maintenance with inhalant or intravenous anesthetics should be considered the standard approach for surgical anesthesia. The use of locoregional anesthetic procedures, and in particular intrathecal anesthesia, can have a dramatic impact on chelonian anesthesia.

DISCLOSURE

The authors have nothing to disclose.

SUPPLEMENTARY DATA

Supplementary data to this article can be found online at https://doi.org/10.1016/j.cvex.2021.08.009.

REFERENCES

1. Farrell AP, Graperil AK, Frances ETB. Comparative aspects of heart morphology. In: Gans C, Gaunt AS, editors. Biology of the reptilia, visceral organs, vol. 19. New York: Society for the Study of Amphibians and Reptiles; 1998. p. 375–424.
2. White FN. Functional anatomy of the heart of reptiles. Am Zoologist 1968;8:211–9.
3. Overgaard J, Stecyk JAW, Farrell AP, et al. Adrenergic control of the cardiovascular system in the turtle Trachemys scripta. J Exp Biol 2002;205:3335–45.
4. Galli G, Taylor EW, Wang T. The cardiovascular responses of the freshwater turtle Trachemys scripta to warming and cooling. J Exp Biol 2004;207:1471–8.
5. Greunz EM, Williams C, Ringgaard S, et al. Elimination of intracardiac shunting provides stable gas anesthesia in tortoises. Sci Rep 2018;8:17124.
6. Hicks JW, Malvin GM. Mechanism of intracardiac shunting in the turtle Pseudemys scripta. Am J Physiol 1992;262:986–92.
7. Goe A, Shmalberg J, Gatson B, et al. Epinephrine or GV-26 electrical stimulation reduces inhalant anesthetic recovery time in common snapping turtles (Chelydra serpentina). J Zoo Wild Med 2016;47:501–7.
8. Hicks JW. Cardiac shunting in reptiles: mechanisms, regulation, and physiological functions. In: Gans C, Gaunt AS, editors. Biology of reptilia, morphology G. Visceral organs. Ithaca, NY, USA: SSAR Press; 1998. p. 425–83.
9. Krosniunas EH, Hicks JW. Cardiac output and shunt during voluntary activity at different temperatures in the turtles, Trachemys scripta. Physiol Biochem Zool 2003;76:679–94.
10. Crossley DA, Wearing OH, Platzack B, et al. Acute and chronic temperature effects on cardiovascular regulation in the red-eared slider (Trachemys scripta). J Comp Physiol B 2015;185:401–11.
11. Holz P, Barker IK, Crashaw GT, et al. The anatomy and perfusion of the renal portal system in the red-eared slider (Trachemys scripta elegans). J Zoo Wild Med 1997;28:378–85.
12. Di Giuseppe M, Faraci L, Luparello M, et al. Preliminary survey on influence of renal portal system during propofol anesthesia in yellow-bellied turtle (Trachemys scripta scripta). J Vet Med Allied Sci 2018;2:1–4.
13. Kummrow MS, Tseng F, Hesse L, et al. Pharmacokinetics of buprenorphine after single dose subcutaneous administration in red-eared sliders (Trachemys scripta elegans). J Zoo Wildl Med 2008;39:590–5.
14. Wood SC, Lenfant CJ. Respiration: mechanics, control and gas exchange. In: Gans C, editor. Biology of the reptilia No. 5. San Diego: Academic Press; 1976.
15. Vigani A. Chelonia (Tortoises, turtles and terrapins). In: West G, Heard D, Caulkett N, editors. Zoo animal and wildlife immobilization and anesthesia. 2nd edition. Ames: Wiley Blacwell; 2014. p. 365–87.
16. Sladky KK, Mans C. Clinical anesthesia in reptiles. J Exot Pet Med 2012;21:17–31.
17. Prange HD, Jackson DC. Ventilation, gas exchange and metabolic scaling of a sea turtle. Respir Physiol 1976;35:369–77.
18. Landberg T, Mailhot JD, Brainerd EL. Lung ventilation during treadmill locomotion in a terrestrial turtle, Terrapene carolina. J Exp Biol 2003;206:3391–404.
19. Glass M, Burggren WW, Johansen K. Ventilation in an aquatic and a terrestrial chelonian reptile. J Exp Biol 1978;72:165–79.
20. Ultsch GR, Andreson JF. Gas exchange during hypoxia and hypercarbia of terrestrial turtles: a comparison of a fossorial species (Gopherus polyphemus) with a sympatric nonfossorial species (Terrapene Carolina). Physiol Zool 1988; 61:142–52.

21. Lutz PL, Bentley TB. Respiratory physiology of diving in the sea turtle. Copeia 1985;3:671–9.
22. Jackson DC. Living without oxygen: lessons from the freshwater turtle. Comp Biochem Physiol A Mol Integr Physiol 2000;125:299–315.
23. McArthur S. Anaesthesia, analgesia and euthanasia. In: McArthur S, Wilkinson R, Meyer J, editors. Medicine and surgery of tortoises and turtles. Oxford: Blackwell; 2004. p. 379–401.
24. Lyson TR, Schachner ER, Botha-Brink J, et al. Origin of the unique ventilatory apparatus of turtles. Nat Commun 2014;(5):5211.
25. Schifino Valente AL, Martinez-Silvestre A, Garcia-Guasch L, et al. Evaluation of pulmonary function in European land tortoises using whole-body plethysmography. Vet Rec 2012;171:154–8.
26. Lutcavage ME, Bushnell PG, Jones DR. Oxygen transport in the leatherback sea turtle Dermochelys coriacea. Physiol Zool 1990;63:1012–24.
27. Hochscheid S, McMahon CR, Bradshaw CJA, et al. Allometric scaling of lung volume and its consequences for marine turtle diving performance. Comp Biochem Physiol A Mol Integr Physiol 2007;148:360–7.
28. Dobby N, Chieveley-Williams S. Respiratory physiology- Part 2 Anaesthesia tutorial of the week 160. Available at: https://www.frca.co.uk/Documents/160%20Respiratory%20physiology%20-%20part%202%20compressed.pdf. Accessed January 3, 2021.
29. Bostrom BL, Jones TT, Hastings M, et al. Behavior and physiology: the thermal strategy of the leatherback turtles. PLoS One 2010. Available at. https://www.ncbi.nlm.nih.gov/pmc/articles/PMC2978089/. Accessed January 4, 2021.
30. Longley LA. Chelonian (tortoise, terrapin and turtle) anaesthesia. In: Anaesthesia of exotic pets. London: Saunders Elsevier; 2008. p. 228–37.
31. Shepard MK, Divers S, Braun C, et al. Pharmacodynamics of alfaxalone after single-dose intramuscular administration in red-eared sliders (Trachemys scripta elegans): a comparison of two different doses at two different ambient temperatures. Vet Anaesth Analg 2013;40:590–8.
32. Kischinovsky M, Duse A, Wang T, et al. Intramuscular administration of alfaxalone in red-eared sliders (Trachemys scripta elegans)- effects of dose and body temperature. Vet Anaesth Analg 2013;40:13–20.
33. Schumacher J. Respiratory medicine of reptiles. Vet Clin Exot Anim 2011;14:207–24.
34. Smits AW, Kozubowski MM. Partitioning of body fluids and cardiovascular responses to circulatory hypovolemia in the turtle, Pseudemys scripta elegans. J Exp Biol 1985;116:237–50.
35. Colon VA, Di Girolamo N. Prognostic value of packed cell volume and blood glucose concentration in 954 client-owned chelonians. J Am Vet Med Assoc 2020;257(12):1265–72.
36. Singer MA. Do mammals, birds, reptiles and fish have similar nitrogen conserving systems? Comp Biochem Physiol B Biochem Mol Biol 2003;134(4):543–58.
37. Sykes JM, Greenacre CB. Techniques for drug delivery in reptiles and amphibians. J Exot Pet Med 2006;15:210–7.
38. Quesada RJ, Aitken-Palmer C, Conley K, et al. Accidental submeningeal injection of propofol in gopher tortoises (Gopherus polyphemus). Vet Rec 2010;167:494–5.
39. Innis CJ, De Voe R, et al. A call for additional study on the safety of subcarapacial venipuncture in chelonians. In: Proceedings association of reptilian and amphibian veterinarians. South Padre Island (TX); 2010. p. 8–10.

40. Emery L, et al. Sedative effects of intranasal midazolam and dexmedetomidine in 2 species of Tortoises (Chelonoidis carbonaria and Geochelone platynota). J Exot Pet Med 2014;23(4):380–3.

41. Schnellbacher RW, Hernandex SM, Tuberville TD, et al. The efficacy of intranasal administration of dexmedetomidine and ketamine to yellow-bellied sliders (Trachemys scripta scripta). J Herp Med Surg 2012;22:91–8.

42. Young BD, Stegeman N, Norby B, et al. Comparison of intraosseous and peripheral venous fluid dynamics in the desert tortoise (Gopherus agassizii). J Zoo Wildl Med 2012;43(1):59–66.

43. Morici M, Interlandi C, Costa GL, et al. Sedation with intracloacal administration of dexmedetomidine and ketamine in yellow-bellied sliders (Trachemys scripta scripta). J Exot Pet Med 2017;26:188–91.

44. Greer LL, Jenne KJ, Diggs HE. Medetomidine-ketamine anesthesia in red-eared slider turtles (Trachemys scripta elegans). Contemp Top Lab Anim Sci 2001; 40:9–11.

45. Scheelings TF, Gatto C, Reina RD. Anaesthesia of hatchling green sea turtles (Chelonia mydas) with intramuscular ketamine-medetomidine-tramadol. Aust Vet J 2020;98:511–6.

46. Harms CA, Eckert SA, Kubis SA, et al. Field anaesthesia of leatherback sea turtles (Dermochelys coriacea). Vet Rec 2007;161:15–21.

47. Chittick EJ, Stamper MA, Beasley JF, et al. Medetomidine, ketamine, and sevoflurane for anesthesia of injured loggerhead sea turtles: 13 cases (1996-2000). J Am Vot Mcd Assoc 2002;221:1019–25.

48. Dennis PM, Heard DJ. Cardiopulmonary effects of a medetomidine-ketamine combination administered intravenously in gopher tortoises. J Am Vet Med Assoc 2002;220:1516–9.

49. Sleeman JM, Gaynor J. Sedative and cardiopulmonary effects of medetomidine and reversal with atipamezole in desert tortoises (Gopherus agassizii). J Zoo Wild Med 2000;31:28–35.

50. Bettschart-Wolfensberger R, Stauffer S, Hassig M, et al. Racemic ketamine in comparison to S-ketamine in combination with azaperone and butorphanol for castration of pigs. Schweiz Arch Tierheilkd 2013;155:669–75.

51. Larenza MP, Althaus H, Conrot A, et al. Anaesthesia recovery quality after racemic kctamine or S-ketamine administration to male cats undergoing neutering surgery. Schweiz Arch Tierheilkd 2008;150:599–607.

52. Bochmann M, Wegner S, Hatt J-M. Preliminary clinical comparison of anesthesia with ketamine/medetomidine and S-ketamine/medetomidine in Testudo spp. J Herp Med Surg 2018;28:40–6.

53. Adetunji VE, Ogunsola J, Adeyemo OK. Evaluation of diazepam-ketamine combination for immobilization of African land tortoise (Testudo graeca). Sokoto J Vet Sci 2019. Available at: https://www.ajol.info/index.php/sokjvs/article/view/185467. Accessed January 7, 2021.

54. Oppenheim YC, Moon PF. Sedative effects of midazolam in red eared slider turtles (Trachemys scripta elegans). J Zoo Wild Med 1995;26:409–13.

55. Emery L, Parson G, Gerhardt L, et al. Sedative effects of intranasal midazolam and dexmedetomidine in 2 species of tortoises (Chelonoidis carbonara and Geochelone platynota). J Exot Pet Med 2014;23:380–3.

56. Sladky KK, Miletic V, Paul-Murphy J, et al. Analgesic efficacy and respiratory effects of butorphanol and morphine in turtles. J Am Vet Med Assoc 2007;9: 1356–62.

57. Kinney ME, Johnson SM, Sladky KK. Behavioural evaluation of red eared slider turtles (Trachemys scripta elegans) administered either morphine or butorphanol following unilateral gonadectomy. J Herp Med Surg 2011;21:54–62.
58. Mans C, Lahner LL, Baker BB, et al. Antinociceptive efficacy of buprenorphine and hydromorphone in red-eared slider turtles (Trachemys scripta elegans). J Zoo Wild Med 2012;43:662–5.
59. Baker BB, Sladky MS, Johnson SM. Evaluation of the analgesic effects of oral and subcutaneous tramadol administration in red-eared slider turtles. J Am Vet Med Assoc 2011;238:220–7.
60. MacLean RA, Harms CA, Braun-McNeill J. Propofol anesthesia in loggerhead (Caretta caretta) sea turtles. J Wildl Dis 2008;44:143–50.
61. Quagliatto Santos AL, Scarpa Bosso AC, Ferreira Alves Junior JR, et al. Pharmacological restraint of captivity giant Amazonian turtle Podocnemis expansa (Testudines, Podocnemididae) with xylazine and propofol. Acta Cir Bras 2008;23: 270–3.
62. Ziolo MS, Bertelsen MF. Effects of propofol administered via the supravertebral sinus in red-eared sliders. J Am Vet Med Assoc 2009;234:390–3.
63. Knotek Z. Alfaxalone as an induction agent for anesthesia in terrapins and tortoises. Vet Rec 2014;175:327–30.
64. Phillips BE, Posner LP, Lewbart GA, et al. Effects of alfaxalone administered intravenously to healthy yearling loggerhead sea turtles (Caretta caretta) at three different doses. J Am Vet Med Ass 2017;250:909–17.
65. Scheelings TF. Use of intravenous and intramuscular alfaxalone in Macquarie River Turtles (Emydura macquarii). J Herp Med Surg 2013;3-4:91–4.
66. Hansen LL, Bertelsen MF. Assessment of the effects of intramuscular administration of alfaxalone with and without medetomidine in Horsfield's tortoises (Agrionemys horsfieldii). Vet Anaesth Analg 2013;40:e68–75.
67. Scarabelli S. TIVA in chelonians. St Louis, MO: Proceedings Exoticscon; 2019.
68. Odette O, Churgin SM, Sladky KK, et al. Anesthetic induction and recovery parameters in bearded dragons (Pogona vitticeps): comparison of isoflurane delivered in 100% oxygen versus 21% oxygen. J Zoo Wildl Med 2015;46:534–9.
69. Bertelsen MF, Mosley C, Crawshaw GJ, et al. Inhalation anesthesia in dumeril's monitor (Varanus dumerili) with isoflurane, sevoflurane and nitrous oxude: effects of inspired gases on induction and recovery. J Zoo Wildl Med 2005;36:62–8.
70. Bello AA, Bello-Klein A. A technique to anesthetize turtles with ether. Physiol Behav 1991;50:847–8.
71. Wyneken J. Normal reptile heart morphology and function. Vet Clin Exot Anim 2009;12:51–63.
72. Camacho M, del Pino Quintana M, Calabuig P, et al. Acid-base and plasma biochemical changes using crystalloid fluids in stranded juvenile loggerhead sea turtles (Caretta caretta). PLoS One 2015;13:e0132217. Available at: https://journals.plos.org/plosone/article?id=10.1371/journal.pone.0132217. Accessed January 10, 2021.
73. Norton TM. Chelonian emergency and critical care. J Exot Pet Med 2005;14: 106–30.
74. Williams CJ, Malte CL, Malte H, et al. Ectothermy and cardiac shunts profoundly slow the equilibration of inhaled anaesthetics in a multi-compartment model. Sci Rep 2020;10(1):17157.
75. Mans C. Clinical technique: intrathecal drug administration in turtles and tortoises. J Exot Pet Med 2014;23(1):67–70.

Sedation and Anesthesia of Lizards

Tatiana H. Ferreira, DVM, MSc, PhD, Dipl ACVAA, Christoph Mans, Dr med vet, Dipl ACZM*

KEYWORDS

• Lizards • General anesthesia • Sedation • Regional anesthesia • Chemical restraint

KEY POINTS

- The effect of drug administration location should be considered for injectable sedation and anesthetic drugs; the cranial body half is recommended.
- Injectable drug protocols are available to offer safe and reliable sedation in a variety of lizard species. Partially or completely reversible protocols will ensure a more predictable recovery.
- Neuraxial anesthesia has been shown to be effective and safe in lizard species using lidocaine or bupivacaine. In addition, neuraxial morphine provides regional analgesia.

INTRODUCTION

Lizards are commonly kept as companion animals and are maintained at zoological and educational facilities. Therefore, various lizard species are routinely evaluated by veterinarians and may require sedation and anesthesia for various invasive, and most nonelective, surgical procedures and for different noninvasive clinical techniques, such as diagnostic imaging or performing a complete physical examination in aggressive or fragile species. The information published on safe and effective protocols in lizards continues to grow. However, interspecies variation in anatomy, physiology, and response to sedative and anesthetic drug protocols limits the ability to extrapolate from a published study performed in one species to another. The anesthetic management of the reptilian patient, including the design of the anesthetic protocol, represents unique challenges due to marked anatomic and physiologic differences between taxa. Commonly, anesthetic protocols, including monitoring techniques to evaluate cardiopulmonary performance derived from domestic animals, are applied to lizard patients. However, these techniques are often of limited value and should be interpreted with caution.

The authors do not have any commercial or financial conflicts of interest, or any funding sources to disclose.
Department of Surgical Sciences, School of Veterinary Medicine, University of Wisconsin–Madison, 2015 Linden Drive, Madison, WI 53706, USA
* Corresponding author.
E-mail addresses: tatiana.ferreira@wisc.edu (T.H.F.); christoph.mans@wisc.edu (C.M.)

Regional, and in particular, neuraxial (spinal) anesthesia and analgesia in lizards has, until recently, received very little attention. However, the regional delivery of anesthetic and analgesic drugs may offer substantial benefits for lizards undergoing various surgical procedures of the caudal body half (eg, tail amputation, cloacoscopy). Studies published have shown that drug doses and efficacy vary between lizards and chelonians, and that effective and safe neuraxial anesthesia can be induced with bupivacaine and lidocaine.

PHYSIOLOGIC AND ANATOMIC CONSIDERATIONS

Lizards are poikilothermic, meaning their body temperature is directly dependent on environmental temperature. Changes in body temperature significantly affect metabolic rate and many other physiologic processes. Drug absorption, distribution, metabolism, and excretion of drugs in reptiles are directly related to environmental temperature.[1] Consequently, it is important to maintain the reptile patient at its preferred optimal body temperature (POBT) to achieve more predictable anesthetic drug effects. POBT is generally considered to be 20 to 25° C (68–77° F) in temperate and aquatic species and 25 to 35° C (77–95° F) in tropical species.[1] In general, at lower temperatures, induction times are prolonged, and reptiles may not achieve the desired anesthetic depth. At higher temperatures, induction times are faster; however, the duration of sedation or anesthesia induced by injectable drugs is shorter due to accelerated drug metabolism and excretion at higher temperatures.[1]

DRUG ADMINISTRATION SITE AND THE HEPATIC FIRST-PASS EFFECT

The hepatic first-pass effect following pelvic limb administration in lizards has been shown to affect anesthetic drug efficacy in lizards and other reptiles.[2,3] The venous blood flow from the pelvic limb drains into the ventral abdominal vein, which either passes directly to the liver or through the hepatic portal vein and into the liver.[2,4] Hence, any drug administered in the pelvic limb first enters the liver before reaching systemic circulation, resulting in a hepatic first-pass effect; that is, if the particular drug undergoes hepatic metabolism or excretion and hence reduced bioavailability of drug with hepatic metabolism, this results in lower plasma concentrations and/or reduced or no clinical efficacy.[2,5,6] In leopard geckos (Eublepharis macularius), pelvic limb administration of dexmedetomidine-ketamine resulted in significantly reduced anesthetic efficacy compared with administration of the same dosages in the forelimb.[2] Because most drugs commonly used in sedation, anesthesia, and analgesia in lizards undergo hepatic metabolism and/or excretion; the injection site becomes clinically relevant. Therefore, it is advised to avoid administering anesthetic drugs in the caudal body half by either intramuscular (IM) or subcutaneous (SC) injection in the pelvic limbs or surrounding areas (Fig. 1). However, the intravenous (IV) administration of anesthetics in the ventral tail vein of lizards does not result in a hepatic first effect since the coccygeal vein in lizards drains directly into the caudal vena cava.[4] Therefore, IV administration of anesthetic drugs in the ventral coccygeal vein is routinely performed (Table 1).

DRUG ADMINISTRATION ROUTE

Historically the IM route of drug administration has been recommended in reptiles because of suspected faster and more predictable drug absorption and therefore faster and more consistent induction of sedation or anesthesia. However, IM injections are considered painful, and in particular, if large drug volumes need to be administered

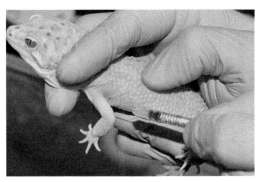

Fig. 1. Parenteral drug administration in the cranial body half of a leopard gecko *(Euble-pharis macularius).* Drugs can be either administered in the forelimb musculature or subcutaneously in the axillary and shoulder region.

(eg, alfaxalone), the SC route should be used.[1] Although the IM injection of anesthetics may result in more rapid and less variable onset times than SC, in most cases, the variation in induction times may not be clinically relevant. Several studies have been published in lizards showing onset times ranging between 5 and 30 minutes after the SC administration of dexmedetomidine-ketamine, dexmedetomidine-midazolam, or alfaxalone-midazolam.[2,7–9] However, recent research in inland bearded dragons *(Pogona vitticeps)* has shown that the SC route is substantially less effective for induction of tiletamine-zolazepam sedation than the IM route.[52] Therefore, further studies evaluating the difference in drug efficacy following IM compared with SC routes in lizards are necessary.

The IV route is excellent for administration of anesthetic agents in many lizard species with a large enough tail, and in species that are not prone to tail autonomy. Intravenous administration results in rapid onset of anesthesia and requires substantially lower drug amounts than SC or IM administration. However, depending on the lizard species, patient size, and cooperation, IV access may be challenging or impossible to obtain, making the SC or IM route more feasible. In lizards, IV injections are most commonly administered into the ventral coccygeal vein (**Fig. 2**).

PREANESTHETIC ASSESSMENT

A preanesthetic assessment, including complete history, visual and physical examination, and diagnostic tests, such as blood work and imaging, should be performed if indicated and feasible. Fasting before anesthesia is recommended for 24 to 48 hours to ensure that gastric emptying is complete. It is crucial to keep lizards at their POBT as it will influence drug metabolism and, therefore, induction and recovery times.[1] If lizards are in compromised conditions (eg, dehydrated), chemical restraint should be delayed until they have received supportive care.

INJECTABLE ANESTHETIC DRUGS

A variety of agents representing different classes of drugs are frequently used, either alone or in combination, depending on the desired level of sedation or anesthesia. It is recommended to avoid administering high dosages of a single anesthetic agent (eg, ketamine, alfaxalone). Instead, protocols in which multiple drugs are combined with synergistic actions, thereby requiring lower dosages for each drug, should be considered. In addition, using readily reversible drug protocols will provide for more rapid

Table 1
Sedation and anesthetic protocols reported in lizards

Drug Protocol	Species	Dose, (mg/kg)	Route	Comments
Alfaxalone	Green iguana (*Iguana iguana*)	5	IV	Light anesthesia within <1 min. Duration of maximum effect: 2–9 min. Intubation possible in all animals. Recovery: 14 ± 4 min.[44]
		10	IM	Light-moderate sedation within 8 ± 2 min. Duration of maximum effect: 11 ± 4 min. Intubation possible in 40% of animals. Recovery: 29 ± 36 min 28–32°C.[23]
		20	IM	Light anesthesia within 5 ± 2 min. Duration of maximum effect 22 ± 7 min. Intubation possible in all animals. Recovery: 45 ± 8 min 28–32°C.[23]
		30	IM	Surgical anesthesia within 4 ± 1 min. Duration of maximum effect 39 ± 12 min. Intubation possible in all animals. Recovery: 68 ± 9 min 28–32°C.[23]
	Veiled chameleon (*Chamaeleo calyptratus*)	5	IV	Light anesthesia within 2 min. Duration of maximum effect: 5–10 min. Intubation possible in all animals. Recovery: 20 ± 5 min. Animals received butorphanol (2 mg/kg IM) before induction.[45] *Butorphanol has no analgesic effects in reptiles and should not be used for premedication or analgesia.*
		15	IV	Light anesthesia, suitable for electroejaculation. No adverse effects after repeated administration in weekly intervals. Animals maintained spontaneous ventilation.[46]

	Dose	Route	Effects
Australian lizards	9	IV	Moderate sedation–light anesthesia in most species; duration of effect <30 min, intubation possible, apnea reported.[47]
Inland bearded dragon (*Pogona vitticeps*)	10	SC	Moderate sedation. Righting reflex maintained in most animals (6/8). No effect on jaw tone. Recovery: 83 (53–94) minutes. 25–27°C.[48]
	20	SC	Deep sedation. Loss of righting reflex: 11 ± 6 min. Return of righting reflex: 83 ± 36 min 25–27°C.[8]
Leopard gecko (*Eublepharis macularius*)	10–20	SC	Light-moderate sedation, inconsistent effects.[7]
Alfaxalone + midazolam Leopard gecko	15 + 1	SC	Moderate-deep sedation. Loss of righting reflex: 10 ± 10 min. Intubation possible in 33%, prolonged recovery (56 ± 29 min) after reversal with flumazenil. 26–28°C.[7]
Dexmedetomidine + ketamine Inland bearded dragon	0.1 + 20	SC	Deep sedation–light anesthesia. Righting reflex and pelvic limb withdrawal reflex lost in most animals Time to effect ~5–10 min. Recovery: 10–20 min after reversal with atipamezole. 25–27°C.[9]
Leopard gecko	0.1 + 10	IM	Deep sedation–light anesthesia. Righting reflex and pelvic limb withdrawal reflex in 7 of 9 and 8 of 9 animals, respectively. Jaw tone absent or reduced in 8 of 9 animals. Onset time within 5–10 min. Recovery: ~10–15 after administration of atipamezole.[2]

(continued on next page)

Table 1
(continued)

Drug Protocol	Species	Dose, (mg/kg)	Route	Comments
Dexmedetomidine + ketamine + midazolam	Inland bearded dragon	1.1 + 10 + 1	SC	Deep sedation–light anesthesia. Righting reflex and pelvic limb withdrawal reflex lost in 8 of 9 animals. Time to effect: ~5–20 min. Recovery: 10–35 min after reversal with flumazenil + atipamezole. 25–27°C.[9]
	Various lizard species	0.05– 0.1 + 3– 5 + 0.5– 1	SC	Moderate sedation–light anesthesia, intubation may be possible, partially reversible; rapid recovery (6 ± 2 min) after reversal with atipamezole.[49]
Dexmedetomidine + midazolam	Leopard gecko	0.1 + 1	SC	Moderate–deep sedation. Loss of righting reflex: 24 ± 12-min intubation possible in 33%, completely reversible; rapid recovery: 6 ± 2 min after reversal with flumazenil + atipamezole. 26–28°C.[7]
	Inland bearded dragon	0.1 + 1	SC	Moderate sedation. Righting reflex and pelvic limb withdrawal reflex maintained. Time to effect: ~15–20 min. Recovery: 5–25 min after reversal with flumazenil + atipamezole. 25–27°C.[9]

Drug	Species	Dose (mg/kg)	Route	Comments
	Various lizard species	0.05–1 + 0.5–1	SC	Mild-moderate sedation, completely reversible; rapid recovery after reversal with flumazenil + atipamezole.[49]
Propofol	Green iguana	5–10	IV, IO	Induction agent, apnea common, requires intubation and intermittent positive pressure ventilation.[16,30]
Tiletamine-zolazepam (Telazol)	Green iguana	10.5 ± 4.2	IM	Light anesthesia, Time to effect: 7 ± 1 min, intubation possible, initial excitement phase, long recovery times.[50]
	Inland bearded dragon	20	IM	Deep sedation–light anesthesia. Righting reflex lost in all animals within 12 ± 8 min. Jaw tone lost in 9 of 10 animals. Recovery: 69 ± 39 min after reversal with flumazenil. 25–27°C. The SC route was less effective than the IM route. Doses between 2 and 10 mg/kg IM did not result in consistent sedation, remained ambulatory, and maintained righting reflex. 25–26°C.[52]

Atipamezole is dosed at 10 times the amount of dexmedetomidine or 5 times the amount of medetomidine in milligrams. The recommended dose of flumazenil is 0.05 mg/kg in most cases. Lower doses (0.01 mg/kg) should be considered in large animals to reduce injection volume.

Abbreviations: IM, intramuscular; IO, intraosseous; IV, intravenous; SC, subcutaneous.

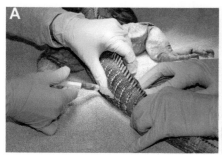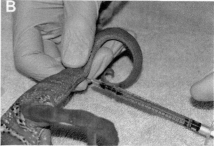

Fig. 2. IV drug administration in the ventral coccygeal using the lateral approach in a green iguana (*Iguana iguana*) (*A*) and the ventral approach in a panther chameleon *(Furcifer pardalis)* (*B*).

recoveries. Reversal of anesthetic drugs is particularly important in diseased lizards that have reduced liver or kidney function. Because most deleterious side effects (eg, prolonged recovery, cardiopulmonary depression) associated with anesthetic and sedative drug administration are dose-dependent, individual drug dosage reduction and reversibility will result in fewer complications and improved recoveries. Similar drugs and drug combinations can also be chosen for sedation, premedication, or induction of general anesthesia. If the patient is scheduled for a painful procedure, it is recommended to include an analgesic agent, such as an opioid, in the preanesthetic protocol. Many injectable protocols in lizards include administering an alpha-2 agonist (eg, dexmedetomidine) with ketamine and/or midazolam. Alternatively, alfaxalone administered IV or SC can be used for chemical restraint. A μ-opioid receptor agonist (eg, morphine, hydromorphone) should be added to the protocol if additional analgesia is required. One must keep in mind that many factors (eg, site of injection, underlying disease, dehydration, body temperature) may affect the onset, recovery, and efficacy of anesthetic drugs.[1] Therefore, an individualized approach to choosing appropriate drug combinations and dosages should be considered.

Injectable agents alone can be used to facilitate a variety of short diagnostic and surgical procedures and induce general anesthesia. Maintenance of a surgical plane of anesthesia for lengthy, invasive procedures is frequently based on administering an inhalation agent, such as isoflurane or sevoflurane. Alternatively, injectable protocols can be used to induce moderate to deep sedation or light anesthesia. It can be combined with locoregional anesthesia to perform various diagnostic (eg, cloacoscopy) or therapeutic procedures (eg, hemipenile or tail amputation). The main benefit of using injectable drug protocols at published doses is that spontaneous ventilation is maintained in most cases. Therefore, endotracheal intubation and intermittent positive pressure ventilation are not required. The administration of supplemental oxygen in spontaneously breathing, sedated bearded dragons has been shown not cause respiratory depression.[8] The lack of supplemental oxygen provision did not result in measurable negative peri-sedative or post-sedative effects.[8] Published injectable sedation and anesthesia protocols are summarized in **Table 1**.

INHALANT ANESTHESIA

Reptiles have unique cardiac and pulmonary anatomy that can influence their cardiopulmonary parameters under anesthesia and their response to inhalant anesthetics. Noncrocodilian reptiles have 2 completely separated atria and 1 ventricle, which is incompletely divided by a septum-like structure (muscular ridge) into *cavum dorsale* and *cavum pulmonale*. The *cavum dorsale* of some noncrocodilians, including lizards, can be further subdivided into 2 compartments (*cavum venosum* and *cavum arteriosum*) by another septum.[10] The incomplete ventricle division allows intracardiac mixing of blood, which could be left-to-right or right-to-left (R-L) shunts. The degree of shunting can be affected by the extent of ventricle division; varanid lizards have a well-developed muscular ridge, allowing better functional separation and less shunting.[10] Breathing pattern (breath-holding) can lead to changes in intracardiac shunting as well; however, lizards are considered continuous breathers, and therefore show fewer fluctuations in blood-gas levels and blood flow distribution than other reptiles, such as turtles (intermittent breathers), with more breathing-apnea periods.[10]

Lizard lungs can vary from compartmentalized and well perfused multichambered lung to unicameral lung (essentially, a large air sac with a vascularized wall), but overall, compared with mammals, lizards have simple and nonalveolated lungs.[11] Their lungs can be associated with inefficient gas exchange, with varying degrees of ventilation-perfusion mismatch and diffusion impairment.[11]

INDUCTION

Induction of general anesthesia in lizards can be achieved by injectable or inhalant anesthetics. Intramuscular, SC, IV (see **Fig. 2**), or intraosseous injection of various sedatives and injectable anesthetics (discussed earlier) can result in an anesthetic plane sufficient for endotracheal intubation.

Inhalant induction is feasible in lizards; however, R-L shunting and potential breath-holding will limit anesthetic uptake, leading to longer and more variable anesthetic induction when compared with mammals. Inhalant inductions can be performed using face masks, chambers, or even small, self-sealing plastic bags depending on the size of the lizard (**Fig. 3**). Environmental contamination is a concern with inhalant inductions and should be taken into consideration.

In inland bearded dragons, the median isoflurane induction time was 8 minutes (interquartile range: 4 minutes).[12] Induction time varied slightly but was not clinically significantly faster with sevoflurane compared with isoflurane in various lizard species.[13–15]

Apnea following induction of anesthesia is common; therefore, intubation followed by assisted or controlled ventilation may be required, especially at a surgical level of inhalant anesthesia.[12,16]

ENDOTRACHEAL INTUBATION

Lizards that are relaxed, without protective airway or oropharyngeal reflexes, and especially if hypoventilating or apneic, should be intubated. Intubation is easily performed in most lizard species because the glottis is rostrally located (**Fig. 4**A), caudal to the base of the tongue. Ideally, a plastic strap or tie gauze should be used to open the mouth gently and avoid damaging the teeth and gingiva (**Fig. 4**B).[1] A drop of diluted lidocaine can be used to desensitize the glottis. The reptile glottis is only open during active inspiration or expiration.

Lizards should be intubated with the largest-diameter tube that can be placed without force or trauma. Mucus plugs can partially or completely obstruct the lumen of the endotracheal tube (ETT) during long anesthetic events, preventing complete deflation of the lungs during expiration, or it may affect both phases of the breathing cycle. Even though lizards have incomplete tracheal rings, uncuffed ETTs are commonly used because of the size required. Small lizards may require sizes as small as 1 mm (internal diameter) or even over-the-needle IV catheters (14–22 gauge). These

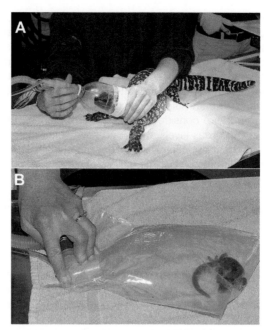

Fig. 3. Induction of gaseous anesthesia in lizards. (*A*) Mask induction of a beaded lizard *(Heloderma horridum)*. (*B*) Chamber induction of a Madagascar day gecko *(Phelsuma madagascariensis)* using a sealable plastic bag.

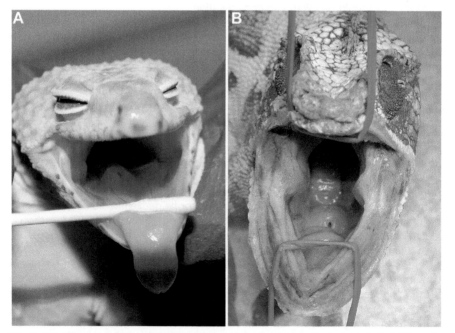

Fig. 4. Visualization of the glottis in a leopard gecko *(Eublepharis macularius)* (*A*) and a panther chameleon *(Furcifer pardalis) (B)*.

smaller ETT (especially <2 mm internal diameter, and the IV catheters) can kink easily, which will lead to airway obstruction. Kinking and obstruction can be prevented by fixating small lizards and the ETT on a tongue depressor to avoid any shifting of the tube during the patient's movement (**Fig. 5**A). Cuffed ETTs can be used in large lizards, but they should be carefully inflated, if necessary, to minimize tracheal trauma.

A mouth gag or a piece of rubber tubing can be used to protect the ETT from the animal biting on it (**Fig. 5**B). Securing the ETT is also important to avoid unintentional extubation, kinks, or movement of the tube within the trachea, which could lead to trauma. For that purpose, tape or elastic/plastic straps can be used around the ETT and the lizard's head (see **Fig. 5**B). Use caution with elastic straps to avoid accidental obstruction of a small ETT.

ANESTHETIC MAINTENANCE

Inhalants are the most common anesthetics used for the maintenance of anesthesia in reptiles. The potency of an inhalant anesthetic is measured as the minimum alveolar concentration of the agent that will prevent gross purposeful movement in response to a supramaximal stimulus in 50% of the population. However, lizards have simple and nonalveolated lungs; therefore, the term minimum anesthetic concentration (MAC) should be used. Determining the MAC of different inhalants can be a challenge in reptiles because of significant slow equilibration and variations in anesthetic depth despite constant anesthetic inhalant concentrations. The cause is likely due to unique cardiopulmonary characteristics, including intracardiac shunting, ventilation-perfusion mismatch, and pulmonary diffusion issues, which can lead to altered anesthetic uptake, distribution, and elimination. Nonetheless, there are few studies assessing MAC in lizards (**Table 2**). The MAC of isoflurane, sevoflurane, and desflurane decreased with increasing duration of the anesthetic event in green iguanas; for instance, isoflurane MAC was 2.4 ± 0.7 at approximately 4 hours of anesthesia and decreased to 1.8% at approximately 10 hours of anesthesia.[15] Very high concentrations may be needed initially, but with time the requirements decrease, so it is important to lower the vaporizer settings over time, especially during long procedures.[15]

There is limited information in the literature regarding the cardiovascular effects of different inhalants in lizards. Heart rate (HR) and blood pressure (BP) decrease with increasing concentrations of isoflurane (1–2 MAC).[17,18] No significant difference was

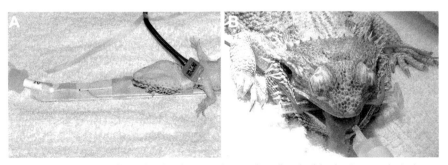

Fig. 5. Securing an endotracheal tube in a leopard gecko *(Eublepharis macularius)* on a wooden tongue depressor (*A*). The animal is secured to the same tongue depressor, therefore minimizing the risk of dislodging or kinking of the endotracheal tube. (*B*) The endotracheal tube is secured using elastic ties and a 1-mL syringe. The syringe also acts as a bite block to prevent damage to the endotracheal tube.

Table 2		
Minimum anesthetic concentration (MAC) of inhalants in lizards		
Inhalant	Species	Minimum Alveolar Concentration (MAC), %
Isoflurane	Green iguana (Iguana iguana)	2.1 ± 0.5^{15}
		$2.0–2.1 \pm 0.6^{21}$
	Dumeril's monitor (Varanus dumerilii)	1.5 ± 0.2^{51}
Sevoflurane	Green iguana	3.4 ± 1.2^{15}
	Dumeril's monitor	2.5 ± 0.5^{20}
Desflurane	Green iguana	8.9 ± 2.1^{15}

found between these parameters when isoflurane, sevoflurane, and desflurane were compared at MAC level.[15]

Assisted or controlled ventilation is required for lengthy procedures or when surgical depth of anesthesia is necessary.[1,16] The frequency of mechanical ventilation necessary is currently unknown in lizards. Most studies ventilate at 4 to 6 breaths/min and 25 to 30 mL/kg.[13–15,17,19–21] However, the clinical impact of these ventilation parameters on their unique lungs, and studies assessing specific guidelines, are not available at this time. In addition, the minute volume requirement to maintain normal carbon dioxide (CO_2) levels may change depending on the species, physical status, body temperature, anesthesia depth, and surgical procedure. Therefore, ideally, ventilator settings should be guided by blood-gas analysis if available. Otherwise, capnography can be used; however, this monitoring technique can be associated with significant limitations in lizards.

MONITORING

Careful monitoring is essential for a safe and effective anesthetic event. However, many monitoring modalities commonly used in domestic species are either not validated or have several limitations when applied to reptiles. In addition, the size of some lizards, the challenges faced with different anatomic variations, and the scarcity of reference values in conscious animals also limit the application and interpretation of different monitoring modalities.

Anesthetic Depth

Clinical evaluation of anesthetic depth is often performed in reptiles by assessing reflexes such as righting, palpebral, corneal, limb withdrawal in response to pinch, and cloacal tone. However, these are not always possible because of anatomic differences between species. For instance, a lack of eyelids and presence of spectacles will preclude the assessment of palpebral and corneal reflexes in most geckos.[1] Adequate surgical depth of anesthesia in lizards has been associated with lack of spontaneous movement, lack of movement in response to toe or tail pinch, good muscle relaxation, no righting reflex, no palpebral reflex, and reduced cloacal tone.[1] The tongue retraction in varanids may still be present, but the corneal reflex should be present at surgical anesthetic depth; otherwise, if lost, it indicates excessive anesthetic depth.[1,22,23] The effect on HR depends on the anesthetic protocol used, but significant respiratory depression leading to apnea must be expected with surgical anesthetic depth in lizards.

Body Temperature

Body temperature can be monitored using the cloaca in a clinical setting. Alternatively, infrared thermometers to measure the skin temperature of small lizards can be used.[24] Anesthetic drug metabolism of reptiles is influenced by temperature, and it is important to keep them at their POBT. For most temperate and tropical lizards, keeping their body temperature between 25 and 30°C during anesthesia and recovery is recommended. This can be accomplished by using heating pads and circulating water or air blankets. Careful monitoring during anesthesia and recovery to avoid overheating is crucial.

Cardiovascular

Monitoring of cardiovascular parameters can be challenging in lizards because of their size. A flat Doppler probe is very useful. It can be placed over the carotid arteries, axillary region, or heart to monitor HR in conscious, sedated, or anesthetized lizards.[1,16] The heart position varies depending on the species of lizard. In iguanids and agamids, it is found close to the pectoral girdle, whereas in varanids it is located more caudally in the coelomic cavity.[16] HR changes can happen due to stress, ambient temperature, metabolism, noxious stimulation, and sedative/anesthetic drugs.

Electrocardiography (ECG) can be used to monitor HR and rhythm (**Fig. 6**). The ECG of lizards is similar to mammalian species; P, QRS, and T waves can be identified.[25] In a study in adult tropical house geckos (*Hemidactylus mabouia*), maximal voltage variation (lead II in mammals) was obtained with the electrodes placed on the neck and coelom (ground on the tail), aligning the electrodes on the mid-longitudinal snout-vent axis, which coincided with the base-apex orientation axis of their ventricle.[25] Voltage was close to zero (flat line) when the electrodes were placed at the forelimbs

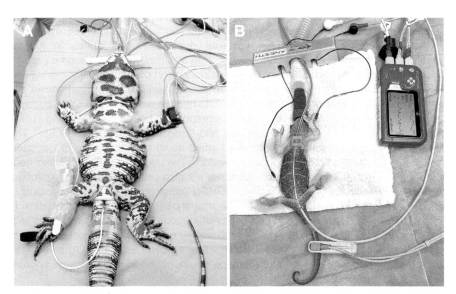

Fig. 6. Anesthetic monitoring using Doppler, electrocardiography, and pulse oximetry in a black-and-white tegu *(Salvator merianae)* (A) and a veiled chameleon (*Chamaeleo calyptratus*) (B). An intraosseous catheter for perioperative fluid and drug administration has been placed in the right tibia of the tegu.

(equivalent to lead I placement). The mean electrical axis in these animals was close to 90°, but this could vary by species.

Invasive BP measurement using arterial catheters is challenging in lizards and therefore not routinely used in the clinical setting as it typically requires a surgical approach with a cut down procedure. Even though noninvasive BP measuring techniques (ie, oscillometric) are possible in some lizard species by placing the cuff in the femoral area, but it does not measure BP consistently. When it does, it is poorly correlated with invasive BP values.[18] The Doppler has also been used by placing the crystal over the medial aspect of the distal portion of the pelvic limb and the cuff around the thigh,[15] but the validity of this technique has not been verified. Nevertheless, inhalant anesthesia can cause significant dose-dependent hypotension in lizards.[17,18] Thus, until more accurate measurement techniques are studied, noninvasive BP measurements can be attempted to monitor trends.

Normal BP values can differ significantly depending on the species and various environmental factors, such as stress, manipulation, and noxious stimulation. In general, lizards have lower arterial BP compared with mammals. The mean arterial pressure (MAP) of conscious unrestrained green iguanas (*Iguana iguana*) was 79 ± 13 mm Hg,[18] whereas black-and-white tegus (*Salvator merianae*) had a mean MAP between 38 and 44 mm Hg.[26] Robust baroreceptor reflex-mediated responses, as well as a similar contribution from vagal and sympathetic efferent to HR changes, have been identified in lizards.[18,26,27]

Respiratory Monitoring

Reptiles, in particular turtles, can tolerate hypoxemia well because of their low metabolism, leading to slow depletion of aerobic reserves.[28] This low oxygen tolerance has also been reported in lizards, such as the green iguana that can stay submerged in water for more than 4 hours, tolerating extremely high lactate levels.[29] Despite this tolerance, reptiles regulate ventilation to avoid anoxia.[28]

Lizards can breath-hold for long periods and have variable RR depending on species, ambient temperature, activity/metabolism, and manipulation/restraint. Anesthetics can produce significant respiratory depression and apnea in lizards, requiring assisted or controlled ventilation.[12,30] In addition, ETT can become partially or completely obstructed, affecting the respiratory effort of the animal.

Capnography is a noninvasive monitor to assess ventilation in anesthetized patients. In smaller patients with limited tidal volume, this can be challenging because the sampling rate of some side-stream capnographs can be too high, resulting in dilution of the sample with fresh gas and low end-tidal carbon dioxide ($ETCO_2$).[31] The dead space of mainstream capnograph adapters could also contribute to inaccuracies in $ETCO_2$ measurements in small patients.[31] The use of uncuffed ETT and non-rebreathing systems with high fresh gas flows will also contribute to sample dilution, resulting in inaccurate (low) $ETCO_2$ values. Furthermore, the measurement of $ETCO_2$ does not always accurately estimate arterial partial pressure of carbon dioxide ($Paco_2$) in reptiles, likely due to the presence of intracardiac shunting. In a study with green iguanas, $ETCO_2$ and $Paco_2$ were similar at 10 minutes of anesthesia. However, at 40 minutes of anesthesia, $ETCO_2$ was significantly lower than $Paco_2$ (gradient was more than 30 mm Hg), making it challenging to use capnography to assess spontaneous or controlled ventilation.[14]

Pulse oximetry is a noninvasive and easy way to monitor oxygen saturation; however, studies have shown that values obtained in lizards do not correlate with values derived from blood-gas machines.[17,27] Pulse oximetry still can be used to provide trends during an anesthetic event. Small reflectance probes can be placed in the cloaca, oral cavity, or esophagus at the level of the carotid artery.[1] The R-L shunting that occurs in reptiles can lead to low oxygen saturation and arterial partial pressure of oxygen (Pao_2), which has been documented in lizards.[11,17,27] Besides the intracardiac shunting affecting Pao_2 levels, large alveolar to arterial oxygen differences can result from ventilation-perfusion mismatch and diffusion impairment.[11,32]

To obtain more accurate information regarding oxygenation, ventilation, and acid-base status, arterial blood-gas analysis is ideal. However, with the challenges in obtaining blood samples, it is not commonly applied in the clinical setting.

RECOVERY

Maintaining lizards at their POBT during recovery is essential, and a temperature-controlled environment, such as incubators, is ideal. However, close monitoring of their RR and effort should be continued until consistent, spontaneous breathing is confirmed, oropharyngeal reflexes have returned, and the patients start ambulating.

Recovery time will depend on the anesthetic used for sedation or induction/maintenance of anesthesia, duration, and level of inhalant anesthesia. Whenever possible, reversal drugs should be administered, although reversal of analgesic drugs may not be indicated if a painful procedure has been performed. Historically, it has been recommended that ventilation can be depressed with oxygen supplementation in reptiles, which could affect recovery time after inhalant anesthesia.[28] However, recent studies have not shown any effect of inspired oxygen (room air or 100% O_2) on ventilation during recovery of lizards.[8,12,13] For example, after 1 hour of isoflurane anesthesia in inland bearded dragons, extubation was possible in 12 $\pm$ 5 minutes in room air and 15 $\pm$ 5 minutes in 100% O_2.[12]

In green iguanas premedicated with butorphanol, recovery time after a short period of anesthesia was significantly longer with isoflurane (35 $\pm$ 27 minutes) when compared with sevoflurane (7 $\pm$ 4 minutes).[14] However, after long anesthetic events, no significant difference was noted between isoflurane and sevoflurane recovery time in Dumeril's monitors (*Varanus dumerilii*; 70 $\pm$ 13 and 62 $\pm$ 19) or between isoflurane, sevoflurane, and desflurane in green iguanas (68 $\pm$ 29, 64 $\pm$ 19, and 48 $\pm$ 25).[13,19] It is challenging to compare different studies because the parameters used to determine recovery time can differ; return of righting reflex, extubation time, and other more subjective measures (level of alertness) are also used in different studies.

The administration of epinephrine has been reported to hasten recovery from inhalant anesthesia in chelonians and American alligators (*Alligator mississippiensis*).[33,34] The mechanism proposed is based on an increase in sympathetic tone leading to a reduction in R-L shunting and a more efficient wash-out of inhalant. However, the effect of epinephrine on the inhalant anesthetic recovery of lizards is unknown.

LOCOREGIONAL ANESTHESIA

Lizards frequently undergo various surgical procedures that require general anesthesia.[35] However, according to a survey, anesthesia in reptiles can be associated with a significant incidence of complications, including respiratory depression or apnea, prolonged recovery, and death.[36] Therefore, the use of locoregional anesthesia may help decrease the requirements for systemically administered sedatives/anesthetics, as well as systemic analgesics, potentially contributing to shortened recoveries and lower incidence of anesthesia-related morbidity and mortality, particularly in debilitated reptiles. The popularity of locoregional anesthesia has been increasing.[37] However, data in lizards regarding pharmacokinetics/pharmacodynamics of local anesthetics and specific techniques and are still limited.

NEURAXIAL ANESTHESIA

In lizards, the spinal meninge that represents the dura mater in mammals, which is the outermost meninge, is closely attached to the vertebral column.[38] This characteristic may render the performance of epidural injections (injectate deposited between the dura mater and the wall of the vertebral canal) unlikely, making intrathecal injections more feasible. Intrathecal anesthesia (or also called spinal anesthesia) is the result of local anesthetic being deposited in the subarachnoid space, which contains cerebrospinal fluid (CSF). Owing to the small size of most lizards, the visualization of CSF to confirm which technique is being performed is unlikely. Therefore, using the term neuraxial anesthesia for these species is recommended.[39]

To date, there are only studies on sacrococcygeal neuraxial anesthesia in inland bearded dragons and a case report in a black-and-white tegu (**Fig. 7**).[39,40] The authors have performed successful neuraxial anesthesia in green iguanas for tail amputation (see **Fig. 7**). Although very limited data have been published, complications have been limited to respiratory depression when excessive doses of local anesthetics were used).[39]

Anesthesia of the caudal aspect of the body (cloaca, pelvic limbs, and up to 25%–50% of the trunk) has been described with sacrococcygeal neuraxial injections.[39] Depending on the volume and total dose used, further cranial migration can be obtained; however, this is not recommended because complications such as respiratory depression and the need for orotracheal intubation may be involved.[39]

Equipment

Some of the equipment required (such as a needle) will depend on the size of the lizard.

- Skin preparation solutions (ie, chlorhexidine, alcohol)
- Needle: for small lizards, such as bearded dragons, a 28-gauge, 13-mm (0.5 inches) needle (permanently attached to a 0.5-mL syringe). For larger lizards, such as iguanas and tegus, 22-gauge to 25-gauge, 25-mm to 38-mm (1–1.5 inch) spinal needles are recommended (**Fig. 8**)
- Syringes: depend on the size of the lizard, but in general, 0.5-mL to 3-mL syringes are appropriate
- Preservative-free local anesthetic (ie, lidocaine or bupivacaine) ± analgesic (ie, morphine)
- Preservative-free saline (NaCl 0.9%) if needed for diluting the local anesthetic
- Sterile gloves

Technique

Anatomic landmarks

The sacrococcygeal space is located by palpating the caudal border of the ilia with one hand and using the other hand to move the tail up and down and side-to-side, finding the mobile portion (coccygeal vertebrae). An imaginary line can be drawn across the midline, just caudal to the caudal border of the ilia, where the tail starts moving. The needle will be inserted in the middle of this line (see **Figs. 7** and **8**).

Step-by-step procedure

- Heavy sedation is required to avoid movement of the animal during the procedure.
- The animal is placed in sternal recumbency, with its limbs in a natural position.
- The needle insertion site is located, and the area should be aseptically prepared.

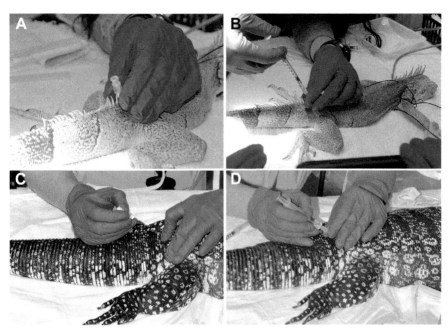

Fig. 7. Neuraxial drug administration for induction of spinal anesthesia in a green iguana *(Iguana iguana) (A, B)* and black-and-white tegu *(Salvator merianae) (C, D)*; 25-gauge spinal needles were used in both cases to perform the neuraxial injection at the sacrococcygeal junction.

- The needle is inserted at approximately 75 degree with the skin, with its bevel facing cranially.
- The needle is slowly advanced until a twitch of the tail and/or pelvic limbs is observed. A twitch is not always required for a successful injection; however, it has been shown to be a good predictor of success.[39] The presence of a tail twitch has also been commonly observed while performing neuraxial anesthesia in cats and has not been associated with adverse effects.[41] Approximately half to two-thirds of a 13-mm needle has been reported to successfully reach the target site in bearded dragons of various sizes (220–520 g).[39] Needle insertion depth will depend on the species and individual.
- Slight adjustments of the needle angle or even the insertion site may be required if the needle tip contacts bone too superficially or the needle is advanced too deeply without eliciting the twitch. The needle always should be inserted at the midline.
- Once the appropriate needle placement is achieved, aspirate to check for the presence of blood. Blood has been aspirated on several occasions during bearded dragon neuraxial injections, which could predispose the animal to systemic toxicity.[39] If blood is aspirated, the injection should be aborted, and the procedure restarted with a new needle/syringe. In larger lizards, there is the possibility of observing CSF while aspirating.
- If no blood is present, injection can be performed.
- If no motor block of the pelvic limbs occurs after neuraxial injection (ie, demonstrating withdrawal when it is pinched), or if cloacal tone is not lost within 5 to

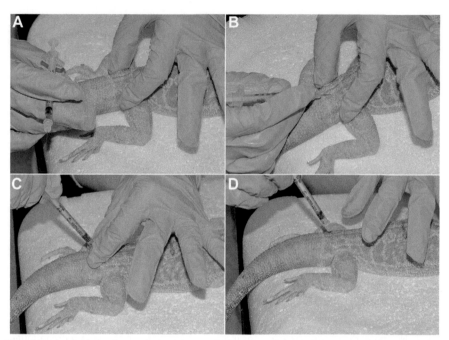

Fig. 8. Neuraxial injection technique in a sedated inland bearded dragon (*Pogona vitticeps*). (*A*) Identification of the sacrococcygeal junction by lateral movement of the tail base. (*B*) Following sterile preparation, the needle is inserted midline at the level of the sacrococcygeal junction in an ~75-degree angle and the bevel facing cranially. The needle is then slowly advanced until a twitch of a pelvic limb or tail occurs. A twitch is not always required for a successful injection; however, it has been shown to be a good predictor of success. Slight adjustments of the needle angle or even the insertion site may be required if the needle tip contacts bone too superficially or the needle is advanced too deeply without eliciting the twitch. (*C*) Aspiration should always be performed before drug administration, to check for the presence of blood. If blood is aspirated, the injection should be aborted, and the procedure restarted with a new needle/syringe. In larger lizards, there is the possibility of observing CSF while aspirating. (*D*). Drug injection should be performed over 2 to 5 seconds, depending on the volume.

10 minutes, another injection at the same dose can be performed. This has been shown to increase the overall success rate from 50% to 75% in one bearded dragon study and from 95% to 100% in another.[39]

Drugs Used for Neuraxial Anesthesia and Analgesia in Lizards

Lidocaine

Lidocaine 2% at 4 mg/kg (0.2 ml/kg) resulted in blockade of forelimbs and apnea of some animals in a pilot study in bearded dragons, which led the authors to test a lower dose but maintain the same injection volume.[39] Lidocaine (1%) at 2 mg/kg (0.2 mL/kg) resulted in blockade onset within 5 minutes in all the successful injections.[39] The blockade extended cranially up to 25% of the trunk length in most bearded dragons, lasting 40 ± 14 minutes at that level; and motor blockade of the pelvic limbs and loss of cloacal tone lasted 48 ± 25 and 49 ± 25 minutes, respectively.[39] A case report of cloacoscopy in a tegu with a colonic urate enterolith described the successful use of

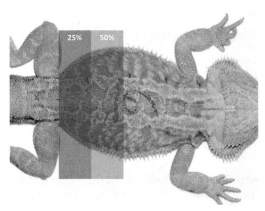

Fig. 9. Trunk spread in a bearded dragon. X = neuraxial injection site at the sacrococcygeal junction.

neuraxial lidocaine (2 mg/kg, 2%) with morphine (0.1 mg/kg, 1%); however, duration and cranial extension of the blockade were not reported.[40]

Bupivacaine

Two doses of bupivacaine 0.5% were evaluated (1 and 2 mg/kg) in bearded dragons.[39] Neuraxial bupivacaine at 1 mg/kg (0.2 mL/kg) resulted in a median cloacal tone loss of 83 (25–135) minutes and pelvic limb blockade of 68 (30–105) minutes. Nine of 10 animals presented sensory blockade of up to 25% of the trunk (lasting 60 [20–90] minutes), and 5 of 10 animals presented sensory blockade of up to 50% of the trunk (lasting 10 [5–90] minutes) (**Fig. 9**).[39] Even though the higher dose/volume (2 mg/kg, 0.4 mL/kg) resulted in more consistent cranial spread (9 of 10, and 6 of 10 animals had sensory blockade up to 50% of the trunk and up to 75% of the trunk, respectively), some animals became apneic. One animal had to be intubated and ventilated.[39] Therefore, the authors do not recommend the high dose for clinical use.

Morphine

Preservative-free opioids, such as morphine, can be used alone or in combination with local anesthetics in neuraxial injections. When used alone, opioids do not produce motor blockade. Neuraxial morphine use has been described in chelonians, and its use is associated with prolongation of analgesia provided by the local anesthetic.[42] In a study in bearded dragons, morphine was administered at 0.5 mg/kg in conjunction with lidocaine (2 mg/kg) and resulted in spinal analgesia lasting at least 12, but less than 24 hours. The duration of motor block induced by lidocaine was not significantly affected by the addition of morphine.[39] Neuraxial morphine (0.1 mg/kg) in a clinical case has been reported in a black-and-white tegu.[40] In this case, morphine was combined with lidocaine for neuraxial administration in the sedated animal to facilitate cloacoscopy. The efficacy and duration of neuraxial morphine in species other than bearded dragons has not been systematically evaluated.

LOCAL INFILTRATION

Local anesthetics can be injected into SC tissue and/or muscular layers around the surgical field to desensitize specific areas for procedures such as skin biopsies, laceration repairs, line blocks before celiotomies, and digit amputations. The toxic dose of specific local anesthetics has not been established in reptiles. Thus the maximum doses used

Table 3
Doses of local anesthetics for local infiltration (extrapolated from domestic species)[43]

Local Anesthetic	Maximum Dose, mg/kg
Lidocaine	4–10
Mepivacaine	2–6
Bupivacaine	1–2
Levobupivacaine	1.5–3
Ropivacaine	1.5–3

are extrapolated from mammalian species (**Table 3**).[43] Owing to the small size of some lizards, dilution of the local anesthetic may be necessary to obtain enough volume to cover the targeted area yet keeping the total dose within a safe range, avoiding overdose and systemic toxicity. In addition, while performing local infiltration, negative aspiration of blood should always be confirmed before injecting the local anesthetic to prevent intravascular administration and potential systemic toxicity.

SUMMARY

The field of lizard sedation, anesthesia, and locoregional anesthesia is advancing with new drug protocols, and new locoregional techniques are being developed and evaluated. Inducing and maintaining effective and safe chemical restraint in lizards can be challenging, particularly in systemically diseased individuals. Understanding the anatomic and physiologic adaptations of lizards, using reversible or partially reversible injectable protocols, and using locoregional anesthesia may increase the quality of chemical restraint, facilitate faster recoveries, and limit anesthesia-related morbidity and mortality.

REFERENCES

1. Mans C, Sladky KK, Schumacher J. General anesthesia. In: Divers S, Stahl S, editors. Mader's reptile medicine and surgery. 3rd edition. Philadelphia: WB Saunders; 2019. p. 447–64.

2. Fink DM, Doss GA, Sladky KK, et al. Effect of injection site on dexmedetomidine-ketamine induced sedation in leopard geckos (Eublepharis macularius). J Am Vet Med Assoc 2018;253:1146–50.

3. Yaw TJ, Mans C, Johnson SM, et al. Effect of injection site on alfaxalone-induced sedation in ball pythons (Python regius). J Small Anim Pract 2018;59:747–51.

4. Benson KG, Forrest L. Characterization of the renal portal system of the common green iguana (Iguana iguana) by digital subtraction imaging. J Zoo Wildl Med 1999;30:235–41.

5. Kummrow MS, Tseng F, Hesse L, et al. Pharmacokinetics of buprenorphine after single-dose subcutaneous administration in red-eared sliders (Trachemys scripta elegans). J Zoo Wildl Med 2008;39:590–5.

6. Olsson A, Phalen D. Preliminary studies of chemical immobilization of captive juvenile estuarine (Crocodylus porosus) and Australian freshwater (C. johnstoni) crocodiles with medetomidine and reversal with atipamezole. Vet Anaesth Analg 2012;39:345–56.

7. Doss GA, Fink DM, Sladky KK, et al. Comparison of subcutaneous dexmedetomidine–midazolam versus alfaxalone–midazolam sedation in leopard geckos (*Eublepharis macularius*). Vet Anaesth Analg 2017;44:1175–83.

8. Ratliff C, Parkinson LAB, Mans C. Effects of the fraction of inspired oxygen on alfaxalone-sedated inland bearded dragons (*Pogona vitticeps*). Am J Vet Res 2019;80:129–34.

9. Mans, C. BA. Evaluation of four different sedation protocols in bearded dragons (*Pogona vitticeps*). In: ExoticsCon 2018 Proceedings. Atlanta (GA), USA, September 22-September 27; 2018. p. 939.

10. Hicks JW, Ishimatsu A, Molloi S, et al. The mechanism of cardiac shunting in reptiles: A new synthesis. J Exp Biol 1996;199:1435–46.

11. Hlastala MP, Standaert TA, Luchtel DL, et al. The matching of ventilation and perfusion in the lung of the tegu lizard, *Tupinambis nigropunctatus*. Respiration Physiol 1985;60:277–94.

12. Odette O, Churgin SM, Sladky KK, et al. Anesthetic induction and recovery parameters in bearded dragons (*Pogona vitticeps*): Comparison of isoflurane delivered in 100 % oxygen versus 21% oxygen. J Zoo Wildl Med 2015;46:534–9.

13. Bertelsen MF, Mosley C, Crawshaw GJ, et al. Inhalation anesthesia in Dumeril's monitor (*Varanus dumerili*) with isoflurane, sevoflurane, and nitrous oxide: Effects of inspired gases on induction and recovery. J Zoo Wildl Med 2005;36:62–8.

14. Hernandez-Divers SM, Schumacher J, Stahl S, et al. Comparison of isoflurane and sevoflurane anesthesia after premedication with butorphanol in the green iguana (Iguana iguana). J Zoo Wildl Med 2005;36:169–75.

15. Barter LS, Hawkins MG, Brosnan RJ, et al. Median effective dose of isoflurane, sevoflurane, and desflurane in green iguanas. Am J Vet Res 2006;67:392–7.

16. Bertelsen MF. Squamates (snakes and lizards). In: West G, Heard D, Caulkett N, editors. Zoo animal and wildlife immobilization and anesthesia. 2nd edition. Ames, IA: Wiley-Blackwell; 2014. p. 351–63.

17. Mosley CAE, Dyson D, Smith DA. The cardiovascular dose-response effects of isoflurane alone and combined with butorphanol in the green iguana (*Iguana iguana*). Vet Anaesth Analg 2004;31:64–72.

18. Chinnadurai SK, DeVoe R, Koenig A, et al. Comparison of an implantable telemetry device and an oscillometric monitor for measurement of blood pressure in anaesthetized and unrestrained green iguanas (*Iguana iguana*). Vet Anaesth Analg 2010;37:434–9.

19. Brosnan RJ, Pypendop BH, Barter LS, et al. Pharmacokinetics of inhaled anesthetics in green iguanas (*Iguana iguana*). Am J Vet Res 2006;67:1670–4.

20. Bertelsen MF, Mosley CAE, Crawshaw GJ, et al. Anesthetic potency of sevoflurane with and without nitrous oxide in mechanically ventilated Dumeril monitors. J Am Vet Med Assoc 2005;227:575–8.

21. Mosley CAE, Dyson D, Smith DA. Minimum alveolar concentration of isoflurane in green iguanas and the effect of butorphanol on minimum alveolar concentration. J Am Vet Med Assoc 2003;222:1559–64.

22. Arena PC, Richardson KC, Cullen LK. Anaesthesia in two species of large Australian skink. Vet Rec 1998;123:155–8.

23. Bertelsen MF, Sauer CD. Alfaxalone anaesthesia in the green iguana (*Iguana iguana*). Vet Anaesth Analg 2011;38:461–6.

24. Chukwuka CO, Virens J, Cree A. Accuracy of an inexpensive, compact infrared thermometer for measuring skin surface temperature of small lizards. J Therm Biol 2019;84:285–91.

25. Germer CM, Tomaz JM, Carvalho AF, et al. Electrocardiogram, heart movement and heart rate in the awake gecko (*Hemidactylus mabouia*). J Comp Physiol B Biochem Syst Environ Physiol 2015;185:111–8.

26. Filogonio R, Orsolini KF, Oda GM, et al. Baroreflex gain and time of pressure decay at different body temperatures in the tegu lizard, *Salvator merianae*. PLoS One 2020;15:7–9.

27. Hernandez SM, Schumacher J, Lewis SJ, et al. Selected cardiopulmonary values and baroreceptor reflex in conscious green iguanas (*Iguana iguana*). Am J Vet Res 2011;72:1519–26.

28. Glass ML, Wood SC. Gas exchange and control of breathing in reptiles. Physiol Rev 1983;63:232–60.

29. Moberly WR. The metabolic responses of the common iguana, *Iguana iguana,* to activity under restraint. Comp Biochem Physiol 1968;27:1–20.

30. Bennett RA, Schumacher J, Hedjazi-Haring K, et al. Cardiopulmonary and anesthetic effects of propofol administered intraosseously to green iguanas. J Am Vet Med Assoc 1998;212:93–8.

31. Dorsch JA, Dorsch SA. Gas monitoring. In: Dorsch JA, Dorsch SE, editors. Understanding anesthesia equipment. 5th ed. Philladephila: Lippincott Willams & Wilkins; 2008. p. 685–727.

32. Mitchell GS, Gleeson TT, Bennett AF. Pulmonary oxygen transport during activity in lizards. Respir Physiol 1981;43:365–75.

33. Gatson BJ, Goe A, Granone TD, et al. Intramuscular epinephrine results in reduced anesthetic recovery time in American alligators (*Alligator mississippiensis*) undergoing isoflurane anesthesia. J Zoo Wildl Med 2017;48:55–61.

34. Balko JA, Gatson BJ, Cohen EB, et al. Inhalant anesthetic recovery following intramuscular epinephrine in the loggerhead sea turtle (*Caretta caretta*). J Zoo Wildl Med 2018;49:680–8.

35. Di Girolamo N, Mans C. Reptile soft tissue surgery. Vet Clin North Am - Exot Anim Pract 2016;19:97–131.

36. Read MR. Evaluation of the use of anesthesia and analgesia in reptiles. J Am Vet Med Assoc 2004;224:547–52.

37. d'Ovidio D, Adami C. Locoregional anesthesia in exotic pets. Vet Clin North Am - Exot Anim Pract 2019;22:301–14.

38. Starck D. Cranio-cerebral relations in recent reptiles. In: Gans C, Northcutt RG, Ulinski P, editors. Biology of the Reptilia, Volume 9. Neurology A. New York, NY: Academic Press; 1979. p. 1–38.

39. Ferreira TH, Mans C. Evaluation of neuraxial anesthesia in bearded dragons (*Pogona vitticeps*). Vet Anaesth Analg 2019;46:126–34.

40. Epstein JJ, Doss G, Yaw T, et al. Diagnosis and successful medical management of a colonic, urate enterolith in an Argentine black and white tegu (*Salvator merianae*). J Herpetol Med Surg 2020;30:21–7.

41. Otero P, Campoy L. Epidural and spinal anesthesia. In: Campoy L, Read R, editors. Small animal regional anesthesia and analgesia. Ames, IA: Wiley-Blackwell; 2013. p. 227–59.

42. Mans C. Clinical technique: Intrathecal drug administration in turtles and tortoises. J Exot Pet Med 2014;23:67–70.

43. Garcia ER. Local anesthetics. In: Grimm K, Lamont L, Tranquilli W, et al, editors. Lumb and Jones' veterinary anesthesia and analgesia. 5th edition. Ames: Wiley-Blackwell; 2015. p. 332–54.

44. Knotek Z, Hrda A, Knotkova Z, et al. Alfaxalone anesthesia in the green iguana (*Iguana iguana*). Acta Vet Brno 2013;82:109–14.

45. Knotek Z, Hrda A, Kley N, et al. Alfaxalone anesthesia in veiled chameleons (Chameleo calyptratus). Proceedings of the Annual Conference of the Association of Reptile and Amphibian Veterinarians, 18th Annual Conference, Seattle WA, 2011.
46. Perry SM, Konsker I, Lierz M, et al. Determining the safety of repeated electroejaculations in veiled chameleons *Chamaeleo calyptratus*. J Zoo Wildl Med 2019; 50:557–69.
47. Kischinovsky M, Duse A, Wang T, et al. Alfaxalone anaesthesia in the green iguana (*Iguana iguana*). Vet Anaesth Analg 2013;40:241–5.
48. Ferreira TH, Mans C, Di Girolamo N. Evaluation of the sedative and physiological effects of intramuscular lidocaine in bearded dragons (*Pogona vitticeps*) sedated with alfaxalone. Vet Anaesth Analg 2019;46:496–500.
49. Budden L, Doss GA, Clyde VL, et al. Retrospective evaluation of sedation in 16 lizard species with dexmedetomidine-midazolam with or without ketamine. J Herpetol Med Surg 2018;28:47–50.
50. Mauthe von Degerfeld M. Personal experiences in the use of association tiletamine/zolazepam for anaesthesia of the green iguana (*Iguana iguana*). Vet Res Commun 2004;28:351–3.
51. Bertelsen MF, Mosley CAE, Crawshaw GJ, et al. Minimum alveolar concentration of isoflurane in mechanically ventilated Dumeril monitors. J Am Vet Med Assoc 2005;226:1098–101.
52. Available at: https://meridian.allenpress.com/jhms/article-abstract/doi/10.5818/JHMS-D-20-00020/467474/Evaluation-of-tiletamine-zolazepam-sedation-in?redirectedfrom–PDf.

Snake Sedation and Anesthesia

Daniel Almeida, MV, MS, DACVAA*, Martin Kennedy, DVM, DACVAA,
Erin Wend-Hornickle, DVM, DACVAA

KEYWORDS

- Snake • Sedation • Anesthesia • Analgesia • Zoo animal
- Zoologic companion animal • Reptile

KEY POINTS

- Sedation and anesthesia in snakes may be required for physical examination, diagnostics, therapeutics, surgical procedures, and euthanasia.
- Due to anatomic and physiologic differences and a wide range of species and sizes, reptiles generally are more challenging to anesthetize compared with other commonly encountered zoologic companion animal species.
- The same principles of anesthetic monitoring that are used in small animals should be employed with snakes.
- The prevention or minimization of pain is a cornerstone of modern veterinary practice and one of the pillars of anesthesia. It is a clinician's responsibility to adopt appropriate pain management strategies when the procedures or interventions performed are associated with pain.

INTRODUCTION

Snakes have become more popular as pets, and therefore it is important for general and exotic animal practitioners to familiarize themselves with the differences between these species and more commonly encountered companion animals. Additionally, with these animals, even something as simple as physical examination might require deep sedation or general anesthesia to be performed. The purpose of this review is to highlight important anatomic and physiologic differences, along with a review of the more commonly used drugs and monitoring techniques in snakes. Although not the focus of this article, a brief discussion about analgesia is included, because it is one of the pillars of anesthesia.

Veterinary Clinical Sciences, College of Veterinary Medicine, University of Minnesota, 1352 Boyd Avenue, Saint Paul, MN 55108, USA
* Corresponding author.
E-mail address: alme0061@umn.edu

Vet Clin Exot Anim 25 (2022) 97–112
https://doi.org/10.1016/j.cvex.2021.08.003
1094-9194/22/© 2021 Elsevier Inc. All rights reserved.

GENERAL CONSIDERATIONS

Despite numerous families, thousands of species, wide-ranging distribution, and great variability in size, snakes are anatomically and physiologically very similar. Reptiles have slow metabolic rates, which vary among them depending on species, size, diet, and ambient temperature. Comparatively, in general, their metabolism is one-fifth to one-seventh that of a similarly sized mammal.[1]

Snakes belong to the largest order of reptiles, Squamata. A majority of snakes are nonvenomous but are capable of inflicting tissue damage with a bite. Venomous snakes primarily use their venom to immobilize their prey rather than defend themselves; however, caretakers need to exercise caution when handling venomous snakes to avoid envenomation. Diagnostics, therapeutics, surgical procedures, and even euthanasia may require immobilization or anesthesia in addition to a snake tube to perform them safely.

Unlike mammals, snakes overall are considered poikilothermic and ectothermic, relying on environmental temperatures to maintain their body temperature. While in the hospital, snakes should be kept in an area that can be heated and maintained at 28°C (82°F) for the perianesthetic period. If a patient is of a species with a higher preferred optimal temperature zone (POTZ), it also is ideal to supply a separate hot-spot in the terrarium it is held in.

All snakes have a strong flight reflex and attempt to escape if given the opportunity. Snakes also may become stressed if other predatory reptiles or animals are housed within their line of sight. Providing hiding areas within the terrarium may reduce the stress of hospitalization.

Reptiles can be more challenging to anesthetize compared with other animals that veterinarians commonly work with.[2] With more reptiles being kept as pets, veterinarians who treat them are faced with an increasing number of situations where sedation or anesthesia may be required. Snakes commonly require sedation or general anesthesia to ensure the safety of personnel and to prevent pain and distress of the patient during examination, diagnostics, and therapeutics; challenges they face derive from anatomic and physiologic differences, wide range of patient sizes, and variable responses to anesthetic agents.[3]

PREFERRED OPTIMUM TEMPERATURE ZONE

Snakes have a POTZ, which varies according to the species' natural environment and, within that, on specific activities, such as predation or digestion. For example, animals found in tropical environments have a preferred body temperature of approximately 28°C (82°F), whereas those in temperate climates prefer 24°C (75°F). High temperatures eventually lead to heat stress (35°C [95°F]) and death (38°C–44°C [100.4°F –111.2°F]); on the other hand, temperatures below 10°C (50°F) lead to torpor, and temperatures below 4°C (39.2°F) can lead to death.[4]

Snakes are reliant on the environment, or other external heat source, to regulate body temperature. This evolutionary trait has advantages, such as having lower energy requirements, and disadvantages, such as limited activity depending on ambient temperature, which can leave them vulnerable.[1] Body temperature affects the anesthetic dose requirement as well as induction and recovery times. Maintenance of body temperature is accomplished with the aid of external heating devices, such as heating pads, circulating warm water blankets, and forced air patient warming systems.

CARDIOVASCULAR

It may be easiest to anatomically describe snakes by dividing the length of their bodies in 3 parts (cranial, middle, and caudal). The heart lies in the caudal aspect of the cranial third of the body, located cranioventral to the bifurcation of the trachea, and it is mobile, not being limited by a diaphragm, and allowing for large ingesta to pass through. There are 2 aortas, right and left, which come together caudal to the heart. Ventrally, at midline, there is a large abdominal vein, which must be avoided when making a celiotomy incision.[4] Snakes have a renal portal system and the potential for hepatic first-pass effect; therefore, some consideration may be given to the potential impact these may have when using the caudal part of the body for injection of drugs.

Snakes have a 3-chambered heart, composed of 2 atria, divided by an atrial septum, and 1 ventricle, which is incompletely divided by a muscular ridge. This incomplete ventricular separation allows for intracardiac (IC) shunting of blood and, as such, plays an important role in the ability of these reptiles to hold their breath, so deoxygenated blood flows through the lungs with ease and blood shunts away from the lungs, toward the systemic circulation. Cardiac shunting is associated with patterns and stage of ventilation; when the animal is breathing, pulmonary resistance is low and there is increased pulmonary blood flow and, conversely, during periods of breath holding, pulmonary vascular resistance increases and there is decreased pulmonary perfusion and a large right-to-left shunting of blood.[1,5]

RESPIRATORY

A snake's glottis is easily visualized, because it is positioned rostrally at the base of the tongue, which makes intubating snakes straightforward; in addition, due to the lack of a cough reflex, potential stimulation of the larynx during intubation does not elicit the same response as in mammals, allowing for intubation even when awake or sedated. Similar to the heart, the trachea is mobile and can move laterally to allow for the passage of large ingesta.[4,5] Snakes lack vocal cords and have a poorly developed mucociliary apparatus.[4]

The trachea is composed of incomplete cartilaginous rings, and the lungs, depending on the species of snake, can be either symmetric, or asymmetrical.[5] Due to evolutionary changes, many snakes, such as viperids and colubrids, evolved to have 1 lung or only 1 functional lung, respectively, whereas some primitive snakes, such as those in the Boidae family, have 2 lungs.[4] The structure of the lungs is such that gas exchange occurs in the cranial portion of the lungs, which has a single chamber and adequate blood supply, whereas the caudal lung functions similar to an air sac and does is not involved in gas exchange.[4,5]

Reptiles exhibit a respiratory pattern of exhalation, followed by inspiration, and a subsequent, variable nonventilatory period. Body temperature can influence the respiratory cycle, with increases in temperature increasing oxygen consumption, which leads to increased ventilation.[5]

If anesthesia leads to hypoventilation and assisted or controlled ventilation is warranted, snakes have fragile lungs, and positive pressure ventilation needs to be performed with caution to avoid causing trauma.

PREPARATION

Snakes should be assessed first without interaction. This is an excellent way to assess respiratory rate and character as well as for any changes in behavior. An external examination can be performed with the snake in a terrarium or snake tube. It is imperative to ensure the diameter of the tube is appropriately sized so the snake cannot turn around within the tube. If manual restraint is safe, a more complete examination may be performed prior to sedation or anesthesia, including heart auscultation and temperature; however, in some patients this may not be possible. Fasting for 1 to 2 feeding cycles prevents compression of the lungs and decreases the chances of regurgitation.

SITES OF INJECTION

Because oral administration of medications or fluids may be challenging or impossible, parenteral administration is necessary in snakes. Subcutaneous (SC) injections are administered between the scales on the dorsal or lateral aspect of the body in the middle third of the length. Using a small-gauge needle is recommended to avoid tissue damage and excessive discomfort. Intramuscular (IM) is the most common route utilized and is achieved best using epaxial muscles on either side of the spine, just cranial to the heart. There is evidence that injections in the posterior third of the body may undergo hepatic metabolism via the renal portal system prior to reaching systemic effects. This may lead to a lesser anesthetic depth and duration but a faster recovery time compared with the same dose injected 1 cm cranial to the heart.[6] The intracoelomic (ICe) route can be used to administer isotonic crystalloids to dehydrated, ill, or anesthetized patients. A small-gauge needle or butterfly is inserted between the lateral and ventral scales in the caudal third of the snake, cranial to the vent. Care must be taken to avoid the lungs and air sac. The needle should be inserted just through the body wall to avoid coelomic organ damage. Aspirating the syringe ensures organ puncture has not occurred before fluids are administered. If in the coelomic cavity, there is no resistance to injection.[7] Alternatively, SC fluid administration can be considered.

The ventral coccygeal vein is the most common intravenous (IV) site utilized in snakes (**Fig. 1**). It can be found on the ventral midline of the tail and accessed caudal to the vent to avoid the hemipenes and anal sacs. Utilization of the jugular vein requires a skin incision to directly visualize the vein and, therefore, is not commonly used. To catheterize the jugular vein, an incision is made 4 to 7 scales cranial to the heart at the junction of the ventral scales and lateral body scales. The vein then is identified with blunt dissection just medial to the tips of the ribs. In large snakes, the palatine vein may be accessible (**Fig. 2**). It is located medially to the palatine teeth. This route usually requires sedation or anesthesia to access safely.[8]

Administration of injectable anesthetic agents is possible via the IC route. Due to the potential for myocardial damage ranging from mild to fatal, this route is considered only when others are not possible. The position of the heart can be seen with the snake in dorsal recumbency. The heart should be immobilized prior to injection with a forefinger and thumb. Some investigators recommend this route be used only in emergencies, however, there is evidence that this route causes minimal lasting tissue damage and is an effective way to induce anesthesia (eg, propofol) in snakes.[3,9,10]

INJECTABLE SEDATIVES AND ANESTHETICS
Alfaxalone

Alfaxalone (3-α-hydroxy-5-α-pregnane-11,20-dione) is a neuroactive steroid that is formulated in a 10-mg/mL solution with a cyclodextrin carrier. It originally was licensed for anesthetic inductions in dogs and cats via IV injection and now has the index Minor Use/Minor Species with labeling for use in more than 50 species, including snakes. Alfaxalone produces central nervous system (CNS) depression by interacting with neuronal γ-aminobutyric acid type A ($GABA_A$) receptors, resulting in increased chloride conductance and hyperpolarization of postsynaptic membranes, thus inhibiting awareness and arousal.[11] The depth and duration of sedation or anesthesia achieved

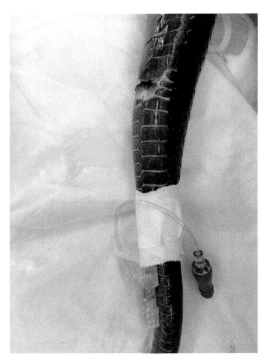

Fig. 1. IV catheter placed in the ventral coccygeal vein of a pine snake (*Pituophis melanoleucus*). (Image courtesy of Dr. Miranda Sadar.)

with alfaxalone administration in snakes depend on the dose, route, site of administration, and the concurrent administration of other drugs. Alfaxalone can be administered IV and slowly titrated to the desired effect; however, a major advantage of alfaxalone is that venous access is not required for sedation or induction of anesthesia. IM, ICe, and SC routes of alfaxalone all have been shown to effectively sedate or anesthetize snakes.[6,7,12–14] Onset is relatively rapid, with signs of sedation in less than 5 minutes after administration and peak effect occurring in less than 15 minutes.

Anesthetic induction with IM administration of alfaxalone at 10 mg/kg, 20 mg/kg, and 30 mg/kg has been explored in the ball python (*Python regius*).[7] When administered in the caudal third of the body, a dose of 30 mg/kg IM was required for successful intubation and resulted in approximately 1 hour of anesthesia time. The 10-mg/kg treatment produced only slight sedation and 20 mg/kg produced deeper sedation with a more consistent loss of the righting reflex (LRR); however, intubation was possible in only 1 of 6 snakes. Respiratory rates decreased with all treatments and some snakes experienced apnea after the 30-mg/kg IM injection. The 20 mg/kg IM treatment also was used to examine the effect of a cranial (1 cm cranial to the heart) versus caudal (posterior third of the body) injection site. Cranial injection produced a significantly increased depth of anesthesia, more successful intubations, an almost 6-times longer duration of intubation, more profound respiratory depression with all snakes experiencing apnea, and significantly longer anesthesia and recovery times compared with caudal injection. A significant effect of cranial versus caudal injection site with alfaxalone administration in ball pythons also has been documented by other investigators,[6] leading to the conclusion that venous blood from caudal tissues may drain to the hepatic portal vein prior to the liver. Therefore, any hepatically metabolized drugs

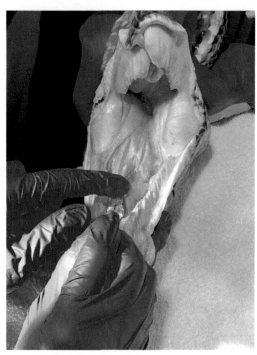

Fig. 2. IV catheter placement in the palatine vein of a reticulated python (*Malayopython reticulatus*). The animal is in dorsal recumbency. (Image courtesy of Dr. Miranda Sadar.)

administered in caudal regions of ball pythons may experience a first pass effect before reaching the CNS.[6,7]

Although the IM route generally is considered superior compared with SC, due to greater perfusion, in snakes with little muscle mass the SC route of administration is easier to perform and well tolerated. Alfaxalone injected SC in corn snakes (*Pantherophis guttatus*) produced anesthesia of variable duration in a dose-dependent manner.[14] Doses of 5 mg/kg, 10 mg/kg, and 15 mg/kg produced anesthesia for 15 minutes to 30 minutes, 25 minutes to 55 minutes, and 50 minutes to 70 minutes, respectively. When these doses were used, respiratory rate decreased significantly at the time of maximal effect compared with baseline, and increasing the dose led to a greater change in respiratory rate. A more consistent loss of reflexes (tongue flick, needle prick, and righting reflex) was observed with the 15-mg/kg dose. Heart rate was unchanged, regardless of the dose used. Injection sites (cranial or caudal) were also compared after a 15-mg/kg dose; there were no significant differences in duration of effect, heart rate, or respiratory rate.

In ball pythons, SC alfaxalone administration at 5 mg/kg resulted in rapid sedation with successful intubation in 7 of 8 snakes when the injection site was located in the cranial third of the body.[6] Cranial injection produced significant sedation for approximately 40 minutes with an accompanying decrease in heart rate and respiratory rate. Caudal injection resulted in slight sedation without any significant changes in heart rate or respiratory rate. A combination of SC alfaxalone (5 mg/kg) and midazolam (0.5 mg/kg) in the cranial injection site also has been reported in ball pythons.[13] The combination allowed for successful intubation in all snakes and resulted in an LRR for a median time of 80 minutes. Heart rate and respiratory rate decreased, and a majority of the snakes exhibited some abnormal spontaneous jaw movements. The combination is partially reversible, and recovery occurred approximately 40 minutes after flumazenil (0.05 mg/kg SC) administration.

The ICe route of injection provides another alternative for alfaxalone administration in snakes of small body size, or when the drug volume may be excessive for IM administration. In common garter snakes (*Thamnophis sirtalis*), the effect of ICe alfaxalone on LRR was investigated at 10 mg/kg, 20 mg/kg, and 30 mg/kg.[12] The low dose failed to produce an LRR in any of the snakes, whereas the 20-mg/kg and 30-mg/kg treatments were successful in 5 of 8 and 8 of 8 snakes, respectively. The median time to LRR with the 30-mg/kg treatment was 3.8 minutes, whereas for the 20-mg/kg treatment it was 8.3 minutes; however, the median time to return of the righting reflex was not significantly different. There was no differences in respiratory rate between the treatment groups. For snakes that experienced an LRR, the heart rate decreased steadily as the anesthetic depth decreased.

Propofol

Propofol (2,6-diisopropylphenol) is a lipid-soluble emulsion containing 1% propofol in an aqueous solution of soybean oil, glycerol, and purified egg phospholipid; the effects of propofol are mediated primarily through its interaction with the $GABA_A$ receptor, increasing the duration of chloride conductance and hyperpolarization of the postsynaptic membrane. With the growing number of reptiles kept as pets, and the fact that these animals may require sedation or anesthesia for physical examinations, diagnostic work-ups, and surgery, a survey published in 2004 found that propofol is 1 of only 2 commonly used injectable anesthetics with more than 40% of respondents reporting having used it in practice.[2]

Propofol gained popularity for its use in reptiles because it affords rapid induction and recovery from anesthesia, with limited negative effects. Benefits of the use of propofol include rapid onset, short duration, physiologic stability, and minimal equipment requirements. Propofol's termination of effect largely is a result of redistribution, which offsets change in metabolic rate.[15] Although favorable in some situations, the relative short duration of action can be seen as a shortcoming of the drug when used as a sole anesthetic agent for longer procedures, because maintenance of anesthesia requires a continuous infusion. With that, as the dose of propofol and the length of anesthetic time increase, so do the potential complications.[15]

In snakes, the coccygeal vein is the most commonly used IV site for drug administration but securing an IV access can be challenging and alternative routes have been used as a result.[2] Propofol was administered in the coccygeal vein of South American rattlesnakes (*Crotalus durissus terrificus*) for induction of anesthesia prior to tracheal intubation. At a dose of 15 mg/kg, spontaneous movements were observed within 60 minutes to 120 minutes after administration.[15]

In ball pythons, IC injections of propofol has been investigated for induction of anesthesia as an alternative to inhalant anesthetics. An IC dose of 10 mg/kg resulted in rapid, uneventful induction of anesthesia (<10 seconds), with no undesirable cardiovascular events appreciated. Compared with isoflurane, propofol use was associated with a significantly shorter induction time and a prolonged recovery after a brief anesthetic episode (less than 30 minutes). On histopathologic examination of the myocardium, there were mild acute inflammatory and some degenerative changes on day 3 after IC injection; those changes were minimal to mild on day 14, and no changes were noted 30 days and 60 days following the procedure.[3] IC propofol also has been used in brown tree snakes (*Boiga irregularis*). A single dose of 5 mg/kg resulted in anesthesia in a majority of animals (78%), lasting an average of 24 minutes. A transient, self-limiting apneic period, lasting no more than 60 seconds, was seen but no significant adverse events were noted.[16] Propofol has no analgesic effect; therefore, if painful procedures are to be performed, additional analgesic drugs need to be administered.

Midazolam

Midazolam is a water-soluble benzodiazepine supplied in a 5-mg/mL solution. Benzodiazepines bind to the $GABA_A$ receptor and alter the receptor conformation, such that the affinity for GABA is increased, producing increased chloride conductance and hyperpolarization of postsynaptic cell membranes.[17] In snakes, midazolam can be administered as a sole agent or combined with other drugs for sedation, anesthetic induction, and/or minimum alveolar concentration (MAC) reduction.[13,18–20]

In ball pythons, moderate to profound sedation has been reported after cranial IM administration of 1 mg/kg and 2 mg/kg of midazolam.[18,19] One investigation compared 1-mg/kg and 2-mg/kg doses and found there was no significant difference between the resulting sedation, muscle relaxation, decrease in heart rate, or change in respiratory rate.[19] With both treatments, signs of sedation were observed 10 minutes to 15 minutes after midazolam administration and 60% of the snakes experienced an LRR, with time to peak effect of approximately 60 minutes. The observed duration of sedation was found highly variable and ranged from 5 hours to greater than 6 days. Flumazenil, 0.08 mg/kg IM, was effective in reversing the sedation in about 10 minutes; however, the reversal was only temporary because all snakes were sedate again within 3 hours of reversal. Other investigators have documented a similar degree of sedation in ball pythons receiving 2-mg/kg midazolam IM at a cranial site; however, the mean recovery time reported was much shorter, at 100 minutes, and this likely is due to differences in methodology.[18] Midazolam, 1 mg/kg IM, injected cranially, also has been shown to reduce isoflurane MAC by 57% in ball pythons.[19]

Lower doses of midazolam can provide effective sedation when combined with other drugs.[13] In ball pythons, 0.5-mg/kg midazolam SC at a cranial site with either 5-mg/kg alfaxalone SC or 0.05-mg/kg dexmedetomidine SC resulted in a similar level of sedation with an LRR and successful intubation in all snakes. Onset was rapid with both treatments and median time to an LRR was not statistically significantly different—5 minutes for alfaxalone-midazolam and 10 minutes for dexmedetomidine-midazolam. The combination of alfaxalone and midazolam resulted in a longer median duration of LRR (80 minutes vs 50 minutes) and a longer median recovery time following administration of reversal agents (42.5 minutes vs 15 minutes). The dexmedetomidine-midazolam combination resulted in more profound decreases in heart rate and respiratory rate, with some snakes even experiencing apnea; however, the combination was fully reversible (flumazenil, 0.05 mg/kg SC, and atipamezole, 0.5 mg/kg SC).[13]

Ketamine

Ketamine is a water-soluble dissociative anesthetic that historically has been used in various animal species, including reptiles. Although ketamine may interact with several different receptors, its main CNS effects are believed to be the result of its interaction with N-methyl-ᴅ-aspartate glutamate receptors.

The available published data on the use of ketamine in snakes are limited and more than 20 years old. The effects of ketamine can be varied, depending on the dose administered, species of snake, metabolic rate, body temperature,[5,21] and influence of previous administration of the drug.[22] Advantages of the use of ketamine include the possibility of IM or IV administration, short duration of action, and a degree of analgesia. Among the disadvantages is prolonged recovery,[5,23] which can be between 6 hours and 24 hours after a sedative dose of ketamine (15 mg/kg) and between 2 days and 3 days after a dose used for anesthesia (40–80 mg/kg).[5] Other disadvantages include inadequate muscle relaxation and insufficient analgesia for invasive procedures.[23] The cardiovascular and respiratory changes than can occur include tachycardia, hypertension, and hypoventilation.[21,23] Ketamine may be administered in combination with other drugs, such as benzodiazepines or α_2-agonists, for muscle relaxation, reduced dose requirements, and shorter recovery times.[5,21,23]

Telazol

Telazol (Zoetis, New Jersey) is an injectable anesthetic combination composed of equal parts by weight of tiletamine and zolazepam. Tiletamine is a dissociative anesthetic and zolazepam is a benzodiazepine. The combination is supplied as a sterile powder and is licensed for use in dogs and cats. Reconstitution of a vial with the recommended 5 mL of diluent produces a 100 mg/mL solution; each mL contains 50 mg of tiletamine base and 50 mg of zolazepam base. A major advantage of Telazol is the relatively low volume of injection needed. There are few published data on the use of Telazol in snakes; however, based on its effects in other reptiles, its administration may provide effective sedation or anesthetic induction, and low doses (2–5 mg/kg) have been recommended.[24] Dose-dependent sedation and anesthesia following Telazol administration at a cranial injection site have been described in ball pythons.[18] Telazol, at 2 mg/kg and 3 mg/kg, resulted in an LRR in 7/10 and 10/10 snakes, respectively, with no significant difference in median time to LRR; 34 minutes for 2 mg/kg versus 44 minutes for 3 mg/kg. With the 2-mg/kg treatment, only 3 snakes lost withdrawal reflex compared with all 10 snakes with the 3-mg/kg treatment. The 3-mg/kg treatment provided significantly longer duration for LRR with a median time of 74.5 minutes versus 41 minutes. Mild decreases in heart rate and respiratory rate were observed and were not significantly different between treatments.

Local Anesthetics

Local anesthetics are a class of drugs capable of interrupting the transmission of noxious stimuli. This is accomplished primarily by blocking voltage-gated sodium channels and their inward currents, which prevents membrane depolarization and the generation of an action potential. The use of local anesthetics may decrease the need for systemic analgesics, can be sufficient to perform minor surgical procedures, or can be in conjunction with general anesthesia to provide adequate analgesia and reduce anesthetic dose requirements.[25] Although commonly used in various animal species, information on their safety and efficacy in reptiles, especially in snakes, is lacking. The authors recognize the benefits of local anesthetics, but, at the time of the writing of this article, a lack of information does not allow for drug or dose recommendations.

Opioids

Opioids are a class of drugs that act as agonists at mu, kappa, or delta opioid receptors in the CNS to modulate nociception. There is evidence that snake species express opioid receptors, which generally are well conserved across species.[26] Currently, the evidence for which opioid and which doses will be most effective for antinociception in snakes is minimal. One study identified that butorphanol, 20 mg/kg SC, increased thermal withdrawal latencies in corn snakes.[27] The same study identified morphine, up to 40 mg/kg, did not alter the thermal withdrawal latencies in this species and it was determined to be an ineffective analgesic.

Another study in ball pythons determined that transdermal fentanyl was an ineffective analgesic even with plasma fentanyl levels over 100 ng/mL.[28] The same plasma levels of fentanyl, however, caused a decrease in respiratory rates. Mu opioid receptor mRNA levels within the CNS were measured. The results confirmed that ball pythons have similar levels of mu opioid expression compared with a species that experiences effective analgesia with mu agonists. These findings suggest that ball pythons have functional mu opioid receptors; however, downstream signaling may be different such that respiration but not nociception is affected.

Because the understanding of opioid effectiveness is unclear in snakes, other drugs with antinociceptive properties should be considered.

α_2-Adrenergic Agonists

α_2-Adrenergic receptor agonists are used frequently in many species for sedation, analgesia, and muscle relaxation. Dexmedetomidine is a dextrorotatory isomer of medetomidine and has relatively high selectivity for α_2-receptors. When used as a sole agent, 1 study showed that dexmedetomidine effectively increases thermal withdrawal latencies in ball pythons without causing sedation, suggesting that it can be used as an effective analgesic.[29] At the doses used in the aforementioned study (0.1 mg/kg and 0.2 mg/kg), dexmedetomidine caused a decrease in respiratory rate, however, not to a degree that required intervention. The effects on respiratory rate can be attenuated by coadministration of doxapram.[30] Evidence on the use of α_2-adrenergic agonists, like many other drugs, is sparse in snakes. More research is needed to gain a better breadth of understanding of how this class of drugs can be used for analgesia in snakes.

INHALANT ANESTHETICS

Inhalant anesthetic agents can be used both for induction and maintenance of general anesthesia in snakes. According to results from a 2002 survey of the Association of Reptile and Amphibian Veterinarians, inhalant anesthesia was the technique used most commonly and isoflurane was the most common agent used.[2] An inhalant induction can be performed using a tight-fitting face mask or an induction chamber, depending on the species of snake. A face mask is appropriate for snakes that can be handled safely and physically restrained, whereas an induction chamber is ideal for venomous or potentially dangerous snakes. The vaporizer initially is set to maximum output until LRR or significant muscle relaxation have been achieved, at which time intubation is performed and the vaporizer output is decreased accordingly for maintenance. Compared with mammals and birds, inhalant inductions in reptiles can be prolonged due to breath holding and right to left shunting of blood resulting in decreased inhalant uptake. In prairie rattlesnakes (Crotalus viridis), the mean time to intubation was 7 minutes with isoflurane and 6 minutes with sevoflurane; however, sevoflurane administration elicited anesthetic gas avoidance behavior during induction.[31] Isoflurane administration resulted in a longer mean time to return of the righting reflex compared with sevoflurane (28 minutes vs 16 minutes, respectively); however, sevoflurane anesthesia resulted in significantly longer mean time to extubation (33 minutes vs 23 minutes). Alternatively, anesthesia can be induced with an injectable drug or drug combination and then maintained with isoflurane or sevoflurane following intubation. In ball pythons, the MAC for isoflurane was determined to be 1.11%; midazolam administration (1 mg/kg IM cranially) reduced isoflurane MAC by 57%, whereas 50% nitrous oxide reduced it by only 17%.[19]

POSITIVE PRESSURE VENTILATION

Overall, general anesthesia is associated with some degree of respiratory depression. Snakes have lower metabolic rates and a lower minute ventilation, which allows snakes to tolerate longer periods of hypoventilation.[5] Therefore, the anesthetist should include an assessment of the adequacy of ventilation and be prepared to provide assisted or controlled ventilation, if needed. In addition to promoting adequate gas exchange and preventing hypoxemia and hypercapnia, adequate ventilation is key in the delivery of inhalant anesthesia.[5]

Ventilation must be appropriate for any given metabolic state (and therefore production of carbon dioxide), and in snakes, metabolism is variable depending on temperature and digestive state, with higher minute ventilation required for higher temperatures and nonfasted animals. Bertelsen and colleagues[15] evaluated the effects of positive pressure ventilation on arterial blood gases and cardiovascular parameters in South American rattlesnakes. The investigators found that, in fasted animals, spontaneous ventilation led to hypercapnia and respiratory acidosis, whereas the institution of mechanical ventilation with a tidal volume of 30 mL/kg and 5 breaths/min was able to maintain the arterial pressure of carbon dioxide within normal limits (14.2 mm Hg $\pm$ 2.7 mm Hg). Over-ventilation and hypocapnia led to respiratory alkalosis and a significant delay in resumption of spontaneous ventilation after anesthesia. With these findings, the investigators concluded that mechanical ventilation with a tidal volume of 30 mL/kg and a respiratory rate of 1 breath/min to 2 breaths/min is appropriate in fasted rattlesnakes; however, these minute ventilation recommendations of 30 mL/kg/min to 60 mL/kg/min may not be applicable to other species of snakes.[32] Thus, the target for optimal minute ventilation likely varies with different species of snakes. Additionally, contrary to what is observed in mammals, positive pressure ventilation was found to increase mean arterial pressure in snakes significantly. A possible explanation for the observed change is the insufflation of the saccular caudal lung led to an increase in venous return and, therefore, an increase in cardiac output and mean arterial pressure.

MONITORING

The same principles of anesthetic monitoring that are used in domestic animals should be used in snakes. Reflexes, respiratory rate, end-tidal carbon dioxide, pulse rate, pulse oximetry, and blood pressure should be included and monitored by a dedicated anesthetist every 5 minutes. Anesthetic depth should be evaluated periodically by carefully assessing the righting reflex, neck tone, and jaw tone when appropriate.[8]

- Respiratory
  - Respiratory rate can be visualized directly via lateral body excursions, reservoir bag movements, or endotracheal tube fogging.[8]
  - Hypoventilation is common in snakes during general anesthesia, and ventilation should be assisted to maintain respiratory rates of 2 breaths/min to 6 breaths/min, tidal volumes of 15 mL/kg to 30 mL/kg, and peak airway pressures less than 10 cm H_2O.[8]
- Cardiovascular
  - Heart rate can be auscultated or audibly monitored using an ultrasonic Doppler device. The Doppler crystal should be positioned and secured directly over the heart. An esophageal stethoscope also may be used for direct auscultation in larger snakes.[33] In large snakes, the palatine artery can be used cautiously to palpate pulses.

○ Heart rhythm can be monitored with an electrocardiogram. Leads can be attached to 25-gauge needles placed transcutaneously cranial and caudal to the heart (**Fig. 3**). Snakes have a sinus venosus wave prior to the P wave, which should not be mistaken for an arrhythmia.[33]

○ Pulse oximetry (**Fig. 4**) has not been validated for use in reptiles; however, it may be used to monitor trends.[34]

○ Blood pressure can be measured indirectly via oscillometry. A cuff can be placed just caudal to the vent.[35] The width of the cuff should be approximately 40% of the circumference at this site. This method overestimates systolic blood pressure at low pressures, underestimates systolic blood pressure at high pressure, and underestimates the diastolic and mean blood pressures; however, it can be useful for monitoring trends. Direct blood pressure monitoring usually is reserved for research settings and involves catheterization of the aortic root or abdominal aorta.

RECOVERY

Recovery can be prolonged in snakes; however, there are some measures that can be taken to hasten it. When using inhalant anesthetics, discontinuation 15 minutes to 20 minutes prior to the end of the procedure may decrease recovery time.[36] Although not investigated in snakes, in some reptilian species, using concentrations of oxygen less than 100% as a carrier gas for inhalant may shorten recovery time, although the evidence is not consistent.[36,37] Recovery can be considered near complete when reflexes in the cranial third of the body return to normal, because, as snakes' reflexes

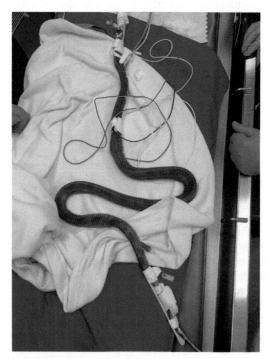

Fig. 3. Placement of electrocardiogram leads in a pine snake (*Pituophis melanoleucus*). (Image courtesy of Dr. Miranda Sadar.)

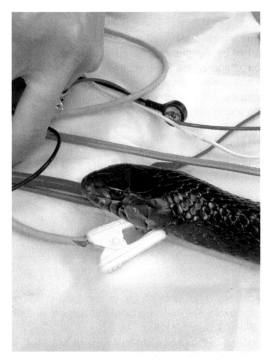

Fig. 4. Pulse oximetry placement in a pine snake (*Pituophis melanoleucus*). (Image courtesy of Dr. Miranda Sadar.)

recover in the opposite manner they become anesthetized, that is, from caudal to cranial.

Finally, because the metabolism of drugs is related to body temperature, snakes should be kept as close to their optimal body temperature as possible to encourage a shorter recovery period. Monitoring should continue throughout the recovery period. To achieve this, it is important to perform procedures requiring anesthesia on snakes early in the day.

PAIN AND ANALGESIA

Although not the core component of this publication, analgesia is an intrinsic part of anesthesia. The prevention or minimization of pain is a cornerstone of modern veterinary practice, and it is a clinician's responsibility to adopt appropriate pain management strategies when the procedures or interventions performed are associated with pain. Snakes possess all neuroanatomic structures necessary for nociception and it generally is accepted that they are able to feel pain.[2] Similar to pain assessment in mammals, it is important to have a systematic approach. Species identification and normal behaviors within a species are important to recognize prior to assessing pain. Changes in normal posture, movement or activity, temperament, and feeding behavior may be identified in snakes exhibiting pain.[38] In the absence of changes in any of these facets, the administration of analgesia should correlate with the amount of tissue damage present or expected with the procedure being performed. In reptiles, evidence-based pain management is limited and much of what is done is anecdotal.

SUMMARY

Although the general principles of anesthesia are the same, anesthetizing snakes presents a different set of challenges compared with mammals. These include understanding the anatomic and physiologic differences of these animals and how they have an impact on anesthetic planning, from handling, restraint, and drug selection, to monitoring techniques. A thorough understanding of the aforementioned is essential for patient safety and quality of care.

ACKNOWLEDGMENTS

The authors would like to thank Dr Miranda Sadar for kindly providing the pictures used in this article.

DISCLOSURE

The authors have no commercial or financial interests to disclose and did not receive funding for this work.

REFERENCES

1. O'Malley B. Anatomy and physiology in reptiles. In: Doneley B, Monks D, Johnson R, et al, editors. Reptile medicine and surgery in clinical practice. Hoboken, NJ: John Wiley & Sons; 2018. p. 15–32.
2. Read MR. Evaluation of the use of anesthesia and analgesia in reptiles. J Am Vet Med Assoc 2004;224(4):547–52.
3. McFadden MS, Bennett RA, Reavill DR, et al. Clinical and histologic effects of intracardiac administration of propofol for induction of anesthesia in ball pythons (Python regius). J Am Vet Med Assoc 2011;239(6):803–7.
4. O'Malley B. General anatomy and physiology of reptiles. In: Clinical anatomy and physiology of exotic species: structure and function of mammals, birds, reptiles, and Amphibians. Philadelphia, PA: Elsevier Saunders; 2005. p. 17–39.
5. Bertelsen MF. Squamates (lizards and snakes). In: West G, Heard D, Caulkett N, editors. Zoo animal and wildlife immobilization and anesthesia. 2nd edition. Aimes, IA: John Wiley & Sons Inc; 2014. p. 351–63.
6. Yaw TJ, Mans C, Johnson SM, et al. Effect of injection site on alfaxalone-induced sedation in ball pythons (Python regius). J Small Anim Pract 2018;59(12):747–51.
7. James LE, Williams CJ, Bertelsen MF, et al. Anaesthetic induction with alfaxalone in the ball python (Python regius): dose response and effect of injection site. Vet Anaesth Analg 2018;45(3):329–37.
8. Mosley C. Anesthesia and analgesia in reptiles. Semin Avian Exot Pet Med 2005; 14(4):243–62.
9. Isaza R, Andrews G, Coke R, et al. Assessment of multiple cardiocentesis in ball pythons (Python regius). Contemp Top Lab Anim Sci 2004;43(6):35–8.
10. Anderson NL, Wack RF, Calloway L, et al. Cardiopulmonary Effects and Efficacy of Propofol as an Anesthetic Agent in Brown Tree Snakes (Boiga irregularis). J Herpetol Med Surg 1999;9(2):9–17.
11. Cottrell GA, Lambert JJ, Peters JA. Modulation of GABAA receptor activity by alphaxalone. Br J Pharmacol 1987;90(3):491–500.
12. Strahl-Heldreth DE, Clark-Price SC, Keating SCJ, et al. Effect of intracoelomic administration of alfaxalone on the righting reflex and tactile stimulus response of common garter snakes (Thamnophis sirtalis). Am J Vet Res 2019;80(2):144–51.

13. Yaw TJ, Mans C, Johnson S, et al. Evaluation of subcutaneous administration of alfaxalone-midazolam and dexmedetomidine-midazolam for sedation of ball pythons (Python regius). J Am Vet Med Assoc 2020;256(5):573–9.

14. Rockwell K, Boykin K, Padlo J, et al. Evaluating the efficacy of alfaxalone in corn snakes (Pantherophis guttatus). Vet Anaesth Analg 2021;48(3):364–71.

15. Bertelsen MF, Buchanan R, Jensen HM, et al. Assessing the influence of mechanical ventilation on blood gases and blood pressure in rattlesnakes. Vet Anaesth Analg 2015;42(4):386–93.

16. Anderson N, Coupe B, Perry G, et al. Field use of propofol: a rapid recovery anesthetic with data from brown tree snakes (Boiga irregularis). Herpetol Rev 2000; 31(3):161.

17. Möhler H, Richards JG. The benzodiazepine receptor: a pharmacological control element of brain function. Eur J Anaesthesiol Suppl 1988;2:15–24.

18. Miller LJ, Fetterer DP, Garza NL, et al. A fixed moderate-dose combination of tiletamine+zolazepam outperforms midazolam in induction of short-term immobilization of ball pythons (Python regius). PLoS One 2018;13(10):e0199339.

19. Larouche CB, Mosley C, Beaufrère H, et al. Effects of midazolam and nitrous oxide on the minimum anesthetic concentration of isoflurane in the ball python (Python regius). Vet Anaesth Analg 2019;46(6):807–14.

20. Larouche CB, Beaufrère H, Mosley C, et al. Evaluation of the effects of midazolam and flumazenil in the ball python (Python regius). J Zoo Wildl Med 2019;50(3): 579–88.

21. Schumacher J, Lillywhite H, Norman W, et al. Effects of Ketamine HCl on Cardiopulmonary Function in Snakes. Copeia 1997;2:395–400.

22. Hill RE, Mackessy SP. Venom yields from several species of colubrid snakes and differential effects of ketamine. Toxicon 1997;35(5):671–8.

23. Heard DJ. Reptile anesthesia. Vet Clin North Am Exot Anim Pract 2001;4(1): 83–117.

24. Bertelsen MF. Squamates (lizards and snakes). In: West G, Heard D, Caulkett N, editors. Zoo animal and wildlife immobilization and anesthesia. Aimes, IA: Blackwell; 2007. p. 233–44.

25. Chatigny F, Kamunde C, Creighton CM, et al. Uses and Doses of Local Anesthetics in Fish, Amphibians, and Reptiles. J Am Assoc Lab Anim Sci 2017; 56(3):244–53.

26. Ng TB, Ng AS, Wong CC. Adrenocorticotropin- and beta-endorphin-like substances in brains of the freshwater snake Ptyas mucosa. Biochem Cell Biol 1990;68(7–8):1012–8.

27. Sladky KK, Kinney ME, Johnson SM. Analgesic efficacy of butorphanol and morphine in bearded dragons and corn snakes. J Am Vet Med Assoc 2008; 233(2):267–73.

28. Kharbush RJ, Gutwillig A, Hartzler KE, et al. Antinociceptive and respiratory effects following application of transdermal fentanyl patches and assessment of brain μ-opioid receptor mRNA expression in ball pythons. Am J Vet Res 2017; 78(7):785–95.

29. Bunke LG, Sladky KK, Johnson SM. Antinociceptive efficacy and respiratory effects of dexmedetomidine in ball pythons (Python regius). Am J Vet Res 2018; 79(7):718–26.

30. Karklus AA, Sladky KK, Johnson SM. Respiratory and antinociceptive effects of dexmedetomidine and doxapram in ball pythons (Python regius). Am J Vet Res 2021;82(1):11–21.

31. Kane LP, Chinnadurai SK, Vivirito K, et al. Comparison of isoflurane, sevoflurane, and desflurane as inhalant anesthetics in prairie rattlesnakes (*Crotalus viridis*). J Am Vet Med Assoc 2020;257(9):945–9.
32. Jakobsen SL, Williams CJA, Wang T, et al. The influence of mechanical ventilation on physiological parameters in ball pythons (*Python regius*). Comp Biochem Physiol A Mol Integr Physiol 2017;207:30–5.
33. Wood SC, L'enfant CJM. Respiration: mechanics, control and gas exchange. In: Gans C, Dawson WR, editors. Biology of the Reptilia. Volume 5. Physiology A. New York, NY: Academic Press; 1976. p. 225–74.
34. Mosley CA, Dyson D, Smith DA. The cardiovascular dose-response effects of isoflurane alone and combined with butorphanol in the green iguana (Iguana iguana). Vet Anaesth Analg 2004;31(1):64–72.
35. Chinnadurai SK, Wrenn A, DeVoe RS. Evaluation of noninvasive oscillometric blood pressure monitoring in anesthetized boid snakes. J Am Vet Med Assoc 2009;234(5):625–30.
36. Odette O, Churgin SM, Sladky KK, et al. Anesthetic induction and recovery parameters in bearded dragons (*Pogona Vitticeps*): comparison of Isoflurane delivered in 100% oxygen versus 21% oxygen. J Zoo Wildl Med 2015;46(3):534–9.
37. Diethelm G. The effect of oxygen content of inspiratory air (FIO2) on recovery times in the green iguana (*Iguana iguana*). Zurich: University of Zurich; 2001.
38. Mosley C. Pain and nociception in reptiles. Vet Clin North Am Exot Anim Pract 2011;14(1):45–60.

Psittacine Sedation and Anesthesia

Mikel Sabater González, LV, CertZooMed, DECZM (Avian), MRCVS[a,b,*],
Chiara Adami, DMV, DACVAA, DECVAA, PhD, MRCVS[c]

KEYWORDS

- Avian anesthesia • Avian anesthetic monitoring • Avian sedation • Psittaciformes

KEY POINTS

- Although psittacine sedation and anesthesia are increasingly advancing, the risk of anesthetic-related death is higher than in small animals.
- Psittacines present anatomic and physiologic peculiarities that should be taken into consideration when performing sedation/anesthesia.
- The preanesthetic physical examination and clinical history are essential tools to detect underlying diseases and identify, for each bird, the anesthetic risk, and develop a patient-specific protocol.
- Minimizing perioperative stress, and therefore its detrimental effects on the cardiovascular and endocrine systems, is an important aspect of the anesthetic management of psittacines.
- Optimization of perioperative pain relief improves quality of patient care and safety; when possible, multimodal analgesia should be preferred over a single-drug approach.
- Continuous monitoring during all the phases of an anesthetic event, including recovery, is paramount for the early detection and prompt treatment of complications.

INTRODUCTION

The increasing knowledge on the anesthetic management of psittacine species has resulted, during recent years, in the development of novel sedation and anesthetic protocols. It has also resulted in a growing awareness of the importance of continuous monitoring of physiologic parameters, extending from premedication to recovery from anesthesia. This article reviews the most important concepts that apply to avian

The authors do not have any commercial or financial conflicts of interest or any funding sources to disclose. The authors contributed to the same extent to the preparation of this article and share first authorship.
[a] Uplands Way Vets Ltd, Low Road, Diss, Norfolk IP222AA, UK; [b] Cambridge Veterinary Group, 89A Cherry Hinton Road, Cambridge, Cambridgeshire CB17BS, UK; [c] School of Veterinary Medicine, Louisiana State University, Skip Bertman Drive, Baton Rouge, LA 70803, USA
* Corresponding author. Marqués de San Juan 23-5, 46015, Valencia, Spain.
E-mail address: exoticsvet@gmail.com

anesthesia with particular focus on psittacine species, the anesthetic/sedative protocols that have been described in the current literature, and the use of equipment. The objective is to provide the reader with useful information to approach psittacine sedation and anesthesia safely and effectively.

SAFETY AND PERIANESTHETIC FATALITIES

The risk of anesthetic-related death in psittacine species remains unknown, but it is expected to be higher than in dogs and cats, which was estimated to be 0.05% and 0.11%, respectively, with fatal complications occurring most frequently in the first 3 hours postoperatively.[1,2] A survey evaluating the management of anesthesia in small animal species included psittacines; however, this work did not focus on perianesthetic mortality.[3] In a more recent study that included 352 birds undergoing inhalational anesthesia, 86% were alive at hospital discharge, 3.4% died during the anesthetic, 4.3% died postoperatively in the intensive care unit, and 6.3% were euthanatized after anesthesia.[4]

Perianesthetic safety is dramatically improved by implementing the routine practice of continuous monitoring and proper planning. The sedation/anesthetic plan should include the anticipated complications, the measures in place to prevent or treat them, and recovery. Complications associated with equipment failure and human error should also be considered and addressed. The use of anesthetic checklists available on dedicated Web sites (eg, www.aaha.org/anesthesia) may help to prevent avoidable errors and improve outcomes.

BEFORE ANESTHESIA
Preanesthetic Evaluation and Planning

The anesthetist should review the clinical history of the patient to identify underlying disorders, previous drug reactions, issues related to recovery from anesthesia, and any other aspect that may be relevant for the procedure and may represent a risk factor. Because of anatomic and physiologic reasons, it is important to know the species, morph variant, age, and sex of the bird.

Some species are prone to develop specific syndromes, such as the hypocalcemic syndrome that is common in Congo and Timneh African gray parrots (*Psittacus erithacus* and *Psittacus timneh*). As a general concept regarding morph variants and level of inbreeding, psittacine mutations and highly inbred individuals may be more sensitive to perianesthetic stress and more prone to be affected by congenital disorders than less selectively bred individuals. Regarding age, certain diseases are more likely to occur in elderly animals, whereas complications, such as hypoglycemia and hypothermia, are more common in neonatal and juvenile parrots. Because psittacines are altricial, chicks are not fully feathered and are more prone to develop hypothermia than chicks of nonaltricial species (**Fig. 1**). Additionally, individuals that are either elderly or very young present a higher anesthetic risk because of potentially altered responses to drugs caused by impairment or immaturity of the cardiovascular, respiratory, hepatic, renal, and nervous systems. The sex and reproductive status are other important factors to consider. Females experiencing dystocia, for example, may be hypocalcemic and have reduced respiratory function because of air sac compression. This is common in females and males with reproductive organomegaly (**Fig. 2**). The size of psittacines limits the suitability and reliability of many pieces of commonly available medical equipment. Moreover, a less precise administration of drug doses may be expected in smaller individuals.

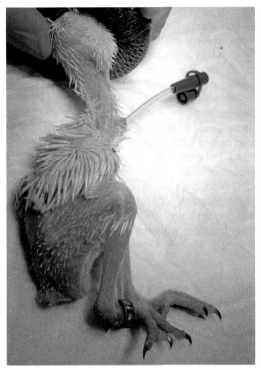

Fig. 1. Inhalational gas anesthesia delivered via face mask in a nonfledged little corella (*Cacatua sanguinea*).

The anesthetist must be aware of the details of the clinical procedure for which the bird is being anesthetized, including estimated duration, anticipated degree of nociception and pain, and technical aspects (eg, patient positioning). In small animals, sedation may be sufficient to perform short and minimally invasive procedures, such as radiographic examinations or blood sampling in young and healthy individuals; however, heavy sedation may not be suitable in older and/or medically compromised patients, for which a brief general anesthetic may be preferred to optimize

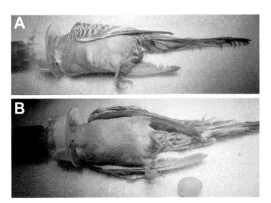

Fig. 2. (*A*) Budgerigar (*Melopsittacus undulatus*) with dystocia. (*B*) Air sac compression decreased significantly after the egg was removed.

monitoring, reduce stress, and decrease the odds for anesthesia-related death.[5] The authors believe this can also be extended to psittacines. For example, ocular and tracheal surgeries may prevent the use of a face mask to deliver inhalational anesthesia and oxygen supplementation, wing surgery may prevent the use of a Doppler and/or intravenous (IV) catheterization of the affected wing, and tracheal surgery may require the delivery of anesthesia and assisted ventilation through the air sac. Moderate to severe blood loss is expected during invasive surgical procedures, such as fracture repairs.

Anamnesis should be finalized to obtain information that is objective and detailed. Nevertheless, the importance of subjective information provided by the owner should not be underestimated. For example, the owner's perception of the bird's temperament, and how it would deal with stress in the hospital setting, helps to determine whether anxiolytics should be administered preventively by the owner to reduce transportation-related stress and facilitate physical examination. Anxious birds often require high doses of sedative and anesthetic agents, which may cause respiratory and cardiovascular depression, whereas in lethargic birds drug dosages should be decreased. All relevant information obtained from the bird's owner should be recorded.

A complete physical examination should always precede the anesthetic event. Failure to perform a physical examination increases the odds for death in dogs.[6] The bird should be examined from a distance and in a safe and quiet environment. Parrots, as prey animals, tend to hide clinical signs of disease. Physical manifestations of disease may include, but are not restricted to, lethargy, standing on the bottom of the cage, hiding or resting the head under the wing, hyperflexed perching, using the beak to hold up the head, prolonged tail bobbing, inability to make loud vocalizations, and altered mentation. Altered mentation may be indicative of intracranial disease.

Complementary diagnostic tests, including hematology, biochemistry, and fecal and urofecal analyses, should be offered to the owner, because these may provide relevant information on the health status of the bird and help to detect potentially life-threatening conditions, such as hypoglycemia and hypocalcemia. Further diagnostics, including electrocardiogram and diagnostic imaging (eg, radiographs, ultrasonography, echocardiography, and computed tomography), may be recommended based on clinical history, anamnesis, and findings of the physical examination.

Transparent communication with the owner is essential to avoid unfulfilled expectations, and to clarify that sedation and anesthesia are never exempt from risks, regardless of the quality of perioperative care. As a consequence, written consent for anesthesia and clinical procedures should be obtained from the bird's owner on admission.

Although emergency procedures cannot be indefinitely delayed, preanesthetic stabilization of the patient's condition is expected to improve the outcome. Nonemergency procedures should not be scheduled out-of-hours, because of the increased perianesthetic risk associated with limited staff availability and/or fatigue.[1,6] Medical training of the bird (eg, tolerance to manual restraint, blood sampling, accepting oral medications) is extremely useful for any medical procedure.[7] If the bird is being treated with medications, the owner should be instructed to either administer them as usual or withdraw them on the day of admission.

Patient Preparation

Obtaining an accurate body weight of the patient on the day of anesthesia is paramount to ensure correct drug dosing. Fasting recommendations depend on the species, age, and clinical condition of the bird. Preanesthetic food withdrawal is recommended because it reduces the risk of perioperative regurgitation and passive reflux; however, prolonged fasting predisposes young and small sized birds to hypoglycemia. If excessive fluid is palpated in the crop, active suction is recommended before premedication. When long anesthetics events are expected (eg, complicated orthopedic procedures), the authors prefer to hospitalize the bird the night before the procedure to stabilize it and provide preemptive analgesia, where applicable. A brief anesthetic procedure may be planned to place an IV or intraosseous (IO) catheter and to prepare the surgical site (eg, plucking feathers), so the duration of the future anesthetic event is reduced. In some bird species, pulling of the feathers results in more intense nociception than a skin incision, because of the clustering of nociceptors and mechanoreceptors around the feather follicles.[8]

Equipment Preparation

Medical equipment (eg, anesthetic machine, oxygen supply, breathing circuit, endotracheal tubes [ETTs], face masks, and monitoring devices) should be routinely checked to ensure proper function (**Fig. 3**). Because of the small size of parrots, nonrebreathing circuits, such as lightweight T-pieces, are preferred to reduce resistance to air flow and minimize dead space, and therefore rebreathing of carbon dioxide (CO_2). For most nonrebreathing systems, the minimum gas flow rate is calculated as three multiples of minute ventilation (tidal volume × respiration rate). Correct setting and functioning of the scavenging system should be verified to minimize personnel exposure to anesthetic gases. The exposure of fractured pneumatic bones, which are part of the respiratory system, results in unavoidable leakage of inhalational anesthetic agents, if used.

Drug Selection and Timing of Administration

Common routes of drug administration in psittacines include intramuscular (IM), subcutaneous, intracelomic, IV, IO, intranasal, oral, and cloacal. When IV catheterization is not possible, an IO catheter may be used instead. Drug dilution is commonly used to facilitate administration of correct dosages to small birds. The use of preanesthetic medications may facilitate handling, provide muscle relaxation and anxiolysis, enhance analgesia, and reduce inhalational anesthetic requirements. Parasympatholytic agents (eg, atropine, glycopyrrolate) reduce the amount of salivary and bronchial secretions but can increase their viscosity; therefore, the authors reserve their use for the treatment of bradyarrhythmias.

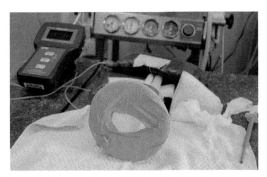

Fig. 3. Capnograph (*left*), face mask (*middle*), Cole ETT (*right*), and anesthetic machine (*background*).

Benzodiazepines and α_2-adrenoreceptor agonists provide sedation and reduce the general anesthetic requirement for induction and maintenance. Some medications (eg, anti-inflammatories, antimicrobials, calcium) may be administered before arrival to the hospital by correctly instructed owners. The authors only consider administration of low-dose anxiolytics (eg, benzodiazepines) by the owner to reduce transport-associated stress in extremely fearful individuals. Prescription of these drugs may be under the supervision of regulatory agencies and should only be provided to clients with a previously established veterinary-patient-client relationship. Deep sedation requires monitoring of physiologic variables, supportive care, and oxygen supplementation, which can only be provided in the hospital setting. Moreover, potential disadvantages of at-home premedication are inaccurate dosing and failure to administer the drug. Sedative agents commonly used in psittacine species are listed in **Table 1**.

The expression "multimodal analgesia" refers to the combined use of different classes of analgesics, with the aim of decreasing its doses and side effects and improving nociception/pain relief by interrupting nociceptive pathways at various levels of transmission. Extensive review of analgesic techniques suitable for parrot species is beyond the scope of this work. However, perioperative analgesia should be optimized through a multimodal approach to improve patient comfort and prevent the detrimental effects of nociception and pain, such as tachycardia, hypertension, reduced gastrointestinal motility, delayed wound healing, plastic changes of nociceptive pathways, and behavioral alterations. Moreover, opioid analgesics can act synergistically with other classes of drugs to potentiate their sedative effect, which is desirable in premedication. For example, in cockatiels (*Nymphicus hollandicus*), the combination of midazolam with butorphanol resulted in deeper sedation than midazolam alone, in restrained and unrestrained birds.[15] For additional information on analgesic drug dosages and combinations, the authors recommend consulting other publications.[18–21]

Resuscitation and emergency drug dosages should be calculated before anesthetic induction to reduce reaction time in case of emergency.

ANESTHETIC INDUCTION

Although literature specific for psittacine species is not currently available, preoxygenation is recommended in every critical patient, especially those with respiratory distress, diagnosed respiratory disease, or air sac compression secondary to intracelomic organomegaly or ascites. In psittacines, oxygen is supplemented via face mask, directing the oxygen flow toward the nostrils, or placing the bird in an induction chamber prefilled with oxygen (**Fig. 4**).

The dose of induction agents depends on the level of sedation achieved with premedication, if it was administered. Therefore, injectable anesthetics should be titrated to effect. A study in quaker parrots (*Myiopsitta monachus*) revealed that 1 mg/kg of midazolam IM combined with 10 mg/kg of alfaxalone IM reduced induction time, but caused prolonged recovery, when compared with the same dose of alfaxalone IM alone.[22] Commonly used injectable anesthetics in psittacine species are listed in **Table 2**.

Inhalational anesthesia is commonly used for induction in avian practice. Isoflurane is traditionally preferred for this purpose; however, sevoflurane and desflurane, although they require a specific vaporizer and are more expensive than isoflurane, are becoming increasingly popular in avian practice.

ESTABLISHMENT OF A PATENT AIRWAY

Regardless of the choice of the anesthetic technique, a patent airway should be established and maintained until recovery. Oxygen, with or without anesthetic gas, is

Table 1
Sedative agents commonly used in psittacine species

Pharmacologic Class	Advantages	Disadvantages	Studies in Psittacines
Benzodiazepines	Minimal cardiorespiratory effects Muscle relaxation Anticonvulsant Reversible with flumazenil Can be administered IN	Lack of analgesic effects Potential dysphoria Diazepam is not suitable IM Avoid if hepatic failure	Hispaniolan Amazon parrots (*Amazona ventralis*) Midazolam (2.0 mg/kg IN). Sedation within 3 min and lasted 15 min. Reduced response to restraint, moderate bradypnea. RecoveBred within 10 min of flumazenil (0.05 mg/kg IN).[9] Blue-fronted and vinaceous-breasted Amazon parrots (*Amazona aestiva* and *Amazona vinacea*) Midazolam (1 mg/kg IN) and ketamine (15 mg/kg IN). Good sedation. IM provoked a slower onset and longer duration.[10] Midazolam (2 mg/kg IN). Sedation with short latency time and fast recovery.[11] Budgerigars (*Melopsittacus undulatus*) Midazolam (13.2 mg/kg ± 1.3 mg/kg IN). Sedation with a more rapid onset and shorter duration (72 min) than diazepam (13.6 ± 1.1 mg/kg IN).[12] Butorphanol (2.5 mg/kg IM) and midazolam (1.25 mg/kg IM). Longer and less consistent sedation than alfaxalone (15 mg/kg IM).[13] Ring-necked parakeets (*Psittacula krameri*)

(continued on next page)

Table 1
(continued)

Pharmacologic Class	Advantages	Disadvantages	Studies in Psittacines
			Midazolam (7.3 mg/kg IN), and combinations of midazolam (3.65 mg/kg IN) and xylazine (10 mg/kg IN) with ketamine (40–50 mg/kg IN). Sedation. Flumazenil (0.13 mg/kg IN) speed recovery.[14] Cockatiels (*Nymphicus hollandicus*) Midazolam (3 mg/kg) and midazolam-butorphanol (3 mg/kg for each drug) IN. Rapid onset of sedation. Midazolam-butorphanol resulted in deeper sedation than midazolam alone.[15] Quaker parrots (*Myiopsitta monachus*) Midazolam (1–2 mg/kg IM). Significant isoflurane-sparing effect in response to a noxious stimulus without observable adverse effects.[16]
α_2-Adrenoreceptor-agonists	Sedative properties Dose-dependent analgesic effect (synergistic effect with opioids) Can be antagonized (atipamezole or yohimbine) Can be administered IN	Dose-dependent cardiorespiratory depression	Amazon parrots (*Amazona* spp) Medetomidine (0.08–2.0 mg/kg IM). Inadequate sedation for handling, and moderate bradypnea and bradycardia.[17] Budgerigars Xylazine (25.6 ± 2.2 mg/kg mg/kg IN). Prolonged sedation when compared with midazolam or diazepam, and insufficient restraint for minor clinical procedures.[12] Ring-necked parrots

Detomidine (12 mg/kg IN), and a combination of xylazine (10 mg/kg IN) with ketamine (40–50 mg/kg IN). Sedation. Prolonged dorsal recumbency with detomidine than with midazolam. Atipamezole (6 mg/kg IN) and yohimbine (12 mg/kg IN) decreased the duration of sedation with detomidine and xylazine, respectively.[14]

Abbreviation: IN, intranasal.

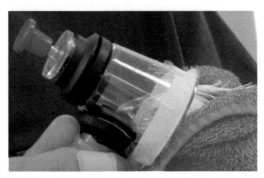

Fig. 4. Anesthetic induction with inhalational gas anesthesia delivered via face mask in a cockatiel (*Nymphicus hollandicus*).

delivered via a face mask, an ETT, or an air sac tube. Face masks of different sizes and materials are commercially available or are customized from commonly available materials (eg, plastic bottles).

Endotracheal intubation ensures surgical access to the head, minimizes the risk of aspiration, allows assisted ventilation, and reduces dead space when compared with face masks. However, it also carries a risk of iatrogenic tracheal damage, such as tracheal stenosis. Avian upper airways include a glottis at the base of the tongue and a trachea with complete cartilaginous rings, which is wider and more mobile compared with mammals of similar body weight. The glottal opening is wider than the distal trachea; this should be considered when selecting the size of the ETT. Craniocaudal narrowing of the tracheal lumen in especially marked in macaws. Endotracheal intubation in psittacines is straightforward (**Fig. 5**). The strong muscular tongue allows for gentle traction and manipulation with blunt forceps during intubation. Noncuffed tubes are preferred because of the complete tracheal rings. In macaws, the use of tubes with a craniocaudal narrowing, such as the pediatric Cole ETT, are recommended. If these are unavailable, an ETT with a diameter smaller than the glottal opening must be used to avoid damaging the trachea. One study investigating risk factors for tracheal strictures in birds revealed that tracheal obstruction occurred in 1.8% of intubated birds and carried a 70% mortality rate. Despite the overrepresentation of parrots in this study, no postintubation tracheal obstructions were identified in psittacines.[24] Local anesthetic sprays (eg, lidocaine) are applied over the glottis before intubation, although they are not strictly necessary.

After intubation, the tube is secured to the rhinotheca, gnathotheca, both, or to other parts of the head. Additional precautions may be necessary to prevent tube damage by the beak. The use of pediatric heat and moisture exchangers with an integrated port for capnography reduces dead space. During repositioning, the ETT should be disconnected from the breathing system to prevent tracheal damage.

Air sac perfusion anesthesia is recommended in cases of tracheal obstruction, requirement of full surgical access to the head, or respiratory arrest in those individuals in which endotracheal intubation is not possible. It is performed through cannulation, with an appropriately sized cannula or customized ETT, of the air sacs, and is usually placed in the caudal thoracic air sacs, of which the left is larger (**Fig. 6**). Cannulation of the abdominal air sac is also possible, although less common. Clavicular air sac intubation was ineffective in providing ventilation or maintaining isoflurane anesthesia in greater sulfur-crested cockatoos (*Cacatua galerita galerita*).[25]

Table 2
Injectable anesthetics commonly used in psittacine species

Pharmacologic Class	Advantages	Disadvantages	Examples of Studies in Psittacines
Cyclodextrin Alfaxalone	Short-acting IV and IM	Muscle tremors and hyperexcitation in quakers[22] Not reversible	Budgerigars 15 mg/kg IM. Sedation. More consistent and shorter duration than butorphanol-midazolam (2.5 mg/kg IM and 1.25 mg/kg IM, respectively).[13] Quaker parrots 10 mg/kg IM. Prolonged induction and decreased recovery time when compared with 25 mg/kg IM.[22] 10 mg/kg combined with 1 mg/kg of midazolam. Reduced induction time but prolonged the recovery time when compared with alfaxalone alone.[22]
Dissociative anesthetics Ketamine	Immobilization Spinal analgesia (on NMDA receptors in the spinal cord) Short-acting IV or IM	Poor muscle relaxation Increased sympathetic tone, with associated increase in arterial blood pressure[8] Direct depressant effect on the myocardium[8] Not reversible	Ring-necked parakeets (*Psittacula krameri*) Ketamine (40–50 mg/kg IN) combined with midazolam (7.3 mg/kg IN) or with combinations of midazolam (3.65 mg/kg IN) and xylazine (10 mg/kg IN). Sedation. Flumazenil (0.13 mg/kg IN) speeds recovery from midazolam.[14]
Propofol	Short acting anesthetic Only IV	Not analgesic Not suitable IM Severe respiratory depression and hypotension Potential agitated recoveries Not reversible	Hispaniolan Amazon parrots (*Amazona ventralis*) 5 mg/kg IV for induction, then CRI (1 mg/kg per min IV). Similar induction times but more respiratory depression (bradypnea, hypercapnia, hypoxemia), prolonged recovery times, and more agitated recoveries than isoflurane. CRI produced only light anesthesia in most birds.[23]

Abbreviations: CRI, continuous rate infusion; IN, intranasal; NMDA; N-methyl-D-aspartate.

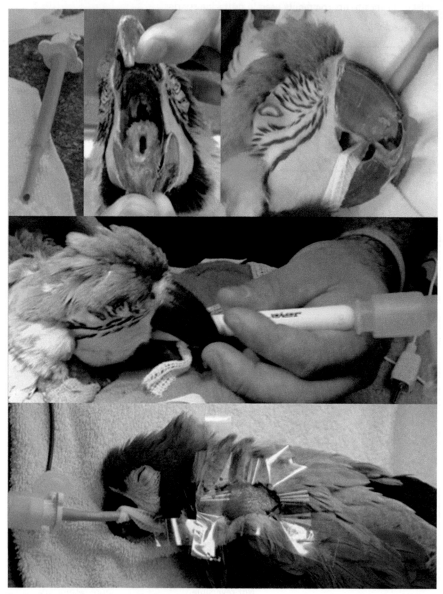

Fig. 5. Composition of images showing ETT intubation in a blue and gold macaw (*Ara ararauna*) and a red-shouldered macaw (*Diopsittaca nobilis*). Note Cole ETTs were used because of their marked craniocaudal narrowing of the tracheal lumen.

Air sac intubation for nonemergency procedures is not recommended in parrots with air sac diseases, severe obesity, ascites, or intracelomic organomegaly. The tube diameter should be similar to the tracheal width, and the recommended length is one-third of the celomic cavity width or less, to avoid damaging intracelomic structures. The anesthetized bird is placed in right lateral recumbency, the skin over the last left ribs at the chondrocostal junction level is aseptically prepared, and a skin

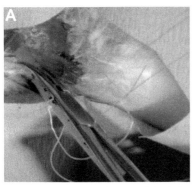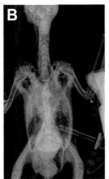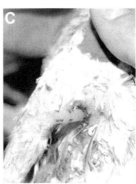

Fig. 6. (A) Air sac intubation of the left caudal thoracic air sac in a Congo African gray parrot (*Psittacus erithacus*). (B) Radiograph confirming correct air sac tube placement. Note the microsidestream probe of the capnograph is connected to the air sac tube. (C) Appearance of the air sac tube after anesthetic recovery.

incision the size of the diameter of the tube is made cranial or caudal to the last rib. The celomic wall is bluntly perforated, the tube is introduced cranially, sutured to the surrounding rib, and secured to the skin with a finger trap suture technique. In cases of tracheal obstruction, the gas flow should be reduced to 0.3 L/min because bypassing the trachea significantly reduces the airways' volume and capacity. Contrarily, if the upper respiratory tract is fully functional, fresh gas flows should be higher because the trachea increases dead space and allows ventilation of respiratory gases. Potential adverse effects of air sac cannulation include subcutaneous emphysema, obstruction, and contamination. Before extubation the sutures should be removed and the muscle and skin layers sutured, although the stoma can be left open to heal by secondary intention.

MAINTENANCE

Anesthesia is maintained using either inhalational or IV techniques, or a combination of both. Inhalational anesthesia is the preferred technique for maintenance, because of greater safety and more rapid recoveries compared with other methods. However, there is limited research on the use of partial and total IV anesthesia in psittacines.

The minimum anesthetic concentration (MAC) is the concentration of inhalational agent required to prevent purposeful movement in response to supramaximal noxious stimulation in 50% of the study subjects. The MAC is agent- and species-dependent; values reported for isoflurane were 1.07% in thick-billed parrots (*Rhynchopsitta pachyrhyncha*); 1.44% in greater sulfur-crested, citron-crested (*Cacatua sulphurea citrinocristata*), and lesser sulfur-crested (*Cacatua sulphurea sulphurea*) cockatoos; and 2.52% in quaker parrots.[16,26,27] One study reported that, in thick-billed parrots, sevoflurane MAC varied depending on the nociceptive model, and was 2.35% when using toe-clamp, but increased to 4.24% with electrical stimulation.[28]

Hypotension during isoflurane anesthesia has been reported in Hispaniolan Amazon parrots (*Amazona ventralis*).[29] Sevoflurane and isoflurane produce similar dose-dependent cardiovascular and respiratory effects, namely hypotension resulting from peripheral vasodilation and myocardial depression, and respiratory depression leading to hypercapnia and potential hypoxemia.[8] Halothane is no longer licensed in most developed countries, and not recommended for avian species because of its side effects.[30]

Premedication can help reduce the inhalational agent's MAC. In blue-fronted Amazon parrots (*Amazona aestiva*), ketamine (10 mg/kg IM), administered alone or in combination with diazepam (0.5 mg/kg IM), decreased the sevoflurane MAC from 2.4% to 1.7% and 1.3%, respectively, and resulted in decreased perianesthetic stress and hypotension when compared with the use of sevoflurane alone.[31] In cockatoos (*Cacatua* spp), butorphanol (1 mg/kg IM) decreased the isoflurane MAC by 25%.[26] Preoperative butorphanol (2 mg/kg IM) did not affect cardiopulmonary parameters in Hispaniolan Amazon parrots anesthetized with sevoflurane.[32] Fentanyl (20 μg/kg IV) significantly reduced isoflurane MAC in healthy Hispaniolan Amazon parrots, but also decreased heart rate (HR) and blood pressure (BP).[33]

IV anesthetics are administered intermittently as boluses or as continuous rate infusions (CRIs). In Hispaniolan Amazon parrots, fentanyl CRIs at 113.4 μg/kg/h, 217.8 μg/kg/h, and 409.8 μg/kg/h after an initial bolus of 20 μg/kg resulted in a reduction in the MAC of isoflurane by 31%, 36%, and 54%, respectively.[33] Also in this species, butorphanol CRI at 75 μg/kg/h after an initial IV bolus of 3 mg/kg resulted in a reduction in the MAC of isoflurane.[34] Lidocaine CRIs at 50 to 100 μg/kg/min have been anecdotally suggested in psittacines (João Brandão, personal communication, 2020); however, MAC-sparing effects and antinociception were not investigated.[35] In Hispaniolan Amazon parrots, propofol CRI at 1 mg/kg/min after a loading dose of 5 mg/kg resulted in significant hypoventilation.[23]

MONITORING

Clinical and instrumental monitoring are useful in psittacines (**Fig. 7**). Regardless of the monitoring technique selected, the small size of many psittacine species limits an easy approach to the patient during surgery. As a result, monitoring devices that allow remote control are preferred. For similar reasons, using transparent surgical drapes facilitates visual assessment of breathing and confirmation of correct placement of monitoring equipment from a distance (**Fig. 8**).

Anesthetic depth is assessed using basic reflexes and responses, such as muscular and cloacal tone, pupil responsiveness, toe pinch, autonomic responses to nociception, such as feather plucking, and palpebral and corneal reflexes (**Fig. 9**). Five stages of avian anesthesia have been described, ranging from light (I) to deep (V), based on reflexes, presence/absence of voluntary movements, responses to postural changes, and breathing pattern.[36] A surgical plane of anesthesia is characterized by a slow corneal reflex, muscle relaxation, lack of purposeful movement, and maintained cloacal tone. Sudden feather erection under anesthesia may indicate cardiac arrest rather than decreased anesthetic depth.[8]

Cardiovascular function is assessed by continuous monitoring of HR and rhythm, intermittent BP measurement, evaluation of capillary refill time, and peripheral pulse palpation. Pulsatile flow detection by placement of a Doppler probe over a peripheral artery is another way of assessing pulse. Esophageal stethoscopes allow HR monitoring with minimal external physical contact with the bird.

Normal ranges for systolic BP in conscious and anesthetized psittacines are 90 to 180 mm Hg and 90 to 150 mm Hg, respectively.[37] BP is measured either directly or indirectly. Direct measurement requires an arterial catheter, usually within the ulnar or metatarsal arteries, connected to a pressure transducer through a noncompliant tubing system filled with heparinized saline. This method is regarded as reliable in birds; nevertheless, its major limitation in psittacines is the small size of the arterial catheter suitable for most species, which leads to technical issues and affects reliability. Contrarily, reliability and accuracy of indirect BP measurements obtained

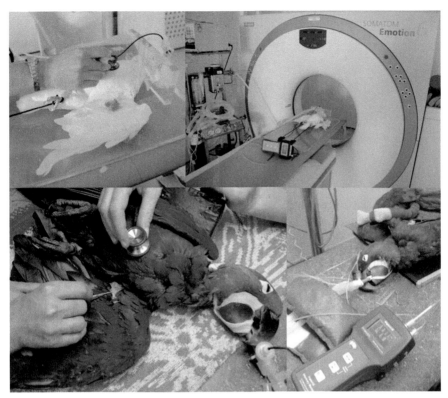

Fig. 7. Hands on and remote anesthetic monitoring in a white cockatoo (*Cacatua alba)* and a hyacinth macaw (*Anodorhynchus hyacinthinus*).

with oscillometry and Doppler in psittacines are debatable.[38] In a study conducted on Hispaniolan Amazon parrots, poor agreement was found between systolic arterial pressure values measured invasively and with Doppler; moreover, attempts to obtain oscillometric BP readings were unsuccessful.[39]

Electrocardiography allows monitoring the HR and heart rhythm. Modules that allow setting of filters and speed may be preferred in small parrots, because of the small size

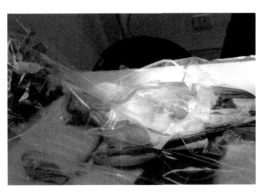

Fig. 8. The use of clear drapes allows visual control of respiration and correct monitoring equipment placement from distance in a galah (*Eolophus roseicapilla*) during a surgical procedure.

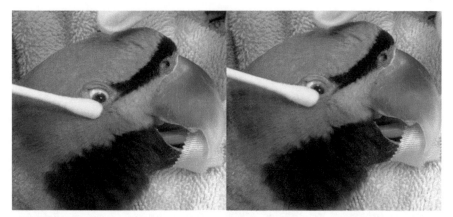

Fig. 9. Corneal reflex in a Derbyan parakeet (*Psittacula derbiana*). The gentle touch of the cornea with a moist cotton bud should induce the prolapse of the third eyelid. The lack of this reflex may indicate too deep of an anesthetic plane or excessive stimulation of the cornea. To differentiate these options, the contralateral corneal reflex must be assessed.

of the deflections to be detected. Alligator clips should not be attached directly to parrots with delicate skin; instead, they should be connected to the end of small-gauge hypodermic needles previously passed through the skin and subcutaneous layer. Alternatively, adhesive electrocardiogram patches or button electrodes are attached to the skin after feather plucking.

Assessment of the respiratory function relies on continuous monitoring of respiratory rate and, with some limitations, of $ETCO_2$. Capnography is a noninvasive monitoring technique that relies on the continuous measurement of end-tidal partial pressure of carbon dioxide ($PETCO_2$) which, in mammals, reflects the $Paco_2$. In birds, gas exchange occurs in fixed parabronchi that use a cross-current system for oxygen uptake and CO_2 release, which often results in a $PETCO_2$ higher than the $Paco_2$. In Timneh African gray parrots, a significant correlation was found between $PETCO_2$ and $Paco_2$; however, $Paco_2$ was consistently overestimated by approximately 5 mm Hg.[40] With this limitation in mind, capnography is used in psittacines as a complementary tool to assess ventilation (**Fig. 10**). The use of microstream capnography, a type of sidestream technology, which allows sampling of very low gas flows (eg, up to 50 mL/min), is recommended in avian species because of their small size.

The use of pulse oximetry in psittacines remains controversial. Current literature shows that, whereas pulse frequency (as detected by commercially available pulse oximeters) and HR correlated well, the agreement between arterial oxygen saturation readings and values derived from blood gas analyzers was poor.[8,41]

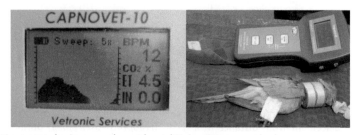

Fig. 10. Capnography in a monk parakeet (*Myiopsitta monachus*).

The use of arterial blood gases measurement and clinical chemistry analysis has gained popularity since affordable portable analyzers (eg, I-Stat [Abbott Laboratories, Abbott Park, IL] or EPOC [Integrated Medcraft, Colchester, CT]) requiring small blood volumes became commercially available. Arterial blood gas analyses may be a complementary tool to assess breathing function, especially in case of respiratory impairment.

Finally, body temperature should be measured before, during, and after anesthesia. Cloacal temperature is measured easily, although it may not represent a reliable estimation of core temperature. Alternative methods include infrared and esophageal thermometry.

SUPPORTIVE CARE

Providing supportive care during anesthesia is essential to maintain adequate respiratory and cardiovascular function, and to prevent/treat hypothermia. Hypoxemia is addressed with oxygen supplementation and intermittent positive pressure ventilation (IPPV), either manual or mechanical. This is especially important in patients with impaired respiratory function (eg, respiratory disease and air sac compression secondary to obesity, intracelomic organomegaly, or ascites). Airway pressure should be carefully monitored during IPPV to avoid iatrogenic barotrauma. It is challenging to provide evidence-based recommendations for IPPV in psittacines. One study reported the use of pressures of 4 cm H_2O in sulfur-crested cockatoos.[42] Mechanical ventilators developed to deliver small tidal volumes and low pressures are commercially available (eg, SAV04 Small Animal Ventilator, Vetronic Services Ltd, Newton Abbot, UK). A study in pigeons revealed that IPPV by means of a pressure-limited mode was not associated with adverse cardiopulmonary effects; however, respiratory alkalemia and cardiovascular depression may occur when air sac integrity is disrupted because the ventilator cannot reach the peak inspiratory pressure and therefore delivers gas constantly.[43]

To maintain adequate BP and organ perfusion, perianesthetic fluid administration is recommended. Fluids are administered as boluses or as CRI. Although rate and mode varies, rates of 5 to 10 mL/kg/h are routinely used for most birds. Fluids must be prewarmed to avoid causing, or worsening, of hypothermia. IV or IO catheterization is mandatory for whole blood, blood derivates, and colloids, and preferred to subcutaneous or intracelomic routes to allow for more efficient crystalloid absorption.

Because of the high metabolic rate of psittacines, which is inversely proportional to size, it is recommended to adopt measures to prevent and treat perianesthetic hypothermia. Thermal losses may be reduced by means of external insulation (eg, bubble wrap, thermal blankets), whereas thermal support may be provided via systems that rely on direct contact with the bird (eg, circulating warm-water/air blankets, such as HotDog [Augustine Surgical Inc, Eden Prairie, MN] or Bair Hugger [3M, Maplewood, MN] system), and remote heating systems (eg, heat lamps, hot pads placed over the breathing circuit to prewarm the inspiratory gases). In ringed turtle-doves (*Streptopelia risoria*) anesthetized with isoflurane, 680-W radiant heat sources placed above the birds were more effective in maintaining core temperature than circulating 40°C warm-water blankets and gas warmer-humidifiers inserted between the vaporizer and the breathing system.[44] However, circulating water blankets decreased heat loss as effectively as 60-W infrared heat emitters in Hispaniolan Amazon parrots undergoing isoflurane anesthesia.[45] Forced-air warming devices are also regarded as effective heating tools. Regardless of the heating system used, precautions should be taken to prevent thermal injuries.

Regarding perianesthetic support, gastrointestinal function should also be considered because various sedative and anesthetic agents may have detrimental effects on the avian digestive system.[46] Midazolam, either alone or with butorphanol, significantly decreased gastrointestinal transit time and motility in cockatiels.[46] Contrarily, a preliminary study conducted in multiple species of psittacines revealed no significant differences in gastrointestinal transit times between birds manually restrained and birds anesthetized with isoflurane.[47]

ANESTHETIC COMPLICATIONS

Common perianesthetic complications in psittacines include hypotension, hypothermia, hypoglycemia, and arrhythmias. Hypotension is challenging to detect, because of the questionable reliability of noninvasive measuring techniques. However, if it is suspected or confirmed, suitable treatment options are adjustment of the anesthetic depth, IV/IO boluses of crystalloids (5–20 mL/kg) and/or colloids (1–5 mL/kg), anticholinergics in case of concomitant bradycardia (eg, atropine, glycopyrrolate), and sympathomimetics (eg, ephedrine). In Hispaniolan Amazon parrots, CRIs of dobutamine (at 5, 10, 15 µg/kg/min) and dopamine (at 5, 7, 10 µg/kg/min) were investigated, and their highest doses were found effective for treating isoflurane-induced hypotension. Second-degree atrioventricular blocks, however, were reported as a common complication of dobutamine infusion.[29] If hypotension persists despite treatment, other potential contributing factors, such as hypoglycemia, hypothermia, anemia, hypoproteinemia, and electrolyte imbalances, should be excluded.

Arrhythmias are detected through cardiac auscultation, preferably concomitant with peripheral pulse palpation and electrocardiography, and should be treated depending on its severity, its effect on hemodynamic stability, and its progression. In birds, arrhythmias are dramatically potentiated by catecholamine release associated with stress or pain, and may result in systolic and diastolic dysfunction, which may culminate in congestive heart failure and, ultimately, death.[48] Sinus tachycardia is often secondary to nociception; hypoxemia; hypercapnia; hypovolemia; and drug administration including alfaxalone, ketamine, atropine, and dopamine. Sinus respiratory arrhythmia, wandering pacemaker, occasional sinus arrest, and sinoatrial blocks are common in anesthetized birds secondary to increased vagal tone. Supraventricular and ventricular premature complexes, and first- and second-degree (Mobitz type 1) atrioventricular blocks, have been reported in apparently healthy parrots under anesthesia.[48,49] Second-degree atrioventricular block was also reported in a healthy Hispaniolan Amazon parrot anesthetized with isoflurane.[49]

Hypoglycemia can cause bradycardia and peripheral vasodilation, leading to hypotension and possible circulatory collapse.[8] Blood glucose levels lower than 150 mg/dL usually warrant medical intervention. The authors dilute 50% dextrose in a 1:1 ratio with lactated Ringer solution or 0.9% saline and administer slowly as an initial bolus of 2 mL/kg IV. Hypoglycemia that is nonresponsive to bolus treatment should be addressed with a 5% dextrose IV infusion until normoglycemia is maintained.

Hypothermia is a common perianesthetic complication in small birds, and it can result in delayed drug metabolism, cardiovascular dysfunction, impaired perfusion, respiratory compromise, cerebral depression, and increased incidence of wound infection.[50]

Tracheal or ETT blockage with mucus secretions may occur, especially in small birds. Airway obstruction may also result from bending of the ETT because of neck flexion, compression by the beak, and aspiration. The latter is more common in birds that were not fasted or positioned so the neck and head were not elevated in relation to the body. Besides complete obstruction and suffocation, aspiration may also cause long-term complications, such as pneumonia and air sacculitis. If esophageal content is detected either in the mouth or in the oral esophagus, it should be suctioned, the pharynx should be packed with swabs, and the head and neck should be elevated with respect to the crop and stomach. Even in the absence of aspiration, gastrointestinal reflux may cause postoperative esophagitis.

RECOVERY

Anesthetic recovery begins when the administration of anesthetics is discontinued, and extends to the moment when the bird is bright and shows normal cardiovascular, respiratory, and neurologic functions. Atipamezole and yohimbine are used to reverse the α_2-adrenoreceptor agonists. Naloxone and naltrexone are opioid antagonists, although opioid agonists/antagonists (eg, butorphanol) may be used to reverse the cardiorespiratory effects of pure opioid agonists. The bird should be extubated when active and vigorous swallowing is observed; at extubation, the distal end of the ETT should be visually inspected for blood or mucus.

The recovery cage should be padded and located in a quiet area of the hospital that is free of predators, excessive noise, and in dim light conditions. Food and water bowls and hard toys should be temporarily removed from the cage to prevent accidental injuries. Thermal support and oxygen supplementation should be continued if needed. Frequent monitoring of physiologic variables is recommended until the bird is alert, normothermic, and ambulatory. Blood glucose must be monitored at regular intervals in patients at a high risk of developing hypoglycemia. To date, pain scores specific for psittacines have not yet been developed; nevertheless, pain should be anticipated and treated preventively after invasive procedures.

The owners should be promptly informed about any perianesthetic complications, including those occurring during recovery. Verbal or, preferably, written discharge instructions detailing what to expect and what to monitor should be given to the owner. Long-term anesthetic-related complications can still occur after discharge from the hospital. For example, traumatic injury of the tracheal mucosa during intubation can cause voice changes or tracheal, and result in tracheal stenosis weeks after the anesthetic.

Finally, data collected from every sedation/anesthetic procedure should be recorded. Performing postanesthetic briefings and morbidity/mortality reports are useful in identifying unexpected complications and improving management of future anesthetic events.

SUMMARY

The anatomic and physiologic characteristics of some species of psittacines limit or impair the anesthetist's capacity to accurately deliver and/or monitor anesthesia. This, combined with the limited amount of scientific studies available when compared with small animal anesthesia, explains, at least to some extent, why the risk of anesthetic-related death in psittacines remains higher than in small animals. Nevertheless, the integration of technological advances and an increasing evidence-based knowledge in psittacine sedation and anesthesia contributes to improve the safety of these procedures. It is the responsibility of the avian anesthetist to remain updated and develop their skills, when possible, in this important field of psittacine medicine.

REFERENCES

1. Brodbelt DC, Pfeiffer DU, Young LE, et al. Results of the confidential enquiry into perioperative small animal fatalities regarding risk factors for anesthetic-related death in dogs. J Am Vet Med Assoc 2008;233:1096–104.
2. Brodbelt D. Perioperative mortality in small animal anesthesia. Vet J 2009;182: 152–61.
3. Clarke KW, Hall LW. A survey of anaesthesia in small animal practice: AV A/BSAVA report. Vet Anaesth Analg 1990;17:4–10.
4. Seamon AB, Hofmeister EH, Divers SJ. Outcome following inhalation anesthesia in birds at a veterinary referral hospital: 352 cases (2004–2014). J Am Vet Med Assoc 2017;251:814–7.
5. Matthews NS, Mohn TJ, Yang M, et al. Factors associated with anesthetic-related death in dogs and cats in primary care veterinary hospitals. J Am Vet Med Assoc 2017;250:655–66.
6. Brodbelt DC, Pfeiffer DU, Young LE, et al. Risk factors for anaesthetic related death in cats: results from the confidential enquiry into perioperative small animal fatalities (CEPSAF). Br J Anaesth 2007;99:617–23.
7. Van Zeeland YRA, Friedman SG, Bergman L. Chapter 5: behavior. In: Speer BL, editor. Current therapy in avian medicine and surgery. St. Louis, MO: Elsevier; 2016. p. 177–251.
8. Heard D. Chapter 19: anesthesia. In: Speer BL, editor. Current therapy in avian medicine and surgery. St. Louis, MO: Elsevier; 2016. p. 601–15.
9. Mans C, Guzman DS-M, Lahner LL, et al. Sedation and physiologic response to manual restraint after intranasal administration of midazolam in Hispaniolan Amazon parrots (*Amazona ventralis*). J Avian Med Surg 2012;26(3):130–9.
10. Bitencourt EH, Padilha VS, de Lima MPA, et al. Sedative effects of the association ketamine and midazolam administered intranasally or intramuscular in parrots (*Amazona aestiva* and *Amazona vinacea*). Pesq Vet Bras 2013;33:1125–9.
11. Schaffer DPH, De Araujo NLLC, Raposo ACS, et al. Sedative effects of intranasal midazolam administration in wild caught blue-fronted Amazon (*Amazona aestiva*) and orange-winged Amazon (*Amazona amazonica*) parrots. J Avian Med Surg 2017;31(3):213–8.
12. Sadegh AB. Comparison of intranasal administration of xylazine, diazepam, and midazolam in budgerigars (*Melopsittacus undulatus*): clinical evaluation. J Zoo Wildl Med 2013;44:241–4.
13. Escalante GC, Balko JA, Chinnadurai SK. Comparison of the sedative effects of alfaxalone and butorphanol-midazolam administered intramuscularly in budgerigars (*Melopsittacus undulatus*). J Avian Med Surg 2018;32(4):279–85.
14. Vesal N, Eskandari MH. Sedative effects of midazolam and xylazine with or without ketamine and detomidine alone following intranasal administration in ring-necked parakeets. J Am Vet Med Assoc 2006;228:383–8.
15. Doss GA, Fink D, Mans C. Assessment of sedation after intranasal administration of midazolam and midazolam-butorphanol in cockatiels (*Nymphicus hollandicus*). AJVR 2018;79(12):1246–52.
16. Zaheer OA, Sanchez A, Beaufrere H. Minimum anesthetic concentration of isoflurane and sparing effect of midazolam in quaker parrots (*Myiopsitta monachus*). Vet Anaesth Analg 2020;47:341–6.
17. Sandmeier P. Evaluation of medetomidine for short-term immobilization of domestic pigeons (*Columba livia*) and Amazon parrots (*Amazona* spp.). J Avian Med Surg 2000;14:8–14.

18. Balko JA, Chinnadurai SK. Advancements in evidence-based analgesia in exotic animals. Vet Clin Exot Anim Prac 2017;20(3):899–915.
19. Hawkins MG, Paul-Murphy J. Avian analgesia. Vet Clin North Am Exot Anim Pract 2011;14(1):61–80.
20. Sanchez-Migallon DG. Advances in avian clinical therapeutics. J Exot Pet Med 2014;23(1):6–20.
21. Hawkins MG, Sanchez-Migallon DG, Beaufrere H, et al. Chapter 5: birds. In: Carpenter JW. Exotics animal formulary. 5th edition. St. Louis, MO: Elsevier; 2018. p. 167–375.
22. Whitehead MC, Hoppes SM, Musser JMB, et al. The use of alfaxalone in quaker parrots (*Myiopsitta monachus*). J Avian Med Surg 2019;33(4):340–8.
23. Langlois I, Harvey RC, Jones MP, et al. Cardiopulmonary and anesthetic effects of isoflurane and propofol in Hispaniolan Amazon parrots (*Amazona ventralis*). J Avian Med Surg 2003;17:4–10.
24. Sykes JMIV, Neiffer D, Terrell S, et al. Review of 23 cases of postintubation tracheal obstructions in birds. J Zoo Wildl Med 2013;44(3):700–13.
25. Jaensch SM, Cullen L, Raidal SR. Comparison of endotracheal, caudal thoracic air sac, and clavicular air sac administration of isoflurane in sulphur-crested cockatoos (*Cacatua galerita*). J Avian Med Surg 2001;15:170–7.
26. Curro TG, Brunson DB, Paul-Murphy J. Determination of the ED50 of isoflurane and evaluation of the isoflurane-sparing effect of butorphanol in cockatoos (*Cacatua* spp). Vet Surg 1994;23:429–33.
27. Mercado JA, Larsen RS, Wack RF, et al. Minimum anesthetic concentration of isoflurane in captive thick-billed parrots (*Rhynchopsitta pachyrhyncha*). Am J Vet Res 2008;69(2):189–94.
28. Phair KA, Larsen RS, Wack RF, et al. Determination of the minimum anesthetic concentration of sevoflurane in thick-billed parrots (*Rhynchopsitta pachyrhyncha*). Am J Vet Res 2012;73(9):1350–5.
29. Schnellbacher RW, da Cunha AF, Beaufrere H, et al. Effects of dopamine and dobutamine on isoflurane-induced hypotension in Hispaniolan Amazon parrots (*Amazona ventralis*). Am J Vet Res 2012;73(7):952–8.
30. Jaensch SM, Cullen L, Raidal SR. Comparative cardiopulmonary effects of halothane and isoflurane in galahs (*Eolophus roseicapillus*). J Avian Med Surg 1999; 13(1):15–22.
31. Paula VV, Otsuki DA, Auler JOC, et al. The effect of premedication with ketamine, alone or with diazepam, on anaesthesia with sevoflurane in parrots (*Amazona aestiva*). BMC Vet Res 2013;9:142–51.
32. Klaphake E, Schumacher J, Greenacre C, et al. Comparative anesthetic and cardiopulmonary effects of pre versus postoperative butorphanol administration in Hispaniolan Amazon parrots (*Amazona ventralis*) anesthetized with sevoflurane. J Avian Med Surg 2006;20:2–7.
33. Hawkins MG, Pascoe PJ, DiMaio Knych HK, et al. Effects of three fentanyl plasma concentrations on the minimum alveolar concentration of isoflurane in Hispaniolan Amazon parrots (*Amazona ventralis*). Am J Vet Res 2018;79:600–5.
34. Litchenberger M, Lennox A, Chavez W, et al. The use of butorphanol constant rate infusion in psittacines. Proc Annu Conf Assoc 2009;73.
35. Schnellbacher R, Comolli J. Constant rate infusions in exotic animals. J Exot Pet Med 2020;35:24pp.
36. Lierz M, Korbel R. Anesthesia and analgesia in birds. J Exot Pet Med 2012;21: 44–58.

37. Lichtenberger M. Determination of indirect blood pressure in the companion bird. Sem Avian Exot Pet 2005;14:149–52.
38. Johnston MS, Davidowsky LA, Rao S, et al. Precision of repeated, Doppler-derived indirect blood pressure measurements in conscious psittacine birds. J Avian Med Surg 2011;25(2):83–90.
39. Acierno MJ, da Cunha A, Smith J, et al. Agreement between direct and indirect blood pressure measurements obtained from anesthetized Hispaniolan Amazon parrots. J Am Vet Med Assoc 2008;233(10):1587–90.
40. Edling TM, Degernes LA, Flammer K, et al. Capnographic monitoring of anesthetized African grey parrots receiving intermittent positive pressure ventilation. J Am Vet Med Assoc 2001;219(12):1714–8.
41. Schmitt PM, Göbel T, Trautvetter E. Evaluation of pulse oximetry as a monitoring method in avian anesthesia. J Avian Med Surg 1988;12:91–9.
42. Chemonges S. Effect of intermittent positive pressure ventilation on depth of anaesthesia during and after isoflurane anaesthesia in sulphur-crested cockatoos (*Cacatua galerita galerita*). Vet Med Int 2014;2014:250523.
43. Touzot-Jourde G, Hernandez-Divers SJ, Trim CM. Cardiopulmonary effects of controlled versus spontaneous ventilation in pigeons anesthetized for coelioscopy. J Am Vet Med Assoc 2005;227:1424–8.
44. Phalen DN, Mitchell ME, Cavazos-Martinez ML. Evaluation of three heat sources for their ability to maintain core body temperature in the anesthetized patient. J Avian Med Surg 1996;10:174–8.
45. Rembert MS, Smith JA, Hosgood G, et al. Comparison of traditional thermal support devices with the forced-air warmer system in anesthetized Hispaniolan Amazon parrots (*Amazona ventralis*). J Avian Med Surg 2001;15:187–93.
46. Martel A, Mans C, Doss GA, et al. Effects of midazolam and midazolam-butorphanol on gastrointestinal transit time and motility in cockatiels (*Nymphicus hollandicus*). J Avian Med Surg 2018;32(4):286–93.
47. Lennox AM, Crosta L, Buerkle M. The effects of isoflurane anesthesia on gastrointestinal transit time. Proc Assoc Avian Vet 2002;53–5.
48. Fitzgerald BC, Beaufrere H. Chapter 6: cardiology. In: Speer BL, editor. Current therapy in avian medicine and surgery. St. Louis, MO: Elsevier; 2016. p. 252–328.
49. Rembert MS, Smith JA, Strickland KN, et al. Intermittent bradyarrhythmia in a Hispaniolan Amazon parrot (*Amazona ventralis*). J Avian Med Surg 2008;22(1):31–40.
50. Haskins S. Monitoring anesthetized patients. In: Tranquilli WJ, Thurmon JC, Grim KG, editors. Lumb and Jones' veterinary anesthesia and analgesia. 4th edition. Ames, IA: Blackwell; 2007. p. 86–105.

Raptor Sedation and Anesthesia

Michelle G. Hawkins, VMD, DABVP (Avian)[a],*, Gregg M. Griffenhagen, DVM, MS, DACVAA[b]

KEYWORDS

• Anesthesia • Sedation • Raptor • Bird of prey

KEY POINTS

• Presedation and anesthetic considerations are essential for successful sedation and anesthesia of a bird of prey.

• Sedation is becoming increasingly popular in avian medicine and anesthesia has long been used in birds of prey for a wide variety of procedures, from obtaining well-positioned radiographs to orthopedic surgeries.

• Understanding the anatomy and physiology of birds of prey is essential for a successful anesthetic or sedative outcome.

• Knowledge on the required equipment for sedation and anesthesia, currently available drugs and drug combinations, as well as drug interactions, is essential for the practitioner.

• Recent advances in avian anesthesia and sedation continue to improve the health and welfare of raptor patients.

PRESEDATION AND ANESTHETIC CONSIDERATIONS

Allowing time for acclimation to new surroundings will reduce stress and unmask clinical disease, although this is not always possible with an acutely injured wild raptor. As many of these patients have not been, and will not ultimately be, held in captivity, many of them will never acclimatize to these artificial surroundings. A complete physical examination including respiratory, cardiac, renal, and hepatic function should be performed, and baseline values recorded for development of an American Society of Anesthesiologists status for the patient as well as for later comparison. A recent study showed that unhealthy avian patients were 19 times more likely to have a mortality event associated with general anesthesia, compared with healthy avian patients.[1]

The bird should first be examined in its hospital/transport cage or flight cage, paying particular attention to respiratory rate (RR) and effort. Record RR before physical

[a] Department of Medicine and Epidemiology and One Health Institute, School of Veterinary Medicine, University of California, Davis, One Shields Avenue Davis, CA 95616, USA;
[b] Department of Clinical Sciences, Colorado State University, Veterinary Teaching Hospital, 300 West Drake Road, Fort Collins, CO 80523, USA
* Corresponding author.
E-mail address: mghawkins@ucdavis.edu

Vet Clin Exot Anim 25 (2022) 135–161
https://doi.org/10.1016/j.cvex.2021.08.011
1094-9194/22/© 2021 Elsevier Inc. All rights reserved.

restraint for comparison with rates under anesthesia. Evaluate the quality of respiration by auscultating the air sacs ventrally and the lungs dorsally for harsh airway sounds or evidence of wheezing. Auscultate and palpate the trachea for abnormalities. Auscultate the heart for murmurs and record the heart rate (HR) for comparison during anesthesia. Pulse quality can be assessed in larger raptors at either the median ulnar or medial metatarsal arteries, evaluating for symmetry and strength. The body weight is recorded for calculating accurate fluid and medication dosages.

Hydration status is evaluated and recorded and dehydration corrected if possible, before anesthesia. Compensatory mechanisms are blunted under anesthesia, exacerbating underlying hypotension and poor peripheral perfusion. Subjective hydration assessment includes examination of the moistness of the cloacal and ocular mucous membranes, and the elasticity of the skin of the eyelids and over the keel. Sunken eyes and cool extremities also indicate dehydration. The venous refill time after digital compression of the median ulnar vein should be immediate; venous refill times of greater than 1 second have been suggested to correlate with greater than 7% dehydration (**Fig. 1** A, B).[2] The packed cell volume (PCV) will often be increased with dehydration. Even though uric acid is secreted through the tubules of the kidney, uric acid values may increase clinically with moderate-to-severe dehydration and will resolve with rehydration.

Ideally, a complete blood cell count and biochemical profile are performed before anesthesia. Any anemias should be characterized as either acute or chronic and regenerative or nonregenerative. Acute anemias are corrected before anesthesia as birds may not be able to compensate for lowered levels of oxygen delivery. Transfusion is indicated if the PCV is less than 15% to 20% and the total solids are less than 2.5 to 3.5 g/dL. If the blood loss is acute, the authors consider transfusion with higher PCVs. The type of surgery to be performed and potential for blood loss are assessed so a fluid plan can be prepared. The PCV may decrease 3% to 5% during anesthesia because of vascular hemodynamic changes associated with certain anesthetic drugs.

Although analgesia is not the focus of this article, appropriate medications should be considered before procedures that would be expected to produce discomfort. Generally, most raptor species should be fasted a minimum of 12 to 24 hours before

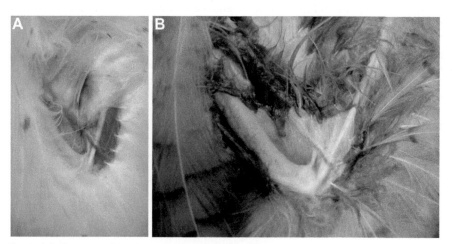

Fig. 1. (A) The most objective way to assess dehydration is evaluating venous refill time of the median ulnar or basilic vein. Filling time should be less than 1 second. (B) Dehydration is often visualized as a thread-like vessel, with a prolonged refill time.

induction, allowing time for passage of casts or pellets. Consideration should be given to performing anesthetic procedures earlier in the day in diurnal birds after an overnight fast. If a crop is present, palpate to be sure it is empty. Ideally, avian patients should be preoxygenated for roughly 5 minutes before induction.

Appropriate restraint is essential to minimize patient stress and time required for anesthetic induction. Stressed birds may die from physical restraint and this risk is magnified in sick or debilitated patients. Appropriate means of physical restraint must be assessed for each patient, and stabilization and supportive care prepared before handling. Nets are used to capture birds in larger enclosures or escapees. They should be sized appropriately for the patient to minimize iatrogenic trauma. Once netted, the bird is gently removed to avoid trauma to the wings, pelvic limbs, or toes. Leather gloves of appropriate size should be used for capture. Covering the head or placement of a hood calms many species of raptors, but care must be taken to ensure adequate airflow. Small species may be captured and controlled using leather garden gloves or a towel placed over them and subsequently grasping around the body to keep the wings from flapping and becoming damaged. Raptors greater than 0.5 kg that are in larger cages, flights, or held "on the glove" may be captured by grasping the legs and allowing them to hang upside down briefly. By reaching quickly under the patient with the palm facing down, the pelvic limbs are grasped between the thumb and index finger and the index and middle fingers. The raptor will fall off the perch and attempt to fly, and the hand is quickly inverted so that the palm is facing up like cupping water, the patient is hanging below the hand, and the feet are controlled. If the legs are jessed (either to the handler's arm or to a perch), the handler can gently "persuade" the bird to fall off of the arm or perch and hang by the jesses, at which point the feet are restrained as described earlier (**Fig. 2**A–D).

Regardless of the physical restraint technique used, care should be taken not to compromise coelomic cage movement or the ability of the anesthetist to monitor the patient. Movement with the bird in hand should be quiet and calm to reduce fright and stress. The capture is performed expeditiously to minimize stress. If a bird should escape and need to be recaptured or is unduly excited, delay anesthesia until the bird has calmed down.

Once the bird is in hand, a towel is initially placed over the dorsum, then wrapped around the wings to restrict flapping and prevent damage to the wings and feathers. If the patient is still hanging, they are righted and the head may be controlled by hooding, placing the towel over the face, or allowed the head to be free for examination (**Fig. 3**C, D). Once adequately restrained by the handler, birds are removed from the towel if possible to prevent hyperthermia that can occur after prolonged restraint. In smaller raptors, the head can be restrained using a "3-point" technique with the thumb and middle finger supporting the mandible and the index finger on top of the head (see **Fig. 3**B). Gentle extension of the bird's neck further limits head movement. Another option is to encircle the bird's neck with the handler's fingers for restraint (see **Fig. 3**A). A third technique places the thumb under the intermandibular space while the other fingers are placed over the top of the head. This is the authors' choice for maintaining full control of the head during restraint. The other hand is placed on the dorsum to secure the wings and legs.

Contrary to many other species of birds, the talons of most raptor species are their main offensive weapon, and as such must be quickly controlled for the safety of the staff and handlers. Their talons are generally long, sharp, and may harbor many types of bacteria found on and in their prey items. Their beaks are also large and sharp, but generally do not have the power that other species have (ie, psittacines). In the authors' experience, bald eagles (*Haliaeetus leucocephalus*), great horned owls (*Bubo*

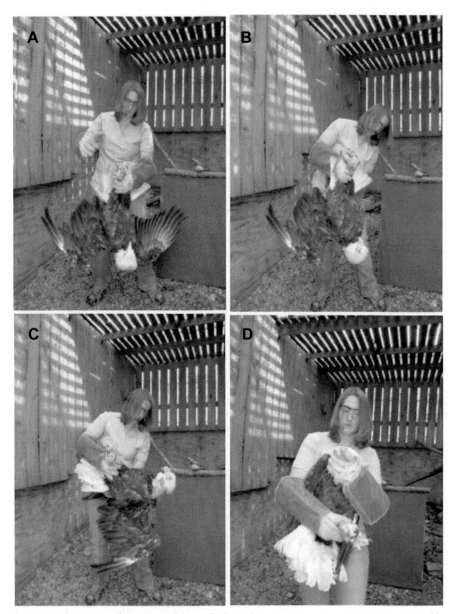

Fig. 2. Hand capture of a raptor within a flight or kennel. The raptor is initially captured by quickly grasping the legs and allowing the patient to hang upside down (*A*). The feet and legs are then secured appropriately in one hand (*B*) while the other hand and arm are used to gently restrain the wings (*C*) and right the bird into an appropriate position facing away from the handler (*D*). (*Courtesy of* Dr Miranda Sadar.)

virginianus), and raptors without talons (ie, vultures and condors) may bite when restrained. This is not to say that one should let down their guard around these dangerous birds, but rather the most dangerous weapon should be neutralized first for the safety of all.

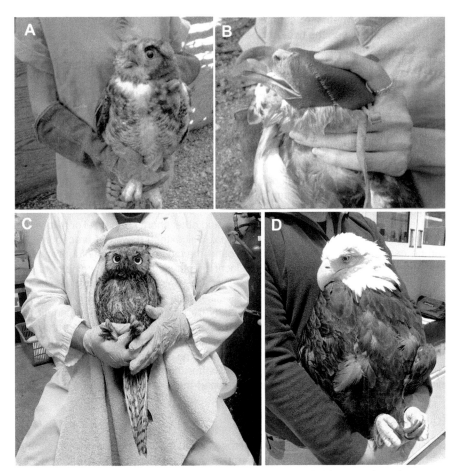

Fig. 3. Examples of raptor restraint. The head may be controlled by encircling the raptor's neck with one hand and gently extending the neck (*A*) or using a "3-point" technique with the thumb and middle finger supporting the mandible and the index finger on top of the head (*B*). Excessive movement of the legs and wings can be prevented by wrapping the raptor in a towel and covering the head (*C*) and using the handler's hands to control the feet and arms to keep the wings from extending (*C, D*). (*Courtesy of* Dr Miranda Sadar [*A, B*] and the Rocky Mountain Raptor Program [*C*].)

SEDATION

Sedation is often necessary for raptor species to safely handle both wild and captive birds. By providing sedation and anxiolysis, many minor, nonpainful procedures can be performed without undue stress for both patient and handler. In one study, evaluating the effects of manual restraint in budgerigars (*Melopsittacus undulatus*), even a short period of restraint for physical examination and blood collection caused a significant increase in plasma lactate concentrations as compared with patients that were sedated before handling[3]; another study in Passeriformes noted similar results.[4] Although these studies were not in raptor species, there is no reason to believe that they would be different, as this effect has been demonstrated in many mammalian species as well.

When deciding whether to sedate or anesthetize a patient, it is important to define the difference between the two. At one author's institution (GG), sedation is generally defined by the magnitude of the patient's response to handling and manipulation. Lightly sedated patients will allow manipulation and positioning with some resistance but will not react violently or with significant force. A heavily sedated patient will allow positioning in dorsal or lateral recumbency or taping without any resistance and will not react or move when no longer stimulated. A patient that can be intubated without resistance should be considered anesthetized and treated accordingly. It is also good to keep in mind that a short general anesthesia may be safer than heavy sedation for many patients, including those that are physiologically unstable or when cardiovascular health status is unknown.

Procedures for which sedation is appropriate include short imaging procedures (computed tomography, radiographs), bandage changes, minor wound care, physical examinations, blood collection, intravenous (IV) or intraosseous (IO) catheter placement (especially before general anesthesia), and other short, nonpainful or mildly painful procedures. The addition of local analgesia will extend the list of procedures that can be carried out to include surgical wound management and painful procedures where nociception can be blocked by a local anesthetic such as lidocaine or bupivacaine. Sedation should not be used for significantly painful procedures where manual restraint would also be necessary, such as initial large wound evaluation/treatment or fracture repair. In addition, more significantly debilitated patients may benefit from general anesthesia rather than sedation to closely monitor physiologic parameters and intervene if necessary (ie, mechanical ventilation, blood pressure support). Sedation is also not appropriate where the duration of the procedure would outlast the expected duration of the agents being used. Rather than redosing sedative drugs, the clinician should convert to general anesthesia at that point.

EQUIPMENT FOR SEDATION

Because of large interindividual and interspecies variability in the response to sedative agents, those that provide minimal sedation in one patient could result in general anesthesia in another. Subsequently, supplies and equipment should be available to convert to general anesthesia any time sedation is being administered. Equipment should include a selection of endotracheal tubes (ETTs) for intubation, Ambu bag, or other methods of mechanical ventilation, towels/blankets/drapes plus an external heat source to support body temperature, oxygen supplementation, and physiologic monitoring including electrocardiography (ECG), noninvasive blood pressure monitoring, pulse oximetry, core body temperature, and capnography if intubated. A Doppler flow probe can be quite valuable for use as an audible indicator of HR, as traditional ECG and pulse oximetry monitors often read incorrectly when high HR is present.

A sedated patient should have a minimum of HR and RR monitored continuously and the respective values recorded every 5 to 15 minutes. HR can easily be monitored using a stethoscope or a Doppler flow probe placed over the metatarsal or ulnar artery. The RR is generally observed passively in the sedated patient. HRs for smaller raptors may range from 200 to 400 bpm, whereas larger species, such as eagles, should have HR between 80 and 150 bpm. RR can vary considerably depending on the size of the patient, but rates of 12 to 20 breaths per minute are typical. The absolute RR is less important than trends over time, and significant decreases should be investigated and treated, whether that is reversal of the sedative agents or intubation and conversion to general anesthesia.

SEDATIVE DRUGS AND DRUG COMBINATIONS

The body of literature concerning sedation and anesthesia in avian species continues to grow, although at a slow pace as compared with other species. Unfortunately, most of the literature centers around species that are easy to house and readily available for researchers. Raptors are not easy research subjects as keeping them in captivity is subject to numerous federal and state rules and regulations, not to mention ethical concerns around keeping wild species in captivity. Therefore, most pharmacokinetic and pharmacodynamic knowledge has been gleaned from other, nonraptor species and should be extrapolated with caution. Recommended doses for drugs and drug combinations are listed in **Table 1**.

Benzodiazepines

Benzodiazepines and their combinations are useful in avian practice and have mostly supplanted other drug combinations for many practitioners. Midazolam and diazepam alone (6–7 mg/kg intramuscularly [IM]) have been used for sedation in canaries[5] with sedation lasting for 17 to 38 minutes, the longer of those times recorded after administration of diazepam. In Northern bobwhite quail (*Colinus virginianus*), midazolam administered at 6 mg/kg IM also produced significant sedation within 10 minutes, with 4 mg/kg also resulting in sedation, but the duration was less than the higher dose. The addition of butorphanol to midazolam results in lower doses of both drugs being needed to produce adequate sedation. In a case series of 3 birds (2 psittacines and 1 chicken), midazolam 0.25 to 1 mg/kg was adequate for wound care when combined with butorphanol 1 to 3 mg/kg and injected IM.[6]

The intranasal (IN) route of administration appears to have similar magnitude and duration of effect as IM injection and may be easier to administer for both the patient and practitioner. Midazolam 7.3 mg/kg IN in ring-necked parakeets caused adequate sedation within 2.7 minutes on average,[7] while reducing the dose to 3.65 mg/kg IN and combining it with ketamine 40 to 50 mg/kg IN also achieved adequate sedation, but resulted in prolonged recovery times. In a field study involving Passeriformes, midazolam 5.6 ± 2.7 mg/kg IN produced significant sedation, but some ventilatory depression was noted as an increase in partial pressure of carbon dioxide.[4] One author (GG) currently recommends midazolam 1 mg/kg and butorphanol 2 mg/kg IN for brief minor procedures and to decrease stress during handling. An additional 1 mg/kg butorphanol ± 0.5 mg/kg midazolam IN can be administered in situations where sedation is inadequate. Flumazenil is a specific benzodiazepine receptor antagonist and can be used to reverse the effects of midazolam or diazepam. When administered IM or IN at doses of 0.05 to 0.1 mg/kg, it can reverse the sedation produced by benzodiazepines and produce smooth and rapid recoveries. The recovery period may be longer if other agents, such as ketamine, are used in combination with the benzodiazepine.

Alpha-2 Agonists

Alpha-2 agonists such as xylazine, medetomidine, and dexmedetomidine are commonly used for sedation in mammalian species but should be used with caution in avian species because of the unpredictability of sedation and potential for significant cardiac depression. Xylazine can no longer be recommended as a sedative unless no other agents are available because of the unreliability of both depth and duration of sedation. Medetomidine has been used with generally good results as both a sole agent[8] and in combination with butorphanol and/or ketamine.[9] Although no longer available commercially, medetomidine is available as a compounded drug

Table 1
Sedative agents for use in raptors[a]

Agent	Dose (IM Unless Otherwise Noted)	Comments
Xylazine	8–10 mg/kg	Generally inconsistent results and poor sedation when used as sole agent; no longer recommended unless no other agents are available.[63]
Xylazine/Ketamine	2 mg/kg (X) + 10–15 mg/kg (K)	Significant species variation in response[64]
Medetomidine	150–350 μg/kg	Wide dose range, must be sourced from compounding pharmacies. Can be reversed with atipamezole IM at 3–5 times the dose of medetomidine.[64]
Medetomidine/ Ketamine	20–100 μg/kg (M) + 2–5 mg/kg (K)	Can replace medetomidine with dexmedetomidine at 0.3–0.5 times the dose of medetomidine
Medetomidine/ Butorphanol	20–80 μg/kg (M) + 0.5–3 mg/kg (B)	
Medetomidine/ Butorphanol/ Ketamine	20–80 μg/kg (M) + 0.5–1 mg/kg (B) + 2–5 mg/kg (K)	
Dexmedetomidine	25–75 μg/kg	Reported to have better sedation than medetomidine at equipotent doses. Can be reversed with atipamezole IM at 4–10 times the dose of dexmedetomidine.[10]
Alfaxalone	5–20 mg/kg	May be associated with excitement and muscle tremors on recovery, sedation variable[3,22,24,25]
Alfaxalone/Midazolam	10 mg/kg (A) + 1 mg/kg (M)	Reduced occurrence of tremors seen with alfaxalone alone, but was associated with significantly longer recoveries[23]

(continued on next page)

Table 1 (continued)		
Agent	Dose (IM Unless Otherwise Noted)	Comments
Midazolam	0.5–7 mg/kg, may be instilled into nares	Doses of up to 7 mg/kg have been used in smaller avian species when used as a sole agent[5,7,65]
Midazolam/ Butorphanol	0.5–1 mg/kg (M) + 1–3 mg/kg (B), may be instilled into nares	Can redose midazolam 1 mg/kg if sedation inadequate
Reversal Agents		
Flumazenil	0.04–0.1 mg/kg IV or IM	Antagonizes benzodiazepines (midazolam/ diazepam)[5,65]
Atipamezole	4–10 times the dose of dexmedetomidine administered/3–5 time the dose of medetomidine	Should only be used IM[10]

[a] These are suggested doses based on published information and the authors' clinical experience. Species and individual variation in response to a given drug can be uncertain, so adjust the dose depending on the clinical response of the animal.

at high concentrations and therefore has the advantage of being dosed at very small volumes.

Dexmedetomidine is the most potent of the alpha-2 agonists, and has been used to good effect in both common buzzards (*Buteo buteo*) and common kestrels (*Falco tinnunculus*), at 25 and 75 μg/kg IM respectively, as a sole sedative agent.[10] Neither species was able to be intubated at these doses, but all lost their righting reflex. Dexmedetomidine can be substituted for medetomidine in most drug combinations at 0.3 to 0.5 times the dose of medetomidine. The alpha-2 agonists can be reversed with administration of atipamezole at 5 to 10 times the administered dose of dexmedetomidine or 3 to 5 times the dose of medetomidine. Atipamezole should only be administered IM to prevent the abrupt circulatory collapse and cardiac arrest that has been associated with IV administration. A potentially revolutionary peripheral antagonist, vatinoxan, has been studied recently in several mammal species that can reverse the peripheral cardiovascular effects without changing the central sedation.[11–13]

Opioids

Opioids, while the mainstay of sedation in many mammalian species, have not been shown to be significant sedatives in many avian species. This has been traditionally ascribed to differing receptor populations, with kappa (κ) opioid receptor being thought to predominate in birds and mu (μ) opioid receptors predominating in mammals. This notion has recently been questioned[14] and the real reasons underlying the difference in response to various drugs not only between classes but also between species are likely more complex than currently understood.

Butorphanol, a κ agonist and μ antagonist opioid, has demonstrated mild sedation for 1 to 2 hours when administered at 0.5 mg/kg IM to red-tailed hawks (*Buteo jamaicensis*) and great horned owls.[15] When administered to American kestrels (*Falco sparverius*), the sedation was considered minimal and some excitement was noted as the dosage was increased to 6 mg/kg IM.[16]

Hydromorphone is a μ opioid agonist that is often used for analgesia and sedation in veterinary medicine. It was evaluated in American kestrels with moderate and somewhat unpredictable sedation results,[17] with only 40% of birds showing significant sedation at a dose of 0.6 mg/kg and minor sedation in a smaller percentage of birds at 0.3 mg/kg. The pharmacokinetics of hydromorphone following IM and IV administration in American kestrels found a high IM bioavailability (75%) and rapid elimination, with a short terminal half-life and a rapid plasma clearance.[18] Hydromorphone should be cautiously used with head injuries, increased intracranial pressure, and acute coelomic conditions because it may interfere with the ability to establish a diagnosis and affect the clinical course of these conditions.[17]

Buprenorphine, considered a partial μ agonist because of the ceiling effect seen with respiratory depression in people, has been evaluated at several doses ranging from 0.1 to 1.8 mg/kg in American kestrels[19,20] and red-tailed hawks.[21] Although minor sedation for up to 24 hours was noted at most doses, the level of sedation was likely not enough to perform procedures more invasive than a physical examination.

Alfaxalone

Alfaxalone is a neuroactive steroid that has shown promise for sedation and induction of general anesthesia across several species. It has the favorable properties of being generally short-acting and its ability to be administered via several routes, including IM. At 10 mg/kg IM in mallard ducks (*Anas platyrhynchos*)[22] and budgerigars,[3] some sedation was noted but was not considered suitable for invasive procedures. In addition, some excitement was noted upon recovery, an observation that is common in many avian species. The addition of 1 mg/kg midazolam to the same dose of alfaxalone in quaker parrots (*Myiopsitta monachus*) reduced the muscle tremors that have been noted with alfaxalone alone, but recovery times were significantly longer.[23] Increasing the dose to 15 to 20 mg/kg resulted in moderate to profound sedation for approximately 30 minutes in budgerigars[24,25] with a more rapid onset and shorter recovery time as compared with butorphanol/midazolam.[25]

GENERAL ANESTHESIA
Preoxygenation

Preoxygenation is performed whenever possible and when hypoxemia may occur (ie, upper respiratory obstruction, cardiac, pulmonary, or air sac disease). It can produce an oxygen reservoir 4 to 5 times normal in the air sacs. The benefits are achieved in ≤1 minute of high inspired oxygen concentration in the healthy bird but may take ≥5 minutes in a bird with compromised respiratory function. Preoxygenation is accomplished with an oxygen cage or an induction chamber in the unrestrained bird, or a facemask in the physically restrained bird. Levels rise slower in an unprimed oxygen cage or induction chamber than a tight-fitting facemask with minimal dead space. In birds breathing room air, the parabronchial oxygen levels can fall precipitously if it becomes apneic.

Intubation and Ventilation

Birds are easily intubated as the laryngeal mound is large and visible at the base of the tongue. ETTs of 2.0 mm inner diameter can be used for small species, and ETTs of 5.0

to 8.0 mm inner diameter for eagles and vultures. Although noncuffed ETTs are most commonly used, there are several disadvantages to their use. These do not provide a sealed airway, thus allowing escape of anesthetic gases. This increases the amount of anesthetic gas required and environmental contamination. Also, airway protection from aspiration of secretions or gastrointestinal contents is reduced. This makes it imperative that the oral cavity be clean before intubation and monitored throughout the procedure. Elevation of the head and neck may reduce the regurgitation of gastrointestinal contents from the crop, proventriculus, or ventriculus into the oral cavity. Cuffed ETTs have been used in larger raptor patients. The cuff is carefully inflated with air to prevent leakage when 10 to 15 cm H_2O pressure is applied. Regardless of whether cuffed or noncuffed ETTs are used, a small amount of blood is commonly evident within the lumen of the tube upon extubation in eagles. Nevertheless, raptors, like other birds, have complete tracheal rings and adverse effects (eg, tracheal stenosis) associated with endotracheal intubation is a well-known fact and clinicians should be extremely careful when inflating a cuff. In one author's experience (MGH), humidification of the gases reduces mucus plug formation. Commercially available ETT humidifiers are available (Humid-Vent Mini, Agibeck Product, Hudson RCI, Temecula, CA, USA; **Fig. 4**). Disadvantages of their use include increased dead space and secretions leading to filter obstruction. The use of an ETT with a Murphy eye, which has both side and end openings, decreases the likelihood of mucus occlusion.

Nonrebreathing systems generally work well for raptors. Nonrebreathing systems, such as the Bain breathing system, are recommended in raptors up to 7 to 8 kg because of their lightweight design. Owing to the high carrier gas flow rates necessary when anesthetizing larger raptors, such as Andean (*Vultur gryphus*) and California condors (*Gymnogyps californianus*) or large vulture species, traditional circle systems are recommended. It is recommended to minimize dead space by having appropriately sized ETT and bags used in the nonrebreathing system. Generally, rates of 1 to 3 L/min are used, depending on whether the patient is intubated.[26]

An air sac cannula may be placed if an alternative airway is necessary. Research has shown that oxygen and anesthesia delivered in this way give comparable blood gas levels compared to endotracheal intubation.[27] Gas can be instilled into an air sac and the anesthetic passes from the air sac through the parabronchi and out through the trachea. The caudal thoracic or abdominal air sacs are generally used. Gases are still delivered at the recommended gas flow rate. Air sac cannulas are also placed for acute, life-threatening obstruction and can be left in place to provide respiratory support for up to 3 to 5 days without replacing tubes. After this point, inflammatory tissue and cells will accumulate on the tube tip.[28] Materials used for air sac cannulas include sterile ETT, large gauge IV catheters (16–18 g), red rubber feeding tubes, and silastic tubing. If the bird is to breathe through the cannula after the anesthetic event, the tube diameter should be at least equal to the patient's tracheal diameter and short enough to minimize dead space and prevent coelomic soft tissue contusion. The most common adverse effects reported with air sac cannulation are apnea, subcutaneous emphysema, obstruction of the tube, and bacterial contamination with associated coelomitis.[27] Ensure meticulous cleaning and inspection of the tube to prevent obstruction. Cleaning is performed with a sterile cotton-tipped applicator or Dacron swab. A filter of small weave gauze (ie, from the inside of an HEPA filter mask) can be placed over the end of the tube to prevent particulate matter from entering.

Both injectable and inhalant anesthetics cause dose-dependent respiratory depression. Sick or debilitated birds may not be able to accommodate these physiologic changes and may require intermittent positive pressure ventilation (IPPV). In mammals, IPPV is associated with reduced cardiac output and hypotension; thus, it is

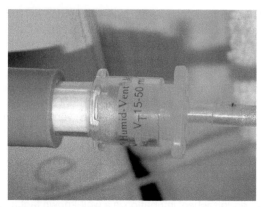

Fig. 4. A Humid-Vent is used to provide moisture to the tracheal epithelium during intubation. The device is placed between the endotracheal tube (right) and the anesthesia circuit (left). This increases dead-space, especially in smaller patients.

recommended that cardiovascular variables be monitored closely during IPPV. The authors recommend initial inspiratory pressures of 8 to 10 cm H_2O and rates of 6 to 10 breaths/min. Thoracic excursions are assessed as soon as ventilation is started, and the tidal volume is adjusted to achieve appropriate coelomic expansion.

PATIENT SUPPORT
Catheters

Placing IV or IO catheters is a simple, quick procedure that every clinician should be able to perform. Most patients expected to undergo anesthesia for more than brief, simple procedures of 15 minutes or less warrant acquiring venous access. For avian patients, there is a variety of IV or IO sites, depending on the species and size of the patient. For wild birds, an IV catheter is generally preferred to avoid potential joint damage, which may complicate release. If an IO catheter is to be placed, pneumatic bones (such as the humerus or femur) must be avoided. Generally, the proximal tibiotarsus or distal ulna are the ideal sites for IO catheterization (**Fig. 5**A, B). Complications associated with IO catheterization include penetration of both cortices, failure to properly enter the medullary cavity, and extravasation of fluids with associated pain. Extravasation has been observed even with proper catheter placement after 1 to 2 days of use. Intraosseous catheterization is contraindicated in septic patients and those with metabolic bone disease. Osteomyelitis may occur because of prolonged use or contamination at the time of placement of the IO catheter. Administration of alkaline or hypertonic solutions may also contribute to osteomyelitis and will cause pain and transient microscopic changes in the bone marrow.[29] These solutions should be diluted before administration and the catheter must be flushed with heparinized saline after any drug injection.

Fluid Therapy

Intravenous fluids are drugs and have an indication, a dose, and expected and unintended effects. Fluid choice remains a controversial topic due largely to inconsistent and opposing results from clinical trials.[30] Resuscitation fluids should be treated with the same level of consideration as any other prescription medication. Choosing the appropriate dose and type of fluid has significant implications for patient outcomes.

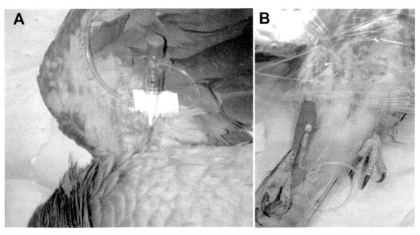

Fig. 5. (*A*) Intravenous catheters can be placed in the median ulnar vein or (*B*) in the medial metatarsal vein.

Crystalloid fluids

Crystalloid fluids, including 0.9% sodium chloride (NaCl), lactated Ringer's solution, Normosol-R, and Plasmalyte-A, are commonly used for IV volume support, maintenance, and rehydration. Fluids are warmed to body temperature (38–39°C) to minimize hypothermia. Fluid rates of 3 to 10 mL/kg/h are recommended for healthy anesthetized patients. Although this is a starting point, rates in small patients may need to be higher, but caution should be exercised to avoid fluid overload. Each patient is assessed individually for their fluid needs. Crystalloid fluid boluses of 10 to 20 mL/kg over 5 to 7 minutes are well tolerated in one author's experience (MGH). For severe hemorrhage, if whole blood transfusion (volume for volume) is not available, it has been recommended to provide crystalloid fluids at 3 times the volume of blood loss. However, this recommendation is based on mammals where the interstitial space is twice the vascular volume. In birds, the interstitial space is 4 times the plasma volume.[31] Replacement fluid volumes may need to be greater than 3 times blood loss. Parenteral dextrose use is minimized to prevent compartmental shifts in electrolytes and water leading to hypovolemia.

Hypertonic saline

Hypertonic saline, or 7.5% NaCl, is used to expand intravascular volume during resuscitation following acute severe hemorrhage when whole blood is not available.[32] The major benefit of hypertonic saline is intravascular volume expansion at one-fourth the volume of isotonic solutions. The mammalian dosage (4 mL/kg) given over 10 minutes is well tolerated in raptors. However, owing to osmotic diuresis and rapid redistribution of sodium cations, the intravascular effect is transient (<30 minutes) and additional fluid therapy must be used. Hypertonic fluids are contraindicated in dehydration, hypernatremia, and head trauma with intracranial hemorrhage. The sustained use of hypertonic saline is not recommended because hypernatremia and hyperchloremic acidemia, increased bleeding, and exacerbation of underlying cardiac and pulmonary disease due to fluid overload may occur.[30]

Synthetic colloids

The use of hydroxyethyl starch solutions (HES) has become controversial after an increasing number of studies in critically ill patients showed that its administration was associated with an increased incidence of acute kidney injury, coagulopathies, and mortality.[30,33,34] Synthetic colloids, such as HES, do not provide albumin, thrombocytes, or coagulation factors. The proposed mechanisms of colloid-induced renal injury include direct toxicity to the nephron and hyperoncotic plasma at the glomerulus leading to reduced glomerular filtration.[30] As synthetic colloids are cleared through the kidneys, they must be used with extreme caution in patients with cardiac and/or renal impairment. For both crystalloid and colloid fluids, coagulation becomes impaired when the induced hemodilution reaches 40%.[33] Coagulopathies are aggravated by coexisting hypothermia.[33] Other potential adverse effects include anaphylactoid reactions. If used, suggested doses should not exceed 20 mL/kg/d.

Blood transfusion

Trauma or disease resulting in hemorrhage is a common emergency presentation of wild raptors. Blood transfusions are rarely used in the early stages of hypovolemic shock except in severe and acute hemorrhage or in some coagulopathies (ie, rodenticide toxicosis).[31] It is indicated when there is a lack of red blood cells, thrombocytes, coagulation factors, or albumin. Hemorrhage is better tolerated than in mammals. However, with loss of greater than 30% blood volume or if the PCV less than 20%, whole blood transfusion is indicated. Heterologous blood cells may last less than 12 hours causing a significant metabolic drain on the recipient as the body uses energy to destroy the foreign cells.[35,36]

The storage of whole blood or blood products has not been studied extensively, and thus transfusions with fresh whole blood are recommended. The anticoagulants citrate phosphate dextrose adenine and acid citrate dextrose are used most commonly at a ratio of 1:9 of anticoagulant:whole blood. If given rapidly, the citrate can decrease ionized calcium and decrease myocardial contractility.[31] It may be necessary to give calcium gluconate or calcium chloride to the patient to reverse this effect. Donors often cannot be screened for infectious diseases when there is an immediate need for whole blood. A major and minor crossmatch should be performed before transfusion when possible. Sixty-six percent of major crossmatches performed between different species were positive for agglutination or hemolysis, whereas between the same species they were all negative.[37] Owing to this, transfusions should ideally be from the same species. However, if a homologous donor is not available, a single heterologous transfusion from a donor of the same genus (ie, Accipiter to Accipiter) may be of some benefit.

Mammalian protocols are presently followed for blood collection and administration. Pediatric blood filters are useful and in one study, an 18 μM filter did not cause hemolysis compared to nonfiltered controls in chickens.[38] Standard microdrip, 60 drop/mL, fluid sets used in small animal veterinary practice will not allow appropriate infusion rates in very small patients. Instead, fluid infusion and syringe pumps are used for accurate fluid administration.

Balanced Anesthesia

Inhalant anesthetics have the advantage of allowing rapid changes in anesthetic depth and rapid recoveries because of their low solubility in tissues and elimination via the respiratory tract. But inhalants also induce dose-dependent cardiopulmonary depression. "Balanced anesthesia" uses multiple drugs at lower overall doses to minimize the adverse effects of each drug while still providing appropriate anesthesia and analgesia. This approach reduces the magnitude of cardiovascular depression and promotes hemodynamic stability. Preanesthetic medications, constant rate infusions (CRIs), and local anesthetic use can reduce the inhalant anesthetic concentrations that are necessary. **Table 2** contains dosing information for several injectable and inhaled anesthetics used in raptors.

Even with balanced anesthetic protocols, morbidity and mortality elevate with increased duration of anesthesia. Minimize anesthesia time by preparing the patient, all drugs, and equipment in advance and provide close patient monitoring so anesthetic adjustments are identified and corrected immediately. Morbidity and mortality also occur during recovery, so it is important to monitor animals until they are fully recovered.

Preanesthetic Medications

Several authors question the necessity of routine administration of parasympatholytics in anesthetic protocols. Atropine and glycopyrrolate reduce mucus production and plug formation but increase its viscosity. In addition, some practitioners avoid using anticholinergics in birds because they increase HR, cardiac work, and myocardial oxygen demand. Therefore, the use of these agents should be weighed against their potential adverse effects.

Sedatives and tranquilizers are used to decrease anxiety and fear during induction, but most tranquilizers lack analgesia. In addition, most require injection and the handling and restraint may be as much as required for anesthetic induction. The merits of premedication must be weighed against this additional stress. For balanced anesthetic protocols, often a benzodiazepine, such as midazolam, can be combined with an opioid medication for sedation and pre-emptive analgesia. Butorphanol 1 to 6 mg/kg IM did not provide antinociception for American kestrels; hyperesthesia or hyperalgesia and agitation was seen in males receiving 6 mg/kg.[16] Hydromorphone 0.1 to 0.6 mg/kg IM to American kestrels had a dose-responsive thermal antinociceptive effect for up to 6 hours.[17] At the higher dosage, some birds were sedated initially and when handled appeared mildly agitated.[17] In red-tailed hawks, a fentanyl CRI produced a dose-related decrease of isoflurane minimum anesthetic concentration with minimal cardiovascular effects[39] If a CRI is to be used during anesthesia, a loading dose of the drug of choice is administered as part of the premedication protocol.

Injectable Anesthetics

Most injectable anesthetic agents are associated with pronounced cardiopulmonary depression and prolonged induction and recovery times; thus, it is recommended to use balanced anesthetic techniques instead of high dosages of individual agents. In addition, reversible anesthetic agents permit faster recovery. Ultimately, the general dosages published for different protocols are adjusted based on individual factors such as species, sex, age, health status, and others. If injectable anesthetics are used, it is vital to have accurate body weights to ensure appropriate drug dosing. Emergency and supportive drug dosages should be calculated and prepared in advance of anesthetic induction, but especially when using injectables. Finally, cardiopulmonary parameters should be monitored closely throughout the anesthetic period and ventilatory equipment, including ETT and a supplemental oxygen supply, should be available if needed.

Alpha-2 agonists

To date, there are few dexmedetomidine studies alone or in combination with midazolam in raptors.[10] Alpha-2 agonists are not recommended for short-term anesthesia in raptors because, in this study, there were inconsistent immobilization, adverse cardiovascular and respiratory effects, unreliable sedative effects, and excitatory reactions. However, with the advent of new peripheral antagonists such as vatinoxan, new

Table 2
Anesthetic and miscellaneous agents for use in raptors[a]

Agent	Dosage	Species/Comments
Alfaxalone	10 mg/kg in 2–4 mg/kg boluses IV	Good anesthesia with smooth recovery; respiratory acidosis resolved on recovery[47]
Atipamezole	4–10 times α_2 adrenergic agonist dose IV	α_2 adrenergic antagonist; 1:1 volume reversal of dexmedetomidine and medetomidine is general rule[10]
Atropine sulfate	0.01–0.02 mg/kg SC, IM, IV 0.04–0.1 mg/kg SC, IM, IV, IO, IT	Most species/premedication Most species/bradycardia; higher doses with CPR
Bupivacaine HCl	2 mg/kg infused SC 2–8 mg/kg perineurally	May be shorter acting in some birds; minimize dose to limit potential toxic effects High plasma levels at 6 and 12 h postadministration so possible for delayed toxicity Variable effectiveness for brachial plexus nerve block
Butorphanol tartrate	0.5–5 mg/kg IM, IV q1-4h 3 mg/kg (premedication) + 75 µg/kg/min IV CRI (maintenance)	Most species, mostly used for premedication
Dexmedetomidine HCl	25–75 µg/kg IM	Common buzzards/kestrels adequate restraint to prevent reaction to handling but did not allow for intubation; no arrhythmias, excitement, or major adverse effects noted; complete reversal with atipamezole[10]
Diazepam	0.05–0.5 mg/kg IV 0.25–0.5 mg/kg IM, IV q24 h x 2–3 d	Most species Raptors/appetite stimulant
Dobutamine	5–15 µg/kg/min IV	β1-Adrenergic agonist used to treat anesthetic-induced hypotension[66]
Dopamine HCl	7–10 µg/kg/min IV	Positive inotrope used to treat anesthetic-induced hypotension[66]
Fentanyl citrate	10–30 µg/kg/h IV	Reduced isoflurane MAC 31%–55% in a dose-related manner in red-tailed hawks[39]
Fentanyl (F)/Midazolam (M)	30 µg bolus (F) + 1–2 mg/kg IM (M) then 30 µg/kg/h IV CRI (F) + 1 mg/kg/h IV CRI (M)	Wild birds/partial IV anesthesia with isoflurane anesthesia for orthopedic surgery. Recovery = 63.2 ± 24.0 min with excellent quality. No

(continued on next page)

Table 2
(continued)

Agent	Dosage	Species/Comments
		significant change in HR detected.[67]
Flumazenil	0.02–0.1 mg/kg IM, IV	Most species- reversal for midazolam
Glycopyrrolate	0.01–0.02 mg/kg IM, IV	Most species
Hydromorphone HCl	0.1–0.6 mg/kg IM q3-6h	American kestrels/doses of 0.1, 0.3, and 0.6 mg/kg IM significantly increased thermal foot withdrawal responses. Appreciable sedation with 0.6 mg/kg[17,18]
Isoflurane	1%–5%	Inhalant anesthetic agent of choice in raptors[68,69]; dose-dependent hypotension with all inhalants; bald eagles may be more likely to exhibit isoflurane-induced arrhythmias[70] No significant differences in ventilation or O_2 transport between dorsal and lateral recumbency in red-tailed hawks.[71]
Ketamine HCl	5–50 mg/kg SC, IM, IV	Seldom used as a sole agent because of poor muscle relaxation and prolonged, violent recoveries; may produce excitation or convulsions in vultures, may fail to produce general anesthesia in some species including great horned owls, snowy owls, Cooper's hawks, sharp-shinned hawks[64] Smaller species require a higher dose; large birds tend to recover more slowly
Ketamine (K)/diazepam (D)	3–8 mg/kg (K) + 0.5–1 mg/kg (D) IM 8–15 (K) mg/kg + 0.5–1 (D) mg/kg IM 10–40 (K) mg/kg IV + 1–1.5 (D) mg/kg IM, IV	Eagles, vultures[72] Falcons[73] Raptors/rapid bolus may produce apnea, arrhythmia, and increased risk of death at higher doses[74]
Ketamine (K)/midazolam (M)	10–40 (K) mg/kg + 0.2–2 (M) mg/kg SC, IM	Most species
Lidocaine	1–4 mg/kg IV	May need to dilute 1:10 in small birds Most species
Midazolam HCl	0.1–3 mg/kg IM, IV	Most species/premedication at lower doses, onset approx.

(continued on next page)

Table 2 (continued)		
Agent	Dosage	Species/Comments
		15 min when administered IM
Naloxone HCl	2 mg IV q4-12h	Most species, including raptors- μ opioid reversal
Propofol	1–5 mg/kg IV 0.25–0.5 mg/kg/min IV	IV sedative-hypnotic agent; give slowly for induction to minimize apnea; intubation and IPPV required. Small boluses allow for quicker recoveries than constant rate infusion. Most species/induction[43] Most species/constant rate infusion[43]
Sevoflurane	3%–8%	Reduced cardiac arrhythmias in bald eagles compared with isoflurane[49]; crested sea eagles had significant decreases in time to induction and recovery.[69]
Tolazoline HCl	15 mg/kg IV	Raptors, including vultures[72]

All opioid agonists and agonist-antagonists may cause respiratory depression; profound bradypnea may occur with potent opioid agonists.

[a] These are suggested doses based on published information and the authors' clinical experience. Species and individual variation in response to a given drug can be uncertain so adjust the dose depending on the clinical response of the animal.

studies in raptors using this antagonist directly with alpha-2 agonists should be evaluated.

Ketamine
Medetomidine/ketamine or xylazine/ketamine combinations have been evaluated in several avian species and often provide a suboptimal plane of anesthesia for painful procedures. Ketamine dosages tend to be higher for smaller birds. When effective, anesthesia occurs within 5 to 10 minutes of IM injection and may last 5 to 20 minutes depending on the dose and size of the bird. In red-tailed hawks, ketamine 30 mg/kg IM produced no significant effect compared to awake birds in arterial blood gas or acid-base values, but did produce mild hyperventilation.[40] A combination of ketamine 30 mg/kg, xylazine 1 mg/kg, and midazolam 0.2 mg/kg IM produced adequate chemical restraint in golden eagles (Aquila chrysaetos).[41] Ketamine has also been reported to cause salivation, excitation, and convulsions when given to vultures, but these signs are rare in other raptor species.[42]

Propofol
Propofol produces a rapid and smooth anesthetic induction, but must be administered intravenously. Because propofol takes about 2 minutes to reach peak effect, one author (MGH) suggests a calculated propofol induction dose be administered in one-quarter increments over 30 to 60 seconds. This will allow more accurate dosing, and minimize apnea and hypotension. Prolonged recovery, with or without moderate to severe central nervous system (CNS) excitatory signs, has been reported after the

use of a CRI in red-tailed hawks and great horned owls[43]; however, others have used boluses of propofol effectively in raptors for anesthesia. Analgesia must be provided because of propofol lacking any analgesic properties.

Alfaxalone

Alfaxalone has a general anesthetic effect by binding to gamma-aminobutyric acid receptors in the CNS. Gamma-aminobutyric acid is a major inhibitory neurotransmitter in the CNS. Alfaxalone is a cardiopulmonary depressant, but at doses needed for sedation and anesthesia, there appears to be minimal depression.[24] One of the major advantages of alfaxalone over propofol is it can be administered IM or SC and still have an effect. Alfaxalone is rapidly metabolized by the liver with no cumulative effect, making it suitable for CRI. Reported doses for small birds (ie, budgerigars, finches, quaker parrots) are in the range of 20 to 30 mg/kg, whereas the dose for pigeons (*Columba livia*, 10 mg/kg) and greater flamingos (*Phoenicopterus roseus*, 2 mg/kg) is lower.[25,44–46] Alfaxalone 10 mg/kg IV in 2 to 4 mg/kg IV boluses produced good to excellent anesthesia in common buzzards with respiratory acidosis that resolved upon recovery.[47] The speed of induction and the degree of relaxation have been improved by the addition of other drugs such as midazolam and butorphanol.[46]

Inhalant Anesthetics

Inhalant anesthetics offer rapid induction and recovery, the ability to rapidly change anesthetic depth, and their use does not require an accurate body weight. Very little is metabolized, reducing hepatic and renal impact, and recovery is independent of both. Inhalant anesthetics can induce life-threatening cardiovascular and respiratory depression. Inhalants are potent negative inotropes; therefore, a dose-related decrease in cardiac output is expected, reflected as a decrease in blood pressure. Thus, the primary goal is to maintain the lightest plane of anesthesia possible allowing for minimal cardiopulmonary depression and completion of the procedure. In some cases, these goals may not be achieved by simply reducing the inhalant, and balanced anesthetic/analgesic protocols or the addition of dopamine or dobutamine (only in the volume-loaded patient) may be necessary to offset inhalant-induced hypotension.

Isoflurane, sevoflurane, and desflurane are the currently available inhalants. Their speed of onset and offset is largely determined by their solubility, with isoflurane having the highest solubility followed by sevoflurane and desflurane. Despite these physiochemical differences, the clinical differences may be fairly small as all 3 agents have similar dose-dependent cardiovascular effects. Cardiac arrhythmias have been noted in 35% to 75% of bald eagles (*H leucocephalus*) anesthetized with isoflurane and sevoflurane.[48,49] In these studies, second-degree AV block was the most prevalent arrhythmia. In one study, they occurred during induction and recovery in 80% of the cases.[48] Catecholamine release was suspected to be the cause. Cardiac arrhythmias are also commonly detected in other bird species,[28,48] but in the authors' experience, arrhythmias are most common in raptors. Sevoflurane has a less pungent odor than other inhalants and is generally more tolerated during mask induction. Many practitioners induce using sevoflurane and maintain anesthesia with the more cost-effective isoflurane.

Constant Rate Infusions

Intravenous CRIs of anesthetic and analgesic drugs are being evaluated in balanced anesthesia protocols.[39,43] Medications administered as CRIs can be titrated to effect. Plasma drug concentrations rise slowly when given as a CRI and thus a loading dose is administered. Disadvantages include a need for IV access and a syringe pump to accurately deliver low dosages. Microdosing of ketamine via CRI can be used to provide effective analgesia. Opioid medications such as fentanyl can be used as CRIs, but μ opioid medications cause respiratory depression and should only be used when a secure airway and ventilation are available.

Local and Regional Anesthetics

Concerns about avian sensitivity to local anesthetics have been attributed to rapid absorption and delayed metabolism. Toxic effects have been previously reported in birds at lidocaine doses of 2.7 to 3.3 mg/kg but in contrast, chickens survive much higher IV doses of lidocaine compared with mammals, with the convulsive dose of lidocaine being approximately 10 times the reported toxic dose.[50,51] A dose of 1.96 mg/kg bupivacaine IV was associated with a 50% probability of a clinically significant change in mean arterial blood pressure and/or HR in isoflurane-anesthetized chickens.[52]

Toxic effects are similar to those reported in mammals and respiratory arrest, seizures, and cardiac arrest have been reported with higher dosages in birds. A single case of hypersensitivity in a chicken after dosing of both lidocaine 4 mg/kg and bupivacaine 0.5 mg/kg administered for femoral and sciatic nerve blocks has been reported.[53] Other adverse effects include depression, drowsiness, muscle tremors, vomiting, hypotension, arrhythmias, and CNS signs including ataxia and nystagmus.

If a surgical procedure such as fracture repair or amputation is being performed, local anesthetics can be used for nerve blocks to minimize pain associated with these procedures. Using these blocks has reduced the perioperative bradycardia seen when manipulating fractured wing bones in birds. The sciatic-femoral nerve block was feasible in raptors undergoing surgery for pododermatitis and the motor responses following electrical stimulation of both nerves were consistent with those reported in mammalian species.[54]

A recent study evaluated the use of preservative-free lidocaine and bupivacaine for spinal anesthesia in chickens.[55] After aseptic preparation, a 23-gauge spinal needle was inserted into the synsacrococcygeal space of the birds; correct needle placement was confirmed by a sudden loss of resistance. Onset of action of 3.33 ± 1.23 minutes was significantly slower with 0.5 mg/kg bupivacaine than 2 mg/kg lidocaine, but the bupivacaine dose provided approximately 55 minutes of spinal anesthesia, whereas lidocaine only provided 18 minutes of duration of action.[55]

High doses of lidocaine, bupivacaine, and ropivacaine have been studied for brachial plexus blocks in ducks without adverse effects.[56–59] Brachial plexus blocks using palpation, ultrasound, or nerve locators have been used with variable degrees of success in avian species, including a recent study on American kestrel cadavers.[56–60] The safe use of transdermal patches, epidural infusions, and intravenous blocks have not yet been reported in birds.

Analgesia

All patients can perceive pain, and appropriate analgesia should be provided. It is important to err on the side of caution and treat pain before the stimulus rather than after. In raptors, a large amount of controversy exists as to which drugs may provide the best analgesia, what dosages are appropriate, and when these agents should be administered. In general, opioids are still considered the mainstay of analgesia in most species, with nonsteroidal anti-inflammatory drugs trailing a close second. The reader is referred to Hawkins and Paul-Murphy (2011)[61] for further reading in addition to a multitude of textbooks on the subject.

Patient Monitoring

The most important factor in patient monitoring is a dedicated anesthetist. A good indicator of the depth of anesthesia is RR and character. Respiration slows and becomes shallower as the anesthetic depth deepens. As apnea rapidly results in death, immediate measures must be taken to lighten anesthesia and provide ventilation if the bird stops breathing on its own. Average RR generally varies inversely with size (ie, the smaller the bird the higher the rate).

HR should also be closely monitored. This can be done with a stethoscope (external or esophageal) or an ECG monitor. Electrocardiogram leads can be placed on the wings and pelvic limbs. HR also varies inversely with size. Small patients may have a rate of greater than 300 beats/min, which may be difficult for oscilloscope monitors. The normal lead II QRS complexes in birds are negative. One of the best ways to monitor HR and character is with a Doppler probe. Direct or indirect blood pressure may also be monitored although few normal reference ranges are established (**Fig. 6**A–C). The palpebral reflex is present only in very light planes, as is reflex movement in response to cere stimulation. The corneal reflex (movement of the third eyelid in response to corneal stimulation) and the pedal reflex (withdrawal of the foot in response to toe stimulation) remain longer and are slow but present at a surgical plane of anesthesia.

The most commonly encountered problem in avian anesthesia is hypothermia. Normal avian body temperature is 104° to 110° F. Birds have a high-surface-to-volume ratio, which predisposes them to heat loss when they are not moving. Hypothermia markedly decreases avian RR and greatly prolongs recovery time. All birds undergoing anesthesia should be kept warm throughout the procedure and the recovery period. This can be accomplished with forced-air warmers, circulating warm water blankets, and warm room temperatures.

Emergencies during anesthesia should be planned for and anticipated. Many can be averted by careful monitoring of RR, HR, and body temperature. Emergency equipment (ie, ETT, oxygen, IV catheters and materials for securing them, ventilatory support, and emergency drugs) should always be close by and prepared for use. It is recommended that emergency drug dosages be calculated and 1 to 2 doses predrawn before induction. Respiratory depression and arrest are treated by turning off the anesthetic and controlling ventilation. Cardiac arrest is usually a result of myocardial hypoxemia and inotropic and chronotropic anesthetic drug effects. Although treatment is often unrewarding, administration of epinephrine IV, intratracheally, or by intracardiac injection is recommended. Cardiac massage should be attempted;

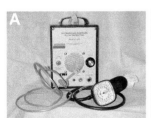 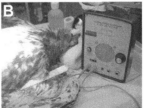 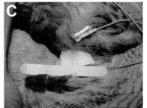

Fig. 6. (A) Indirect blood pressure can be assessed in raptors using a Doppler, blood pressure cuff, and sphygmomanometer. (B) The most accurate placement is over the brachial artery. (C) A #1-3 blood pressure cuff is placed around the humerus and the Doppler is placed over the brachial artery and held in place by two tongue depressors taped together that are opened and placed across the patagium on each side of the wing.

the authors recommend compressing each side of the thoracic coelom dorsolaterally, instead of via keel compression. Severe bradycardia is treated with atropine, assuming it is due to increased parasympathetic tone.

Cardiopulmonary-Cerebral Resuscitation

Cardiopulmonary-cerebral resuscitation (CPCR) is a comprehensive term used to describe the basic principles of cardiopulmonary resuscitation (CPR) as well as advanced life support and post-resuscitation care. Cerebral was added to CPR to identify the importance of being alive with complete neurologic function. The prognosis for respiratory arrest in birds, especially when caused by inhalant anesthetic overdose, is fairly good. Cardiac arrest in avian species carries a poor prognosis because direct compression of the heart is difficult because of the overlying sternum. A recent study evaluating thoracic compression for euthanasia identified an anatomic location for performing direct cardiac compressions in an emergency setting.[62] The bird is held with the thumb and index or middle finger of the dominant hand (approaching from the dorsum) just under the bird's wings. The thumb and finger are positioned on either side of the body cavity so that they are opposite each other in the triangular region formed by the pectoral muscle (ventrally), coracoid (cranially), and scapula (dorsally).[62]

The goal is to use monitoring devices to identify cardiovascular instability early. Early recognition of cardiovascular instability is the key to success in avian anesthesia. If the bird arrests on anesthesia, stop the anesthetic gas administration. Place an ETT and start positive pressure ventilation with 100% oxygen. Epinephrine (0.01 mg/kg) and atropine (0.04 mg/kg) can be given IV, IO, or via the intratracheal route (using a Tomcat catheter inserted down the ETT and doubling the dose used for IV). Intracardiac injections should be attempted only in extreme cases and with care, because of risk for laceration of the coronary vessels. An electrocardiogram, Doppler blood pressure, end-tidal carbon dioxide monitor, and reflexes can be used to evaluate the effectiveness of CPCR resuscitation.

Recovery

Recovery complications are usually associated with long anesthetic procedures (≥0.5–1.0 h). This emphasizes the importance of minimizing anesthetic time. The vaporizer is turned off at the end of the procedure and circle breathing systems are flushed with oxygen. Flushing is generally unnecessary with a nonrebreathing system when oxygen flows are increased. The patient should remain connected to the breathing system and oxygen as long as possible. Signs of recovery include muscle fasciculations followed by wing and leg movement. Once beak tone returns, the bird is extubated. Once extubated, an anesthetic face mask, with or without the rubber diaphragm, is placed over the bird's head to continue oxygen supplementation. Most birds are placed loosely in a towel and held upright to minimize self-trauma and regurgitation. Respiration is monitored during towel restraint to ensure adequate sternal movement. Once recovered, the bird is placed in a warm, well-oxygenated environment for continued recovery. A quiet dark environment minimizes stress and movement.

SUMMARY

Sedation and anesthesia are used routinely in raptors for a plethora of conditions. Understanding the restraint and handling of these patients, and knowing the specific anatomic differences is important for the handler's safety. Because few drugs have been evaluated to date specifically in raptors, extrapolation of drug doses is often necessary for these patients. Complications occur most commonly when anesthetic or sedation times are prolonged and when there is a lack of patient monitoring. Complications are minimized when a patent airway and intravenous catheterization are provided.

DISCLOSURE

The authors have nothing to disclose.

REFERENCES

1. Hollwarth AJ, Pestell ST, Dominic H, et al. Mortality outcomes in avian patients undergoing isoflurane general anaesthesia in a veterinary referral and first opinion practice. J Exot Pet Med 2021. https://doi.org/10.1053/j.jepm.2021.07.001.
2. Steinohrt LA. Avian fluid therapy. J Avian Med Surg 1999;13:83–91.
3. Balko JA, Lindemann DM, Allender MC, et al. Evaluation of the anesthetic and cardiorespiratory effects of intramuscular alfaxalone administration and isoflurane in budgerigars (Melopsittacus undulatus) and comparison with manual restraint. J Am Vet Med Assoc 2019;254:1427–35.
4. Heatley JJCJ, Kingsley L, Beaufrere H, et al. Midazolam sedates Passeriformes for field sampling but affects multiple venous blood analytes. Vet Med (Auckl) 2015;16:61–9.
5. Vesal N, Zare P. Clinical evaluation of intranasal benzodiazepines, alpha-agonists and their antagonists in canaries. Vet Anaesth Analg 2006;33:143–8.
6. Lee ALA. Sedation and local anesthesia as an alternative to general anesthesia in 3 birds. J Exot Pet Med 2016;25:100–5.
7. Vesal N, Eskandari MH. Sedative effects of midazolam and xylazine with or without ketamine and detomidine alone following intranasal administration in Ring-necked Parakeets. J Am Vet Med Assoc 2006;228:383–8.
8. Lawton M. Anesthesia and soft tissue surgery. In: Samour J, editor. Avian medicine. 2nd edition. Philadelphia: Mosby-Elsevier.; 2008. p. 137–54.
9. Hawkins MG, Sanchez-Migallon Guzman D, Beaufrere H, et al. Birds. In: Carpenter JW, Marion CJ, editors. Exotic animal Formulary. 5th edition. St. Louis: Elsevier; 2018. p. 181–376.
10. Santangelo B, Ferrari D, Di Martino I, et al. Dexmedetomidine chemical restraint in two raptor species undergoing inhalation anaesthesia. Vet Res Commun 2009; 33:S209–11.
11. Einwaller J, Painer J, Raekallio M, et al. Cardiovascular effects of intravenous vatinoxan (MK-467) in medetomidine–tiletamine–zolazepam anaesthetised red deer (Cervus elaphus). Vet Anaesth Analg 2020;47:518–27.
12. Honkavaara JM, Raekallio MR, Syrja PM, et al. Concentrations of medetomidine enantiomers and vatinoxan, an α2-adrenoceptor antagonist, in plasma and central nervous tissue after intravenous coadministration in dogs. Vet Anaesth Analg 2020;47:47–52.
13. Pypendop BH, Ahokoivu H, Honkavaara J. Effects of dexmedetomidine, with or without vatinoxan (MK-467), on minimum alveolar concentration of isoflurane in cats. Vet Anaesth Analg 2019;46:443–51.
14. Duhamelle A, Raiwet DL, Langlois I, et al. Preliminary findings of structure and expression of opioid receptor genes in a peregrine falcon (Falco peregrinus), a snowy owl (Bubo scandiacus), and a blue-fronted Amazon parrot (Amazona aestiva). J Avian Med Surg 2018;32:173–84.

15. Riggs SM, Hawkins MG, Craigmill AL, et al. Pharmacokinetics of butorphanol tartrate in red-tailed hawks (Buteo jamaicensis) and great horned owls (Bubo virginianus). Am J Vet Res 2008;69:596–603.

16. Guzman DS, Drazenovich TL, KuKanich B, et al. Evaluation of thermal antinociceptive effects and pharmacokinetics after intramuscular administration of butorphanol tartrate to American kestrels (Falco sparverius). Am J Vet Res 2014; 75:11–8.

17. Guzman DS, Drazenovich TL, Olsen GH, et al. Evaluation of thermal antinociceptive effects after intramuscular administration of hydromorphone hydrochloride to American kestrels (Falco sparverius). Am J Vet Res 2013;74:817–22.

18. Guzman DS, KuKanich B, Drazenovich TL, et al. Pharmacokinetics of hydromorphone hydrochloride after intravenous and intramuscular administration of a single dose to American kestrels (Falco sparverius). Am J Vet Res 2014;75:527–31.

19. Ceulemans SM, Guzman DS, Olsen GH, et al. Evaluation of thermal antinociceptive effects after intramuscular administration of buprenorphine hydrochloride to American kestrels (Falco sparverius). Am J Vet Res 2014;75:705–10.

20. Guzman DS, Ceulemans SM, Beaufrère H, et al. Evaluation of the thermal antinociceptive effects of a sustained-release buprenorphine formulation after intramuscular administration to American kestrels (Falco sparverius). J Avian Med Surg 2018;32:1–7.

21. Gleeson MD, Guzman DSM, Knych HK, et al. Pharmacokinetics of a concentrated buprenorphine formulation in red-tailed hawks (Buteo jamaicensis). Am J Vet Res 2018;79:13–20.

22. Kruse TN, Messenger KM, Bowman AS, et al. Pharmacokinetics and pharmacodynamics of alfaxalone after a single intramuscular or intravascular injection in mallard ducks (Anas platyrhynchos). J Vet Pharmacol Ther 2019;42:713–21.

23. Whitehead MC, Hoppes SM, Musser JMB, et al. The use of alfaxalone in quaker parrots (myiopsitta monachus). J Avian Med Surg 2019;33:340–8.

24. Romano J, Hasse K, Johnston M. Sedative, cardiorespiratory, and thermoregulatory effects of alfaxalone on budgerigars (Melopsittacus undulatus). J Avian Med Surg 2020;34:214–6.

25. Escalante GC, Balko JA, Chinnadurai SK. Comparison of the sedative effects of alfaxalone and butorphanol-midazolam administered intramuscularly in budgerigars (Melopsittacus undulatus). J Avian Med Surg 2018;32:279–85.

26. Hawkins MG, Zehnder A, Pascoe PJ. Cagebird anesthesia. In: West G, Heard D, Caulkett N, editors. Zoo animal and Wildlife immobilization and anesthesia. Ames, IA: Wiley Blackwell; 2014. p. 399–434.

27. Jaensch SM, Cullen L, Raidal SR. Comparison of endotracheal, caudal throacic air sac, and clavicular air sac administration of isoflurane in sulphur-crested cockatoos (Cacatua galerita). J Avian Med Surg 2001;15:170–7.

28. Korbel R, Burike S, Erhardt W, et al. Effect of nitrous oxide application in racing pigeons (Columba livia gmel., 1979, var. dom) - A study using the airsac perfusion technique. Isr J Vet Med 1996;51:133–9.

29. Lamberski N, Daniel GB. Fluid dynamics of intraosseous fluid administration in birds. J Zoo Wildl Med 1992;23:47–54.

30. McLean DJ, Shaw AD. Intravenous fluids: effects on renal outcomes. Br J Anaesth 2018;120:397–402.

31. Martinho F. Indications and techniques for blood transfusion in birds. J Exot Pet Med 2009;18:112–6.

32. Leary AM, Roberts JR, Sharp PJ. The effect of infusion of hypertonic saline on glomerular filtration rate and arginine vasotocin, prolactin and aldosterone in the domestic chicken. J Comp Physiol [B] 1998;168:313–21.

33. Boer C, Bossers SM, Koning NJ. Choice of fluid type: physiological concepts and perioperative indications. Br J Anaesth 2018;120:384–96.

34. Hahn RG. Adverse effects of crystalloid and colloid fluids. Anaesthesiol Intensive Ther 2017;49(4):303–8.

35. Sandmeier P, Stauber EH, Wardrop KJ, et al. Survival of pigeon red blood cells after transfusion into selected raptors. J Am Vet Med Assoc 1994;204:427–9.

36. Finnegan MV, Daniel GB, Ramsay EC. Evaluation of whole blood transfusions in domestic pigeons (Columba livia). J Avian Med Surg 1997;11:7–14.

37. Stauber E, Washizuka A, Wilson E, et al. Crossmatching reactions of blood from various avian species. Isr J Vet Med 1996;51:143.

38. Jankowski G, Nevarez J. Evaluation of a pediatric blood filter for whole blood transfusions in domestic chickens (Gallus gallus). J Avian Med Surg 2010;24:272–8.

39. Pavez JC, Hawkins MG, Pascoe PJ, et al. Effect of fentanyl target-controlled infusions on isoflurane minimum anaesthetic concentration and cardiovascular function in red-tailed hawks (Buteo jamaicensis). Vet Anaesth Analg 2011;38:344–51.

40. Kolias GV Jr, McLeish I. Effects of ketamine hydrochloride in red-tailed hawks (Butoo jamaicensis) 1 - arterial blood gas and acid base. Comp Biochem Physiol 1978;60C:57–9.

41. Sadegh AB, Shafiei Z, Mahmoudi T, et al. Ketamine-xylazine with diazepam or midazolam anesthesia in eagles (Aquila chrysaetos). J Vet Res 2011;15:414–9.

42. Samour JH, Jones DM, Knight JA, et al. Comparative studies of the use of some injectable anaesthetic agents in birds. Vet Rec 1984;115:6–11.

43. Hawkins MG, Wright BD, Pascoe PJ, et al. Pharmacokinetics and anesthetic and cardiopulmonary effects of propofol in red-tailed hawks (Buteo jamaicensis) and great horned owls (Bubo virginianus). Am J Vet Res 2003;64:677–83.

44. Villaverde-Morcillo S, Benito J, Garcia-Sanchez R, et al. Comparison of isoflurane and alfaxalone (Alfaxan) for the induction of anesthesia in flamingos (Phoenicopterus roseus) undergoing orthopedic surgery. J Zoo Wildl Med 2014;45: 361–6.

45. Susanti L, Kang S, Park S, et al. Effect of three different sedatives on electroretinography recordings in domesticpPigeons (Columba livia). J Avian Med Surg 2019;33:115–22.

46. Perrin KL, Nielsen JB, Thomsen AF, et al. Alfaxalone anesthesia in the Bengalese finch (Lonchura domestica). J Zoo Wildl Med 2017;48:1146–53.

47. Kılıç N. Clinical evaluation of alfaxalone in cyclodextrin as an intravenous anesthetic in the common buzzards (Buteo buteo). Iran J Vet Surg 2021;16:24–8.

48. Aguilar RF, Smith VE, Ogburn P, et al. Arrhythmias associated with isoflourane anesthesia in bald eagles (Haliaeetus leucocephalus). J Zoo Wildl Med 1995; 26:508–16.

49. Joyner PH, Jones MP, Ward D, et al. Induction and recovery characteristics and c ardiopulmonary effects of sevoflurane and isoflurane in bald eagles. Am J Vet Res 2008;69:13–22.

50. Imani H, Vesal N, Mohammadi-Samani S. Evaluation of intravenous lidocaine overdose in chickens (Gallus domesticus). Iranian J Vet Surg 2013;8:9–16.

51. Brandao J, da Cunha AF, Pypendop B, et al. Cardiovascular tolerance of intravenous lidocaine in broiler chickens (Gallus gallus domesticus) anesthetized with isoflurane. Vet Anaesth Analg 2015;42:442–8.

52. DiGeronimo PM, da Cunha AF, Pypendop B, et al. Cardiovascular tolerance of intravenous bupivacaine in broiler chickens (Gallus gallus domesticus) anesthetized with isoflurane. Vet Anaesth Analg 2017;44:287–94.

53. Silva HRAD, Nunes N, Gering AP, et al. Hypersensitivity in Chicken (Gallus gallus domesticus) due to the Association of Lidocaine and Bupivacaine in Neural-Guided Femoral and Sciatic Nerve Block. Acta Scientiae Veterinariae 2021;49.

54. d'Ovidio D, Noviello E, Adami C. Nerve stimulator-guided sciatic-femoral nerve block in raptors undergoing surgical treatment of pododermatitis. Vet Anaesth Analg 2015;42:449–53.

55. Khamisabadi A, Kazemi-Darabadi S, Akbari G. Comparison of anesthetic efficacy of lidocaine and bupivacaine in Spinal anesthesia in chickens. J Avian Med Surg 2021;35:60–7.

56. Brenner DJ, Larsen RS, Dickinson PJ, et al. Development of an avian brachial plexus nerve block technique for perioperative analgesia in mallard ducks (Anas platyrhynchos). J Avian Med Surg 2010;24:24–34.

57. Figueiredo JP, Cruz ML, Mendes GM, et al. Assessment of brachial plexus blockade in chickens by an axillary approach. Vet Anaesth Analg 2008;35:511–8.

58. Cardozo LB, Almeida RM, Fiuza LC, et al. Brachial plexus blockade in chickens with 0.75% ropivacaine. Vet Anaesth Analg 2009;36:396–400.

59. D/Otaviano de Castro Vilan RG, Montiani-Ferreirra F, Lange RR, et al. Brachial plexus block in birds. Exot DVM 2006;8:86–91.

60. Micieli F, Mirra A, Santangelo B, et al. Ultrasound-guided dorsal approach for the brachial plexus block in common kestrels (Falco tinnunculus): a cadaver study. Vet Anaesth Analg 2021;48:617–21.

61. Hawkins MG, Paul-Murphy J. Avian analgesia. Vet Clin North Amer Exot Anim Pract 2011;14:61–80.

62. Paul-Murphy JR, Engilis A Jr, Pascoe PJ, et al. Comparison of intraosseous pentobarbital administration and thoracic compression for euthanasia of anesthetized sparrows (Passer domesticus) and starlings (Sturnus vulgaris). Am J Vet Res 2017;78:887–99.

63. Huckabee JR. Raptor therapeutics. Vet Clin North Am Exot Anim Pract 2000;3:91–116, vi.

64. Bailey TA, Apo MM. Pharmaceutics commonly used in avian medicine. In: Samour J, editor. Avian medicine. 3rd edition. Edinburgh: Mosby Elsevier; 2016. p. 637–78.

65. Day TK, Roge CK. Evaluation of sedation in quail induced by use of midazolam and reversed by use of flumazenil. J Am Vet Med Assoc 1996;209:969–71.

66. Schnellbacher RW, da Cunha AF, Beaufrere H, et al. Effects of dopamine and dobutamine on isoflurane-induced hypotension in Hispaniolan Amazon parrots (Amazona ventralis). Am J Vet Res 2012;73:952–8.

67. Paesano FRC, Briganti A. Partial intavenous anaesthesia (PIVA) with infusion of fentanyl and midazolam during orthopedic surgery in wild birds. Intl Conf Avian Herp Exot Mammal Med 2015;332.

68. Seok SH, Jeong DH, Hong IH, et al. Cardiorespiratory dose-response relationship of isoflurane in cinereous vulture (Aegypius monachus) during spontaneous ventilation. J Vet Med Sci 2016;79(1):160–5.

69. Chan FT, Chang GR, Wang HC, et al. Anesthesia with isoflurane and sevoflurane in the crested serpent eagle (Spilornis cheela hoya): minimum anesthetic concentration, physiological effects, hematocrit, plasma chemistry and behavioral effects. J Vet Med Sci 2013;75:1591–600.
70. Carpenter JW, Marion CJ. Exotic animal formulary. 4th edition. St. Louis, Mo: Elsevier; 2013.
71. Hawkins MG, Malka S, Pascoe PJ, et al. Evaluation of the effects of dorsal versus lateral recumbency on the cardiopulmonary system during anesthesia with isoflurane in red-tailed hawks (Buteo jamaicensis). Am J Vet Res 2013;74:136–43.
72. Allen JL, Oosterhuis JE. Effect of tolazoline on xylazine-ketamine-induced anesthesia in turkey vultures. J Am Vet Med Assoc 1986;189:1011–2.
73. Molero C, Bailey TA, Di Somma A. Anaesthesia of falcons with a combination of injectable anaesthesia (ketamine-medetomidine) and gas anaesthesia (Isoflurane)17. Falco: Newsletter of Middle East Falcon Research Group; 2007.
74. Redig PT, Duke GE. Intravenously administered ketamine HCl and diazepam for anesthesia of raptors. J Am Vet Med Assoc 1976;169:886–8.

Backyard Poultry and Waterfowl Sedation and Anesthesia

Christine Molter, DVM, Dipl. ACZM[a],*,
André Escobar, DVM, MS, PhD, Dipl. CBAV (Anesthesiology)[b],
Carrie Schroeder, DVM, Dipl. ACVAA[c]

KEYWORDS

- Anesthesia • Chicken • Duck • Poultry • Sedation • Waterfowl

KEY POINTS

- Anatomy for backyard poultry and waterfowl is similar to other avian species.
- Both injectable and inhalant anesthetic options are available for backyard species.
- The anesthetic plan should be balanced with the procedural and patient needs to have a safe and successful event.

INTRODUCTION

Backyard poultry (chicken [*Gallus gallus domesticus*], turkey [*Meleagris gallopavo domesticus*], helmeted guineafowl [*Numida meleagris*]) and waterfowl (ducks and geese [Anatidae]) are rapidly expanding avian populations in the United States.[1] One US Department of Agriculture study found that 0.8% of all households in the United States own chickens and 4% of households without chickens were planning to obtain them within 5 years.[2] These birds are maintained as food for home use (meat, eggs, or both), gardening partners (pest control, manure for fertilizer), pets, or a combination.[3] Veterinarians are presented with these animals for a variety of conditions, commonly including trauma, lameness, and disease involving the reproductive, nervous, and gastrointestinal systems, which may require anesthesia to properly diagnose and treat.[4]

The authors do not have any commercial or financial conflicts of interest or any funding sources to disclose.
[a] Animal Health Department, Houston Zoo, Inc., 1513 Cambridge Street, Houston, TX 77030, USA; [b] Department of Clinical Sciences, Ross University School of Veterinary Medicine, PO Box 334, Basseterre, St. Kitts, West Indies; [c] Department of Surgical Sciences, University of Wisconsin School of Veterinary Medicine, 2015 Linden Drive, Madison, WI 53706, USA
* Corresponding author.
E-mail address: cmolter@houstonzoo.org

SPECIES ANATOMIC PARTICULARITIES RELEVANT TO SEDATION AND OR ANESTHESIA

The anatomy of backyard poultry and waterfowl is similar to that of other avian species and this should be clinically considered. Most backyard species are highly terrestrial and heavy bodied, and some domestic chicken breeds are also well muscled. For intramuscular (IM) injections, the pectoral musculature is the most common site. The pelvic limb musculature, although abundant in some, is generally not used to avoid the sciatic nerve and associated vasculature, and to avoid partial elimination of drugs by the renal portal system. For venipuncture, intravenous (IV) injections, or IV catheter placement, the medial metatarsal and brachial (also called the ulnar or wing) veins are reasonable options. Jugular veins may be used, although the right jugular vein is often reserved for venipuncture, as it is larger than the left; other peripheral venous sites are more common for catheter placement. In obese domestic chickens or turkeys, the jugular vein may be challenging to identify and profuse adipose tissue may need to be manipulated away from the vessel for visualization. For intraosseous catheter placement, the nonpneumatic distal ulna or tibiotarsus are options though in some species, like large domestic chickens, the greater bone density makes placement more difficult.[5]

For endotracheal intubation and administration of volatile anesthetics, considerations given to other birds should be applied to poultry and waterfowl. These species have a glottis at the base of the tongue (**Fig. 1**), which may be set deep within the oral cavity and require the use of a laryngoscope or transilluminator to visualize, and the oral cavity may contain abundant thick, stringy saliva that needs to be removed from the glottis before intubation and after extubation. The oral cavity is a favorable location to evaluate mucous membrane color and the comb, when present in gallinaceous species, may be blanched to assess capillary refill time.[6] The respiratory tract consists of nares, a trachea with complete cartilaginous rings, a syrinx (where vocalizations are produced), and 2 lungs firmly attached to the dorsal body wall. Domestic chickens have 9 air sacs, including paired cervical, cranial thoracic, caudal thoracic, abdominal, and a single interclavicular air sac.[7] The air sacs are not involved with significant gas exchange, but do connect to the lungs and pneumatic bones, including the humerus and femur. Care should be taken with injections in birds to avoid

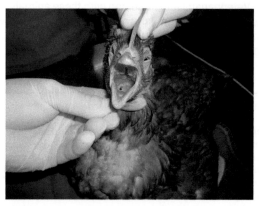

Fig. 1. A domestic chicken under a surgical plane of anesthesia, ready for intubation and with the oral cavity carefully opened. The glottis is in the center of the oropharynx at the base of the tongue, ventrally.

improper needle placement into an air sac by aspirating to ensure no air enters the syringe before injection administration.

It is important to note that, as with other avian species, air sac cannulation may be performed to provide oxygen supplementation and/or administration of inhalational agents in the event of tracheal obstruction or difficulty in endotracheal intubation. Indications and techniques have been described elsewhere.

Obese domestic chickens, turkeys, and geese may have a tremendous amount of coelomic adipose tissue that will reduce air sac space and potentially impede air sac cannulation, and this should be taken into consideration before anesthesia. Obese birds may become hyperthermic, dyspneic, tachypneic, or open-mouth breathe while under stress, during manual restraint, or in warm conditions. Anxiolytic medication, preoxygenation, and working in a temperature-controlled space will help to mitigate the challenges of working with obese birds.

As birds do not have a diaphragm, respiration is mechanically driven by the movement of the sternum and this should not be restricted during manual restraint or during anesthesia. Auscultation of the lungs is best achieved with a stethoscope over the dorsum between the wings and the air sacs over the caudal aspect of the keel. The heart is 4-chambered, analogous to mammals, and located deep to the cranial aspect of the sternum. Auscultation of the heart is best achieved with a stethoscope placed over either side of the sternum. Alternatively, an esophageal stethoscope may be used in large species under general anesthesia.

Most backyard poultry species have a crop, which may be quite large and pendulous, particularly in domestic chickens and especially those with crop stasis or ileus. The crop must be palpated before anesthesia and, if full, should be given time to empty or the bird's head kept elevated to prevent regurgitation and aspiration. Endotracheal intubation will aide in protecting the airway as well. In general, birds do not require fasting from food or water for more than 2 hours.

SEDATION AND PREMEDICATION

Advantages to preanesthetic sedation are numerous and include anxiolysis, decreased requirement for induction agents and maintenance anesthetics, and amnesia.[8–12] Compared with nondomestic avian orders such as Psittaciformes, poultry and some waterfowl are generally more placid and amenable to handling and short-term restraint without significant stress responses. These species generally lack tools for inducing significant harm on handlers and, in the case of pet poultry and waterfowl, are often more forgiving for subsequent veterinary visits as compared with parrots. However, despite the relative ease of veterinary care in poultry and waterfowl, these animals are subject to stress responses as a result of perturbations in their routine and environment, such as a trip to the veterinary clinic or a visit by a veterinarian. These perturbations can cause stress responses that induce adverse effects ranging from changes in the leukogram on a complete blood cell count to dramatic increases in heart rate, respiratory rate, and body temperature.[13,14] As such, mitigation of stress to the avian patient is of the utmost importance and sedation is a component of this effort.

At the time of publication, there is a paucity of evidence for the efficacy of oral sedatives in avian patients. For instance, pigeons administered the serotonin receptor antagonist and reuptake inhibitor, trazodone (30 mg/kg), via the oral route under experimental conditions exhibited no sedation.[15] For greater predictability of response, parenteral means of sedation are typically recommended. IV access generally requires more significant handling and restraint and is, therefore, generally not recommended unless an indwelling IV catheter is in place. Intramuscular administration is a commonly used route for administration of sedatives, offering a relatively predictable absorption and onset time. Pectoral muscles are commonly used to potentially avoid the elimination of drugs by the renal portal system. Most poultry and waterfowl are well muscled and of adequate size to tolerate IM administration of a moderate volume.

The intranasal (IN) route of administration has been described in a number of bird species and is an effective alternative to IM administration.[8,16–20] This route offers rapid uptake through the richly vascularized nasal cavity both through rapid absorption into the blood and along the olfactory and trigeminal nerves into the cerebral spinal fluid.[21] Onset is generally rapid, within 5 to 10 minutes, due to this direct route. Advantages include avoidance of potential muscle trauma caused by injections, increased ease of administration in poorly muscled or conditioned birds, and a potential for improved client/owner perception by administering sedatives less invasively. Disadvantages include a need for increased restraint of the head, a limit to the total volume of administration, potential for aerosolized drug exposure for those administering the agent, and potential for incomplete administration or absorption. Both IM and IN routes are effective means of administration and choice of route is often based on individual circumstances and veterinarian preference.

Midazolam is a benzodiazepine that exerts sedation via facilitation of the inhibitory actions of gamma aminobutyric acid (GABA) at the $GABA_A$ receptor.[12] The result is anxiolysis, sedation, anterograde amnesia, and muscle relaxation of moderate duration. Midazolam is characterized by its favorable safety profile, with minimal adverse effects on the cardiovascular or respiratory system as a sole agent. As with all benzodiazepines, midazolam exerts a synergistic effect with other sedative and anesthetic agents, including opioids and alpha-2 adrenergic receptor agonist agents.[12] Sedation with midazolam via IM and IN routes has been extensively described in a variety of avian species with overwhelmingly favorable results.[8,16–20,22] For instance, IN administration of midazolam in the diving duck surf scoter (*Melanitta perspicillata*) before the induction of general anesthesia with isoflurane resulted in a significantly increased postsurgical survival.[20] Preanesthetic administration of midazolam will not only reduce the stress associated with anesthetic induction and recovery, but will decrease the amount of inhalant needed for maintenance of anesthesia, as measured by minimal anesthetic concentration (MAC) in birds. Intramuscular administration of midazolam (1–2 mg/kg) in quaker parrots (*Myiopsitta monachus*) resulted in a dose-dependent decrease in the MAC of isoflurane of 19% to 28%.[10] Although the MAC of volatile anesthetics such as isoflurane and sevoflurane may vary widely (see the section Inhalant Anesthetics), it can be expected that the preanesthetic administration of sedatives, such as midazolam, will decrease the required concentration of inhaled anesthetic in a dose-dependent manner. The pharmacokinetics of midazolam have been studied with variable results.[23] Based on these studies, as well as evaluations of the duration of clinical sedation, the duration of midazolam is expected to be of brief to moderate duration, lasting from 30 minutes to 2 hours. The dosage range in avian species is large, and dosage should be based on allometric scaling, level of patient stress, and the desired level of sedation. In general, a 1 to 2 mg/kg IM or IN dosage is a starting point with most domestic poultry and waterfowl, but a range of up to 6 mg/kg has been described.[20,24]

A distinct advantage of midazolam is the availability to antagonize sedative effects with the benzodiazepine antagonist flumazenil.[8,16,17,22] This agent can be administered via IN or IM routes (0.01–0.1 mg/kg). Adverse effects are uncommon at clinical dosages in most patients and have not been described in avian patients. Onset of recovery is generally within approximately 10 minutes and the duration of flumazenil is 30 to 60 minutes.[12] Because of the potential for the duration of the agonist to outlast that of the antagonist, patients should be monitored for recurrence of sedation for 1 to 2 hours. Caution should be exercised to avoid access to submersible water and elevated perches until recovery is complete from sedation, at least 2 hours.

When analgesia or an increased level of sedation is required, the addition of butor- phanol is recommended. The combination of butorphanol and midazolam in cocka- tiels resulted in a deeper level of sedation as compared with midazolam as a sole agent,[20] and this combination used in a variety of psittacines for preanesthetic seda- tion resulted in a reduction in duration and an improvement in quality of anesthetic in- duction with no adverse effects.[25] It is important to note that the synergistic combination of an opioid with a benzodiazepine may result in respiratory depression in mammalian species. Although decreased respiratory rates have been reported[20] under sedation, this is likely due to a decreased stress response rather than a true decrease in minute ventilation. The administration of midazolam as a sole agent in passerine birds did result in a modest increase and decrease in the partial pressures of venous carbon dioxide and oxygen, respectively[26]; however, clinically significant respiratory depression as evidenced by arterial blood gas tensions has not been reported.

Naloxone is an opioid antagonist that will reverse the sedation of butorphanol and has been described in mammals at 0.02 to 0.0.4 mg/kg; its use in avian species has been described but not fully evaluated at the time of publication. Although in the past butorphanol was considered the opioid of choice in birds, this concept has been changing, and full-opioid agonists have been used when a higher level of anal- gesia is required. The presence of μ-opioid receptors has been described in the cen- tral nervous system (CNS) of birds,[27] including chickens,[28] and it is expected that the analgesic effect of those drugs is similar than those reported in mammals.

Although midazolam and butorphanol are the most commonly administered agents for sedation in poultry and waterfowl, the use of alpha-2 adrenergic receptor agonists for sedation has been described in avian species.[16–18,29] Alpha-2 adrenergic receptor agonists have the potential to result in profound, dose-dependent sedation that may be better suited for larger and more challenging-to-restrain birds such as ostrich (*Stru- thio* sp.) or emu (*Dromaius novaehollandiae*). Significant bradycardia, increased sys- temic vascular resistance, and decreased cardiac output are typical adverse effects of these agents in mammalian species.[30] Indeed, IN administration of dexmedetomi- dine in pigeons resulted in significant sedation and restraint but was accompanied by a significant decrease in heart rate (median 128 beats per minute).[18] Although these agents offer excellent sedation and chemical restraint that may be required under certain circumstances, caution must be exercised with their administration, and car- diovascular monitoring and supplemental oxygen should be available. Dexmedetomi- dine is readily antagonized by atipamezole given via IM or IN routes. Dosing of atipamezole is based on an agonist-antagonist ratio; atipamezole should be given at an equal volume (based on usage of 0.5 mg/mL dexmedetomidine and 5 mg/mL atipamezole) or at 10 times the agonist dose (eg, 1 mg atipamezole per 0.1 mg dexmedetomidine).

INDUCTION

Anesthetic induction is a critical period that can be associated with increased odds of anesthetic-related morbidity and mortality. Anesthesia-related mortality has been re- ported to be higher in birds (3.6%) than in other animals, and the higher risk should be informed to the owners.[31] In chickens and waterfowl, adverse events such as excitement, arrhythmias, hypothermia, hypotension, regurgitation and aspiration, endotracheal tube obstruction, apnea, and sudden death have been reported during general anesthesia.[32–39]

Preoxygenation is crucial to prevent hypoxemia in case apnea occurs during induction, although this should be avoided in cases of severe distress or stress due to potential risk of arrhythmias associated with increased myocardial oxygen consumption. Birds have minimal to absent functional residual capacity, and preoxygenation will increase the time to oxygen desaturation. A variety of sizes and shapes of facemasks should be readily available due to the differences in beak shapes (**Fig. 2**). Alternatively, creatively adapted masks, such as syringe cases and plastic soda bottles sealed with a stretched procedure glove or plastic bag containing a small slit in the center can be used in waterfowl with long bills. Masks should contain the nares at the base of the upper bill or completely enclose the head, and ideally should be made of a clear material to visualize the nares to ensure they are not being obstructed and to monitor eyelid closure (**Fig. 3**). Oxygen flow rates of at least 1 to 2 L/min are recommended to guarantee high inspired fractions, especially if the mask is not appropriately sealed around the bill. Preoxygenation with 100% oxygen should be done with caution in breath-holding birds because apnea can occur when inspired fractions of oxygen greater than 40% are used during induction, which is attributed to desensitization of O_2-chemoreceptors.[31] In breath-holding birds, apnea and bradycardia also can occur when placing pressure or a mask over their beaks due to the diving reflex.[33] This reflex is induced by stimulation of nasal receptors during forced dives, and is eliminated in redhead ducks (*Aythya Americana*) by breathing 100% oxygen for at least 3 minutes.[40] Although there is a higher risk of apnea in breath-holding birds, preoxygenation should always be performed and airway equipment should be promptly available before induction of anesthesia.

Placing a Doppler probe over the metatarsal artery in premedicated animals before induction is recommended to monitor changes in heart rate and detect irregular pulses associated with dysrhythmias (**Fig. 4**). Removing the feathers before placing the Doppler probe increases the contact with the skin and improves the signal. Intubation should be performed with uncuffed endotracheal tubes after birds show signs of a surgical plane of anesthesia, including loss of palpebral, righting, and toe pinch

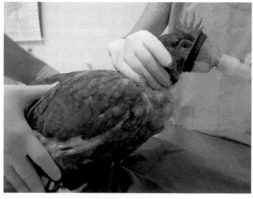

Fig. 2. A domestic chicken being manually restrained on a padded table with the wings gently held against the body with care not to compress the keel. The beak, including the nares, fits snuggly within a face mask for preoxygenation and inhalant anesthesia.

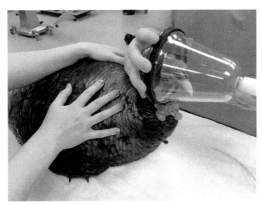

Fig. 3. A large and snug fitting face mask is used to fit over the beak of a domestic turkey. Note that the nares are completely within the mask and are not obstructed.

withdrawal reflexes, and muscle relaxation of the wings and neck. A laryngoscope (eg, size 0 Miller blade) or transilluminator should be used to assist with rapid and accurate intubation (**Fig. 5**). A tracheal seal can be achieved using a Cole tracheal tube with inner diameter 4 mm in chickens weighing between 1.5 and 2.5 kg.

Rebreathing circuits offer higher resistance to ventilation and should be avoided in chickens and waterfowl weighing less than 5 kg during preoxygenation and anesthesia under spontaneous ventilation. Mapleson D and Bain circuits are commonly used because of their light weight and low mechanical dead space, which allow a rapid adjustment of the fresh gas inflow and change in the anesthetic depth when inhalant anesthetics are used.

INJECTABLE ANESTHETICS

Propofol is the most commonly used injectable anesthetic owing to its rapid and smooth induction, and minimal accumulation in the body. In birds, the pharmacokinetics of propofol has only been described in great horned owls (*Bubo virginianus*) and showed a rapid initial distributional half-life (1.5 ± 0.6 minutes), slow elimination

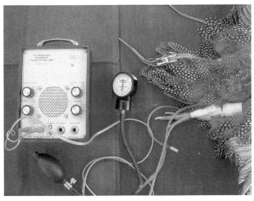

Fig. 4. A Doppler probe is secured over the medial metatarsal artery to assess heart rate in a domestic chicken.

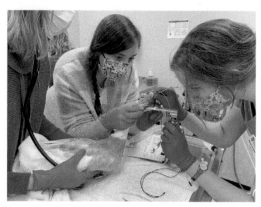

Fig. 5. A domestic duck is intubated while being manually restrained in a surgical plane of anesthesia. A laryngoscope is used to visualize the glottis and aid in rapid, accurate intubation with a noncuffed endotracheal tube.

half-life (40.7 ± 14.2 minutes), and a low volume of distribution at steady state (0.99 ± 0.18 L/kg).[41] However, extrapolating pharmacokinetic data to chickens and waterfowl should be performed with caution because of differences in body composition, especially for drugs that are highly lipid soluble, and have a longer half-life and volume of distribution in birds with higher body fat content.[42]

Studies describing induction of anesthesia with propofol in avian species have been performed in non-premedicated animals and titration of the drug to effect is recommended to avoid profound cardiopulmonary depression. In mute swans (*Cygnus olor*), induction with propofol (8 mg/kg IV) was smooth, and without signs of excitation or apnea.[43] In canvasback ducks (*Aythya valisineria*), propofol (10 mg/kg IV) provided a smooth induction and induced apnea in most of the animals, but signs of excitation, such as generalized tremors, paddling, and opisthotonos were observed. The propofol induction dose was significantly different between males (9.2 ± 1.6 mg/kg IV) and females (7.4 ± 1.6 mg/kg IV) in spectacled eiders (*Somateria fischeri*).[44] In chickens, induction apnea was observed in some animals after administration of propofol (9 mg/kg IV).[39] In a different study, propofol induced arrhythmias in most chickens, and when administered at 3 times the induction dose (6.8 mg/kg IV), all animals died, demonstrating a relative low anesthetic index.[45] Short-term apnea and a smooth induction were reported after administration of propofol (5 mg/kg IV) in turkeys.[46] Overall, propofol may be used as an induction agent with caution. Dosages should be carefully titrated to effect and patients should be closely monitored for adverse effects.

Alfaxalone is a neurosteroid that, similar to propofol, induces depression of the CNS by stimulation of $GABA_A$ receptors.[47] The biggest advantage of alfaxalone over propofol is the ability to administer it as an IM sedative. The pharmacokinetics of alfaxalone in birds have only been described in mallard ducks (*Anas platyrhynchos*), and the IM bioavailability was greater than 100%.[48] After IV administration, the volume of distribution, total body clearance, and elimination half-life were 3 ± 1.93 L/kg, 139 ± 67 mL/kg/min, and 15 ± 7.4 minutes, respectively.[48] Administration of 10 mg/kg IV or IM in unpremedicated mallard ducks was associated with poor induction quality, especially when administered IM, as animals exhibited signs of muscle spasms.[48] In chickens, alfaxalone administration (5 mg/kg IV) induced signs of excitation and muscle rigidity, and additional boluses (5–10 mg/kg IV) were required to induce muscle relaxation and allow endotracheal intubation.[49]

Ketamine is a noncompetitive antagonist of NMDA receptors and also exerts actions on opioid, monoaminergic, and muscarinic receptors.[47] Induction of anesthesia can be performed with either IV or IM administration and should be combined with a muscle relaxant, such as a benzodiazepine or an alpha-2 adrenergic receptor agonist, to avoid muscle stiffness and excitation. Ketamine can induce cardiac arrhythmias and prolonged recoveries, and is not considered a good alternative to induce anesthesia in most avian species.[33,50] Induction and maintenance with ketamine-diazepam-xylazine has been described in chickens undergoing typhlectomy; however, ketamine doses may vary significantly depending of the route of administration, and doses of the concomitant drugs.[51,52] Sinus tachycardia and ventricular tachycardia were observed in chickens anesthetized with medetomidine-midazolam-ketamine and maintained with sevoflurane.[53] Anesthetic-related deaths were reported after administration of medetomidine-midazolam-ketamine in ducks and elegant-crested tinamous (*Eudromia elegans*)[33,50]; these studies suggest that ketamine should be avoided to induce anesthesia if other options are available.

INHALANT ANESTHETICS

Inhalant anesthetics are considered the drug of choice to induce and maintain anesthesia in avian species because of rapid and smooth induction, easy control of anesthetic depth, elimination with minimal reliance on metabolic pathways, and better oxygenation provided by concurrent administration of oxygen.[54] Sevoflurane may be considered a superior induction option over isoflurane because its odor is less pungent and it has a lower blood gas partition coefficient, which possibly allows a faster induction; however, no significant differences in induction times were found between isoflurane and sevoflurane in different avian species.[55–57] Clinicians often choose an inhalational agent based on individual circumstances and preference.

Induction can be performed using 2 different techniques. The first technique uses small, incremental increases in the vaporizer settings of 0.5% every 30 seconds, to a maximum of 5% isoflurane or 8% sevoflurane, until the bird becomes unconscious and can be intubated. The second technique uses a fixed vaporizer concentration of isoflurane (3.5%–5.0%) or sevoflurane (6.0%–8.0%) until the bird can be intubated. In chickens, the induction time is significantly shorter when 5% isoflurane is used (0.87 ± 0.15 minutes) compared with 4% (2.37 ± 0.18 minutes) or 3.5% (5.83 ± 0.33 minutes).[58] Other studies reported a median induction time of 2 minutes with 5% isoflurane,[38,59] and 2 to 3 minutes when 5% sevoflurane[60] was used in chickens. In helmeted guineafowls induced with 8% sevoflurane, the median induction time was 3 minutes.[61] Studies with chickens and backyard fowl do not report induction apnea when inhalant anesthetics were used. It is important to note, however, that premedication with sedatives or analgesics may significantly decrease the inhalant anesthetic requirement and induction times. Regardless of preanesthetic sedation level, birds should be closely monitored during induction of anesthesia to detect apnea, bradycardia, and dysrhythmias.

Ducks are more sensitive to respiratory depression induced by inhalant anesthetics and are more likely to become apneic during induction compared with chickens.[62] This has been shown by the difference of the isoflurane respiratory anesthetic index (AI) between ducks (1.65) and chickens (2.80).[62,63] The isoflurane AI is calculated as a ratio between the expired concentration necessary to induce apnea and its MAC; higher AI values mean less respiratory depression is induced. It has been hypothesized that breath-holding birds are more sensitive to apnea induced by inhalant anesthetics due to physiologic differences, such as enhanced oxygen storages and production of energy via anaerobic metabolism.[64] Most of the canvasback ducks induced with isoflurane using the small increment technique developed apnea after 4.7 ± 3.4 minutes and required assisted ventilation.[33] When working with waterfowl, it is important to anticipate unexpected periods of apnea and be prepared to endotracheally intubate and administer positive-pressure ventilation as necessary.

MAINTENANCE

Fresh gas flow rates between 200 and 400 mL/kg per minute should be selected when non-rebreathing circuits are used to avoid carbon dioxide rebreathing. Inspired fractions of oxygen greater than 40% induced mild hypoventilation attributed to a reduction in tidal volume in pekin ducks (A platyrhynchos domestica) anesthetized with isoflurane.[65] Ventilatory support should be available when oxygen concentrations greater than 21% are used. Mechanical ventilation is recommended for most cases, especially anesthetic procedures longer than 1 hour. The peak inspiratory pressure should not exceed 15 cm H_2O in ducks and chickens and the respiratory rate should be adjusted to maintain an $ETCO_2$ between 30 and 40 mm Hg.

The effect of body position under isoflurane anesthesia has been assessed in raptors, and, although dorsal recumbency results in greater compression of the lungs and air sacs,[66] it also resulted in lower dead space ventilation and higher tidal volume compared with lateral recumbency.[67] Nevertheless, raptors in dorsal recumbency became progressively more hypercapnic compared with lateral recumbency, but those results should be extrapolated with caution to chickens and waterfowls because they have a relatively larger pectoral muscle mass. The amplitude of breathing in chickens in dorsal recumbency is reduced by 40% to 50% compared with erect posture,[68] and careful attention should be paid to positioning, especially in more heavily conditioned birds. Visual assessment should accompany monitoring of respiratory rate and $ETCO_2$ to aid in evaluation of an increase in respiratory effort with positional changes.

INJECTABLE ANESTHETICS

Total intravenous anesthesia (TIVA) may be required in a variety of clinical scenarios, including open air sacs or open fractures of pneumatic bones. TIVA with propofol has been reported in chickens at a rate of 0.81 ± 0.15 mg/kg per minute.[39] Administration of methadone (6 mg/kg IM), nalbuphine (12.5 mg/kg IM), and fentanyl (30 µg/kg loading dose, followed by 30 µg/kg per hour IV) reduced the propofol requirement by 41% to 47%, 43% to 51%, and 8% to 17%, respectively. However, administration of fentanyl was performed in the metatarsal vein and part of the drug could have been eliminated by the renal portal system. In mute swans, a propofol constant rate infusion of 0.85 mg/kg per minute IV provided adequate anesthesia without apnea. Administration of propofol may result in satisfactory and safe anesthesia of avian patients, but careful titration to effect and judicious monitoring of cardiovascular and respiratory parameters are keys to success.

INHALANT ANESTHETICS

The MAC (minimum anesthetic concentration) of an inhalant anesthetic is the dose that prevents movement in 50% of the animals exposed to a supramaximal stimulation and describes the difference in potency between agents and species. MAC values in Galliformes and ducks are described in **Table 1**. It has been shown that opioids have a short anesthetic-sparing effect in Galliformes. In helmeted guineafowls, butorphanol

| Table 1 | | |
| Minimum anesthetic concentration of isoflurane and sevoflurane in Galliformes and ducks | | |
Species	Isoflurane, %	Sevoflurane, %
Chicken (Gallus gallus domesticus)[38,59,63,76–78]	1.10–1.25 ± 0.09–0.20	2.21 ± 0.32
Helmeted guineafowl (Numida meleagris)[61]	—	2.90 ± 0.10
Pekin duck (Anas platyrhynchos)[62]	1.30 ± 0.23	—

(4 mg/kg IV) decreased the MAC of sevoflurane by 20% after 15 minutes of administration, but this effect was insignificant after 30 minutes[61]; however, this dose and route of administration induced ventricular fibrillation in 2 animals and was considered unsafe.[69] In chickens, methadone (6 mg/kg IM) reduced the isoflurane MAC by 30% after 15 minutes of administration, but this effect was also insignificant after 30 minutes.[59] Methadone induced occasional atrioventricular blocks and ventricular premature complexes, decreases in heart rate, and increases in systemic blood pressure. The pharmacokinetics of methadone in chickens anesthetized with isoflurane was characterized by a large volume of distribution at steady state (5.42 L/kg), elimination half-life of 177 minutes, and an IM bioavailability of 79%.[70] Fentanyl (30 µg/kg IV over 1 minute) had the greatest anesthetic-sparing effect in chickens and reduced the isoflurane MAC by 40% after 5 minutes of administration; however, this effect was short-lived and no arrhythmias were observed.[38] The authors suggest a fentanyl loading dose of 20 to 30 µg/kg and a constant rate infusion of 20 to 30 µg/kg per hour in chickens. Because opioids have shown to induce arrhythmias in different MAC studies in birds,[59,69,71] a slow IV loading dose or IM injections along with electrocardiogram (ECG) placement before the opioid administration is recommended. Although opioids may induce a small, or no, MAC-sparing effect in birds, this effect is not necessarily related to their analgesic effect.[72] Tramadol, for example, did not induce a MAC-sparing effect in a white-eyed parakeets (Psittacara leucophthalmus) study,[71] but it is an effective analgesic in Muscovy ducks (Cairina moschata domestica).[73]

MONITORING

Immediately after endotracheal intubation, a capnometer should be connected to the endotracheal tube to confirm intubation. Cardiovascular status can be assessed by the presence of the capnograph wave, Doppler pulse sounds, and cardiac auscultation. An appropriate anesthetic depth is characterized by loss of jaw tone, palpebral and toe pinch withdrawal reflexes, presence of corneal reflex, and adequate muscle relaxation. Sudden bradycardia during anesthesia indicates a profound anesthetic depth, which can be associated with administration of MAC-sparing drugs, hypothermia, and hypovolemia.

Heart rate and rhythm can be monitored using cardiac auscultation, Doppler flow probe, pulse oximeter, or an ECG (**Figs. 6** and **7**). Heart rate and mean arterial blood pressure of gallinaceous birds and waterfowl, anesthetized under 1 MAC of isoflurane or sevoflurane, range between 150 and 300 beats per minute and 80 to 140 mm Hg, respectively.[59,61,62] Blood pressure can be assessed directly by placing a catheter in the ulnar or brachial artery, or indirectly using a Doppler flow probe coupled with a sphygmomanometer. Systolic blood pressure measured using the Doppler method should be interpreted with caution, as it can be underestimated in birds.[74]

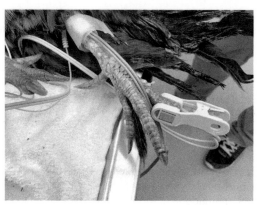

Fig. 6. A pulse oximeter may be secured to various nonfeathered portions of a bird's body, including the toe, as pictured here.

Birds have nucleated red blood cells and pulse oximetry underestimates values of oxygen saturation due to a greater absorption ratio.[75] However, observation of oxygen saturation trends is still valuable, and placement of the pulse oximeter is a simple and practical monitoring tool. Pulse oximetry probes may be placed on a variety of sites, dependent on the size of the bird. Transmittance-style ("clamp") probes may be placed on toes, combs, or wattles; caution is advised against placement on the tongue

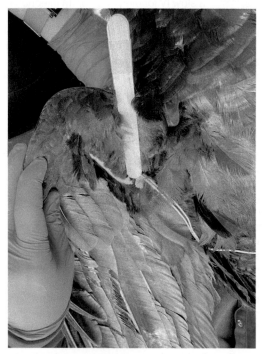

Fig. 7. A Doppler probe is secured against the ulnar artery using a tongue depressor on the inner aspect of the wing of a domestic turkey.

because of the risk of tongue necrosis. Reflectance-style ("flat") probes, depending on the probe size, may be placed against any pulsatile vascular bed, in the dorsal oropharynx, or, cautiously, in the cloaca.

Body temperature should be measured using an esophageal thermometer and attempts to maintain normothermia using a warm water blanket, radiation lamp, and forced-air warming devices should be done immediately after induction. Hypothermia can lead to arrhythmias, profound anesthetic depth, and may substantially prolong the recovery and extubation times.

RECOVERY

Recovery is a sensitive stage of anesthesia that should be monitored closely to avoid self-injury from emergence delirium and flopping behavior. Manual restraint or gently wrapping the bird with a towel can prevent this behavior. Excitation and opisthotonos has been reported in chickens and mute swans recovering from propofol.[39,43] In ducks, propofol provided a smooth recovery, and with isoflurane they tended to struggle.[33] Extubation times in Galliformes anesthetized with isoflurane or sevoflurane administered a single dose of butorphanol (2–4 mg/kg IV), fentanyl (10–30 µg/kg IV) or methadone (3 mg/kg IM) were an average of 5 minutes; however, higher doses of methadone (6 mg/kg IM) increased the extubation time to more than 20 minutes.[38,59,61] Regurgitation has been reported in chickens anesthetized with isoflurane, and recovery in sternal recumbency is suggested to avoid aspiration.[59]

SUMMARY

As with any other species, a balanced and well-informed approach to sedation and general anesthesia in backyard poultry and waterfowl is critical to ensure a safe and successful procedure. Anatomy in these species is similar to other birds and there are multiple injectable and inhalant anesthetic options that should be carefully considered.

REFERENCES

1. Centers for Disease Control. Backyard poultry. Available at: https://www.cdc.gov/healthypets/pets/farm-animals/backyard-poultry.html. Accessed February 6, 2021.

2. United States Department of Agriculture. Urban chicken ownership in four U.S. cities. Available at: https://www.nal.usda.gov/exhibits/ipd/frostonchickens/exhibits/show/backyardchickens/usdaresearchbackyard. Accessed February 6, 2021.

3. Elkhoraibi C, Blatchford RA, Pitesky ME, et al. Backyard chickens in the United States: a survey of flock owners. Poult Sci 2014;93(11):2920–31.

4. Vaught ME, Gladden JN, Rozanski EA, et al. Reasons for evaluation on an emergency basis of and short-term outcomes for chickens from backyard flocks: 78 cases (2014-2017). J Am Vet Med Assoc 2019;254(10):1196–203.

5. Heard D. Anesthesia. In: Speer BL, editor. Current therapy in avian medicine and surgery. 1st edition. St. Louis, Missouri: Elsevier; 2016. p. 601–15.

6. Khamas W, Rutllant-Labeaga J, Greenacre CB. Physical examination, anatomy, and physiology. In: Greenacre CB, Morishita TY, editors. Backyard poultry medicine and surgery: a guide for veterinary practitioners. Hoboken, New Jersey: John Wiley and Sons, Inc; 2015. p. 95–116.

7. O'Malley B. Avian anatomy. In: O'Malley B, editor. Clinical anatomy and physiology of exotic species: structure and function of mammals, birds, reptiles, and amphibians. Philadelphia: Saunders Ltd; 2005. p. 97–161.

8. Mans C, Guzman DSM, Lahner LL, et al. Sedation and physiologic response to manual restraint after intranasal administration of midazolam in Hispaniolan Amazon parrots (*Amazona ventralis*). J Avian Med Surg 2012;26(3):130–9.

9. Concannon KT, Dodam JR, Hellyer PW. Influence of mu- and kappa-opioid agonist on isoflurane minimal anesthetic concentration in chickens. Am J Vet Res 1995;56(6):806–11.

10. Zaheer OA, Sanchez A, Beaufrere H. Minimum anesthetic concentration of isoflurane and sparing effect of midazolam in Quaker parrots (*Myiopsitta monachus*). Vet Anaesth Analg 2020;47(3):341–6.

11. Gilbert DB, Patterson TA, Rose SP. Midazolam induces amnesia in a simple, one-trial maze-learning task in young chicks. Pharmacol Biochem Behav 1989;34(2):439–42.

12. Rathmell JP, Rosow CE. Intravenous sedatives and hypnotics. In: Flood P, Rathmell JP, Shafer S, et al, editors. Stoelting's pharmacolgy and physiology in anesthetic practice. 5th edition. Philadelphia: Wolters Kluwer Health; 2014. p. 160–203.

13. Greenacre CB, Lusby AL. Physiologic responses of Amazon parrots (*Amazona* species) to manual restraint. J Avian Med Surg 2004;18(1):19–22.

14. Blas J. Stress in birds. In: Scanes CG, editor. Sturkie's avian physiology. 6th edition. Waltham: Academic Press; 2015. p. 769–810.

15. Desmarchelier MR, Beaudry F, Ferrek ST, al at. Determination of the pharmacokinetics of a single oral dose of trazodone and its effect on the activity level of domestic pigeons (*Columba livia*). Am J Vet Res 2019;80(1):102–9.

16. Vesel N, Eskandari MH. Sedative effects of midazolam and xylazine with and without ketamine and detomidine alone following intranasal administration in ring-necked parakeets. J Am Vet Med Assoc 2006;228(3):383–8.

17. Vesal N, Zare P. Clinical evaluation of intranasal benzodiazepines, alpha-agonists, and their antagonists in canaries. Vet Anaesth Analg 2006;33(3):143–8.

18. Hornak S, Liptak T, Ledecky V, et al. A preliminary trial of the sedation induced by intranasal administration of midazolam alone or in combination with dexmedetomidine and reversal by atipamezole for a short-term immobilization in pigeons. Vet Anaesth Analg 2015;42(2):192–6.

19. Doss GA, Fink DM, Mans C. Assessment of sedation after intranasal administration of midazolam and midazolam-butorphanol in cockatiels (*Nymphicus hollandicus*). Am J Vet Res 2018;79(12):1246–52.

20. Net RL, Mulcahy DM, Santamaria-Bouvier A, et al. Intranasal administration of midazolam hydrochloride improves survival in female surf scoters (*Melanitta perspicillata*) surgically implanted with intracoelomic transmitters. J Zoo Wildl Med 2019;50(1):167–75.

21. Crowe TP, Greenlee MHW, Kanthasamy AG, et al. Mechanism of intranasal drug delivery to the brain. Life Sci 2018;195:44–52.

22. Day TK, Roge CK. Evaluation of sedation in quail induced by use of midazolam and reversed by use of flumazenil. J Am Vet Med Assoc 1996;209(5):969–71.

23. Cortright KA, Wetzlich SE, Craigmill AL. Plasma pharmacokinetics of midazolam in chickens, turkeys, pheasants, and bobwhite quail. J Vet Pharmacol Ther 2007;30(5):429–36.

24. Martel A, Mans C, Doss GA, et al. Effects of midazolam and midazolam-butorphanol on gastrointestinal transit time and motility in cockatiels (*Nymphicus hollandicus*). J Avian Med Surg 2018;32(4):286–93.

25. Kubiak M, Roach L, Eatwell K. The influence of a combined butorphanol and midazolam premedication on anesthesia on anesthesia in psittacid species. J Avian Med Surg 2016;30(4):317–23.

26. Heatley JJ, Cary J, Kingsley L, et al. Midazolam sedates Passeriformes for field sampling but affects multiple venous blood analytes. Vet Med (Auckl) 2015; 6:61–9.

27. Khurshid N, Agarwal V, Iyengar S. Expression of mu- and delta-opioid receptors in song control regions of adult male zebra finches (*Taenopygia guttata*). J Chem Neuroanat 2009;37(3):158–69.

28. Csillag A, Bourne RC, Stewart MG. Distribution of mu, delta, and kappa opioid receptor binding sites in the brain of the one-day-old domestic chick (*Gallus domesticus*): an in vitro quantitative autoradiographic study. J Comp Neurol 1990; 302(3):543–51.

29. Santangelo B, Ferrari D, Di Martino I, et al. Dexmedetomidine chemical restraint of two raptor species undergoing inhalation anesthesia. Vet Res Commun 2009; 33(Supl 1):209–11.

30. Murrell JC, Hellebreker LJ. Medetomidine and dexmedetomidine: a review of cardiovascular effects and antinociceptive properties in the dog. Vet Anaesth Analg 2005;32(3):117–27.

31. Seamon AB, Hofmelster EH, Divers SJ. Outcome following inhalation anesthesia in birds at a veterinary referral hospital: 352 cases (2004–2014). J Am Vet Med Assoc 2017;251(7):814–7.

32. Ludders JW. Minimal anesthetic concentration and cardiopulmonary dose-response of halothane in ducks. Vet Surg 1994;21(4):319–24.

33. Machin KL, Caulkett NA. Evaluation of isoflurane and propofol anesthesia for intraabdominal transmitter placement in nesting female canvasback ducks. J Wildl Dis 2000;36(2):324–34.

34. Mulcahy DM. Free-living waterfowl and shorebirds. In: West G, Heard D, Caulkett N, editors. Zoo animal and wildlife immobilization and anesthesia. Ames: Willey Blackwell; 2014. p. 481–505.

35. Naganobu K, Haglo M, Sonoda T, et al. Arrhythmogenic effect of hypercapnia in ducks anesthetized with halothane. Am J Vet Res 2001;62(1):127–9.

36. Brenner DJ, Larsen RS, Pascoe PJ, et al. Somatosensory evoked potentials and sensory nerve conduction velocities in the thoracic limb of mallard ducks (*Anas platyrhynchos*). Am J Vet Res 2008;69(11):1476–80.

37. O'Kane PM, Connerton IF, White KL. Pilot study of long-term anaesthesia in broiler chickens. Vet Anaesth Analg 2016;43(1):72–5.

38. Rocha RW, Escobar A, Pypendop BH, et al. Effects of a single intravenous bolus of fentanyl on the minimum anesthetic concentration of isoflurane in chickens (*Gallus gallus domesticus*). Vet Anaesth Analg 2017;44(3):546–54.

39. Santos ER, Monteiro ER, Herrera JR, et al. Total intravenous anesthesia in domestic chicken (*Gallus gallus domesticus*) with propofol alone or in combination with methadone, nalbuphine or fentanyl for ulna osteotomy. Vet Anaesth Analg 2020; 47(3):347–55.

40. Furilla RA, Jones DR. The contribution of nasal receptors to the cardiac response to diving in restrained and unrestrained redhead ducks (*Aythya Americana*). J Exp Biol 1986;121:227–38.

41. Hawkins MG, Wright BD, Pascoe PJ, et al. Pharmacokinetics and anesthetic and cardiopulmonary effects of propofol in red-tailed hawks (*Buteo jamaicensis*) and great horned owls (*Bubo virginianus*). Am J Vet Res 2003;64(6):667–83.

42. Pascoe PJ, Pypendop BH, Pavez Phillips JC, et al. Pharmacokinetics of fentanyl after intravenous administration in isoflurane-anesthetized red-tailed hawks (*Buteo jamaicensis*) and Hispaniolan Amazon parrots (*Amazona ventralis*). Am J Vet Res 2018;79(6):606–13.

43. Muller K, Holzapfel J, Brunnberg L. Total intravenous anesthesia by boluses or by continuous rate infusion of propofol in mute swans (*Cygnus olor*). Vet Anaesth Analg 2011;38(4):286–91.

44. Mulcahy DM, Tuomi P, Larsen S. Differential mortality of male spectacled eiders (*Somateria fisheri*) and kind eiders (*Somateria spectabilis*) subsequent to anesthesia with propofol, bupivacaine and ketoprofen. J Avian Med Surg 2003; 17(3):117–23.

45. Lukasik VM, Gentz EJ, Erb HN, et al. Cardiopulmonary effects of propofol anesthesia in chickens (*Gallus gallus domesticus*). J Avian Med Surg 1997; 11(2):93–7.

46. Schumacher J, Citino SB, Hernandes K, et al. Cardiopulmonary and anesthetic effects of propofol in wild turkeys. Am J Vet Res 1997;58(9):1014–7.

47. Berry SH. Injectable anesthetics. In: Grimm KA, Lamont LA, Tranquilli WJ, et al, editors. Veterinary anesthesia and analgesia. The fifth edition of Lumb and Jones. Ames: Willey Blackwell; 2015. p. 277–96.

48. Kruse TN, Messenger KM, Bowman AS, et al. Pharmacokinetics and pharmacodynamics of alfaxalone after a single intramuscular or intravascular injection in mallard ducks (*Anas platyrhynchos*). J Vet Pharmacol Therap 2019;42(6):713–21.

49. White DM, Martinez-Taboada F. Induction of anesthesia with intravenous alfaxolone in two Isa Brown chickens (*Gallus gallus domesticus*). J Exot Pet Med 2019;29:119–22.

50. Ronaldson HJ, Monticelli P, Cuff AR, et al. Anesthesia and anesthetic-related complications of 8 elegant-crested tinamous (*Eudromia elegans*) undergoing experimental surgery. J Avian Med Surg 2020;34(1):17–25.

51. Maiti SK, Tiwary R, Vasan P, et al. Xylazine, diazepam and midazolam premedicated ketamine anaesthesia in White Leghorn cockerels for typhlectomy. J S Afr Vet Assoc 2006;77(1):12–8.

52. Mostachio GQ, de-Oliveira LD, Carciofi AC, et al. The effects of anesthesia with a combination of intramuscular xylazine–diazepam–ketamine on heart rate, respiratory rate and cloacal temperature in roosters. Vet Anaesth Analg 2008;35(3): 232–6.

53. Celik Y, Atalan G, Gune V, et al. Use of medetomidine, midazolam, ketamine, and sevoflurane as an anesthetic protocol for domestic chickens. Vet Mex 2020; 7(1):1–12.

54. Ludders JW. Inhaled anesthesia for birds. In: Gleed R, Ludders JW, editors. Recent advances in veterinary anesthesia and analgesia: companion animals. International Veterinary Information Service; 2001. Available at: https://www.ivis. org/library/recent-advances-veterinary-anesthesia-and-analgesia-companion-animals. Accessed April 1, 2021.

55. Joyner PH, Jones MP, Ward D, et al. Induction and recovery characteristics and cardiopulmonary effects of sevoflurane and isoflurane in bald eagles. Am J Vet Res 2008;69(1):13–22.

56. Granone TD, de Francisco ON, Killos MD, et al. Comparison of three different inhalant anesthetic agents (isoflurane, sevoflurane, desflurane) in red-tailed hawks (*Buteo jamaicensis*). Vet Anaesth Analg 2012;39(1):29–37.

57. Chan FT, Chang GR, Wang HC, et al. Anesthesia with isoflurane and sevoflurane in the crested serpent eagle (*Spilornis cheela hoya*): minimum anesthetic concentration, physiological effects, hematocrit, plasma chemistry and behavioral effects. J Vet Med Sci 2013;75(12):1591–600.

58. Deori P, Sarma KK, Nath PJ, et al. Physiological alteration, quality of anesthesia and economy of isoflurane in domestic chickens (*Gallus domesticus*). Vet World 2017;10(5):493–7.

59. Escobar A, da Rocha RW, Pypendop BH, et al. Effects of methadone on the minimum anesthetic concentration of isoflurane, and its effects on heart rate, blood pressure and ventilation during isoflurane anesthesia in hens (*Gallus gallus domesticus*). PLOS One 2016;11(3):e0152546.

60. Naganobu K, Ise K, Miyamoto T, et al. Sevoflurane anesthesia in chickens during spontaneous and controlled ventilation. Vet Rec 2003;152(2):45–8.

61. Escobar A, Valadao CA, Brosnan RJ, et al. Effects of butorphanol on the minimum anesthetic concentration of sevoflurane in guineafowl (*Numida meleagris*). Am J Vet Res 2012;73(2):183–8.

62. Ludders JW, Mitchell GS, Rode J. Minimal anesthetic concentration and cardiopulmonary dose response of isoflurane in ducks. Vet Surg 1990;19(4):304–7.

63. Midon M, Escobar A, Yamada DI, et al. Isoflurane respiratory anesthetic index in chickens (*Gallus gallus domesticus*). J Zoo Wildl Med 2021,52(1).327–31.

64. Butler PJ, Jones DR. Physiology of diving of birds and mammals. Physiol Rev 1997;77(3):837–99.

65. Seaman GC, Ludders JW, Erb HN, et al. Effects of low and high fractions of inspired oxygen on ventilation in ducks anesthetized with isoflurane. Am J Vet Res 1994;55(3):395–8.

66. Malka S, Hawkins MC, Jones JH, et al. Effect of body position on respiratory system volumes in anesthetized red-tailed hawks (*Buteo jamaicensis*) as measured via computed tomography. Am J Vet Res 2009;70(9):1155–60.

67. Hawkins MG, Malka S, Pascoe PJ, et al. Evaluation of the effects of dorsal versus lateral recumbency on the cardiopulmonary system during anesthesia with isoflurane in red-tailed hawks (*Buteo jamaicensis*). Am J Vet Res 2013;74(1):136–43.

68. King AS, Payne DC. Normal breathing and the effects of posture in *Gallus domesticus*. J Physiol 1964;174:340–7.

69. Escobar A, Valadao CA, Brosnan RJ, et al. Cardiopulmonary effects of butorphanol in sevoflurane-anesthetized guineafowl (*Numida meleagris*). Vet Anaesth Analg 2014;41(3):284–9.

70. Escobar A, Barletta M, Pypendop BH, et al. Pharmacokinetics and pharmacodynamics of methadone administered intravenously and intramuscularly to isoflurane-anesthetized chickens. Am J Vet Res 2021;82(3):181–8.

71. Escobar A, da Rocha RW, Midon M, et al. Effects of tramadol on the minimum anesthetic concentration of isoflurane in white-eyed parakeets (*Psittacara leucophthalmus*). J Zoo Wildl Med 2017;48(2):380–7.

72. Brosnan RJ, Pypendop BH, Siao KT, et al. Effects of remifentanil on measures of anesthetic immobility and analgesia in cats. Am J Vet Res 2009;70(9):1065–71.

73. Bailey RS, Sheldon JD, Allender MC. Analgesic efficacy of tramadol compared with meloxicam in ducks (*Cairina moschata domestica*) evaluated by ground-reactive forces. J Avian Med Surg 2019;33(2):133–40.

74. Zehnder AM, Hawkings MG, Pascoe PJ, et al. Evaluation of indirect blood pressure monitoring in awake and anesthetized red-tailed hawks (*Buteo jamaicensis*): effect of cuff size placement, and monitoring equipment. Vet Anaesth Analg 2009;36(5):464–79.

75. Schmitt PM, Gobel T, Trautvetter E. Evaluation of pulse oximetry as a monitoring method in avian anesthesia. J Avian Med Surg 1998;12(2):91–9.

76. Naganobu K, Hagio M. Dose-related cardiovascular effects of isoflurane in chickens during controlled ventilation. J Vet Med Sci 2000;62:435–7.

77. Naganobu K, Fujisawa Y, Ohde H, et al. Determination of the minimum anesthetic concentration and cardiovascular dose response for sevoflurane in chickens during controlled ventilation. Vet Surg 2000;29:102–5.

78. Martin-Jurado O, Vogt R, Kutter AP, et al. Effect of inhalation of isoflurane at end-tidal concentrations greater than, equal to, and less than the minimum anesthetic concentration on bispectral index in chickens. Am J Vet Res 2008;69:1254–61.

Rabbit Sedation and Anesthesia

Sara Gardhouse, DVM, DABVP (ECM), DACZM[a],*, Andrea Sanchez, DVM, DVSc, DACVAA[b]

KEYWORDS

- Rabbit • *Oryctolagus cuniculus* • Anesthesia • Monitoring • Premedication
- Induction • Local anesthesia • Recovery

KEY POINTS

- Rabbits (*Oryctolagus cuniculus*) are prey animals with several behaviors that make them unique anesthetic candidates that require special considerations in the preanesthetic, anesthetic, and postanesthetic periods.
- As prey animals, the preoperative assessment of the rabbit patient is critical, as they instinctually hide any signs of illness and disease.
- Multimodal anesthesia (balanced anesthesia) using various drugs and routes of administration helps to provide the safest anesthetic plan for rabbits.
- There are various ways to obtain airway access in rabbits, each of which has its advantages and disadvantages.
- The recovery period following anesthesia in rabbits is as critical as the preanesthetic and anesthetic periods, and should not be ignored for its importance.

INTRODUCTION

Increasingly, rabbits are presented to veterinarians for evaluation, diagnostics, and treatment, and with them on the rise as one of the most common domestic pets in North America, owners expect high-level medical and surgical care.[1] Deep sedation is often necessary for procedures requiring restraint, evaluation, or minor medical needs, and general anesthesia is frequently required for medical and surgical procedures. Successful management of the rabbit anesthetic case requires understanding of basic anesthetic principles, awareness of the limitations, and the necessary requirements to ensure high standards of anesthetic care for the patient.

Disclosure: The authors have nothing to disclose.
[a] Department of Clinical Sciences, Kansas State University, 1800 Denison Avenue, Manhattan, KS 66506, USA; [b] Department of Clinical Studies, Ontario Veterinary College, 55 Stone Road East, Ontario N1G 2W1, Canada
* Corresponding author.
E-mail address: sgardhous@vet.k-state.edu

ANAMNESIS

A thorough history and husbandry evaluation is critical to the understanding of rabbits.[2] Evaluation must include a thorough evaluation of the husbandry and a chronologic report of the presenting complaint.[2] Asking detailed questions is key to the assessment of the patient, and open-ended questions tend to provide better information.[2]

PREANESTHETIC ASSESSMENT AND CONSIDERATIONS

Rabbits have a reputation of being difficult or dangerous to anesthetize.[3–5] As a prey species, they are adept at concealing illness, and suitability as an anesthetic candidate may not be as ideal as initially perceived on presentation. As a result, a thorough preanesthetic evaluation is key to a good outcome. A complete physical examination including cardiac, respiratory, and gastrointestinal assessment (**Table 1**), and preanesthetic bloodwork may reveal underlying disease that has been concealed.[2] If there is suspicion for fluid deficits or gastrointestinal ileus, stabilization should be performed before sedation or anesthesia. An accurate body weight is critical to successful anesthesia and to ensure accurate dosing of drugs.

Overall anesthetic mortality reported in healthy rabbits ranges from 1.39%[3] to 4.8%.[4] Prevalence is even higher when evaluating anesthetic and sedation-related deaths in systemically ill rabbits with a 7.37% risk of death in one of these studies' populations.[3] Although the mortality associated with anesthesia is generally considered to occur during the anesthetic event, this study also revealed that rabbits are as likely to die in the immediate 3 hours following anesthesia, and that these deaths can occur up to 48 hours postanesthetically.[3]

Owing to rabbits' prey nature, a crucial consideration to reduce stress before anesthesia is ensuring suitable accommodations away from cats, dogs, ferrets, and birds of prey that are their predators in natural settings.[6] This can be enhanced with the provision of privacy shelters and hides, and administration of anxiolytics and/or sedatives such as benzodiazepines.[6] Other strategies to reduce stress include providing a litter tray and housing with their bonded mate when possible.[6]

Another important consideration is the large surface-area-to-volume ratio and poor thermal tolerance that makes small mammals, like rabbits, susceptible to hypothermia during general anesthesia. Inhalant anesthetics can also alter thermoregulatory thresholds for compensatory responses in a dose-dependent fashion and also have a cooling effect on the respiratory membranes.[7] Thermoregulatory systems can be further depressed by other drugs used in the perioperative period such as opioids.[8]

Hypothermia has the potential to create substantial impairment in cardiovascular performance, slow recovery from anesthesia, impair coagulation, and decrease metabolism of anesthetic drugs.[9,10] A significant association between hypothermia at the time of admission and mortality has been demonstrated in rabbits.[11,12] Therefore, measurement of body temperature and thermal support during the perioperative period are critical to improve outcomes.

Table 1 Normal vital parameters in the rabbit[13]	
Parameter	**Reference Range**
Heart rate (beats/min)	200–300
Respiratory rate (breaths/min)	32–60
Temperature (°C [°F])	38.5–39.5 [101.3–103.1]

PREOPERATIVE BLOOD TESTS

It is straightforward to obtain a blood sample from most rabbits without the aid of sedation.[6] At a minimum, a packed cell volume (reference interval 34%–43%),[13] total protein (5.0–7.5 g/dL),[13] and blood glucose (4.1–8.2 mmol/L; 74–148 mg/dL)[13] should be performed before anesthesia, but ideally, a complete blood cell count and biochemistry profile should be performed to provide a more complete picture of overall health.[6] Additional diagnostics such as a urinalysis and diagnostic imaging may be indicated depending on the reason for anesthesia.[6]

Blood glucose can be used as a prognostic indicator in rabbits.[14] A significant relationship between blood glucose and food intake, signs of stress, and severity of clinical disease has been demonstrated.[14] Stressed rabbits demonstrate a higher blood glucose than those with no signs of stress, and complete anorexia results in a higher blood glucose than those with normal food intake or hyporexia.[14] Severe hyperglycemia (>20 mmol/L, 360 mg/dL) has been associated with a poor prognosis.[14] In addition, in cases of diagnosed intestinal obstruction, the mean blood glucose was higher (24.7 mmol/L, 444.6 mg/dL) compared with nonobstructive gastrointestinal ileus (8.5 mmol/L, 153 mg/dL).[14] Based on these results, blood glucose can be used as an indicator of the severity of a rabbit's condition on presentation, and aid in differentiation of gastrointestinal ileus versus true gastrointestinal obstruction.[14]

In addition to blood glucose, cholesterol, non–high-density lipoprotein cholesterol, and triglycerides are also indicators of disease in rabbits and are associated with evidence of severe infection or sepsis, renal failure, and hepatopathy.[15] These parameters should be taken into consideration before anesthesia and included as part of the conversation with the owner regarding prognosis and risks.

FASTING

Rabbits are unable to vomit because of a highly developed and muscular cardiac sphincter.[16] Contrary to other species, long fasting times are contraindicated and it is typically recommended to provide access to food and water close to the time of anesthesia to ensure ongoing gastrointestinal motility; however, removing food 1 to 2 hours before anesthesia and after premedication reduces the risk of finding food in the oral cavity during intubation that could be aspirated into the respiratory tract.[17] Following an anesthetic event, food should be available as soon as the rabbit is ambulatory and feeding support should be considered when alert and swallowing.[17,18]

FLUID THERAPY

Preoperative assessment of hydration can be challenging in rabbits and intraoperative monitoring of blood pressure can also present unique challenges; however, preoperative assessment of packed cell volume, total protein, blood urea nitrogen, creatinine, and urine specific gravity can provide some assessment with respect to overall hydration.[8] An important consideration is to ensure constant hydration of the gastrointestinal tract to ensure there is normal gastrointestinal motility and function; without attention to this detail, potential consequences such as a functional ileus can be fatal.[18,19]

In human and small animal medicine, it is becoming more widely acknowledged that intravenous (IV) fluid therapy should not be all encompassing as a volume per hour, but rather as a goal-oriented therapy titrated to the needs of the individual.[20] As significant as hypovolemia and hypoperfusion can be, overhydration and fluid overload can be as detrimental.[20]

Water intake in rabbits is comparatively higher than in other mammals.[21,22] The average daily water intake has been reported to range from 50 to 150 mL/kg of body weight.[2] In addition, with decreased food intake, polydipsia develops and water intake may increase by as much as 6.5 times, which is an important consideration in anorexic patients.[2] This unique physiologic response, combined with their specialized gastrointestinal anatomy, makes fluid therapy a critical part of the perianesthetic management plan.

INTRAVENOUS CATHETERS

Intravenous access should be obtained in any rabbit undergoing anesthesia and can typically be achieved with adequate premedication/sedation protocols. The use of topical, local anesthetic creams containing lidocaine 2.5% and prilocaine 2.5% over the IV site 20 minutes before placement of a catheter can provide vasodilation and comfort through full-thickness analgesia.[23] Common locations for IV catheters include the cephalic vein, lateral saphenous vein, and in certain situations, the marginal ear vein.[24] It is important to note that there is the potential for ear necrosis and sloughing if certain medications leak perivascularly when the marginal ear vein is used.[24] The most common size of catheters that are appropriate are 22, 24, or 26 gauge, depending on the size of the vein and the rabbit (**Fig. 1**).[24]

INTRAOSSEOUS CATHETERS

In certain situations, such as very small or severely hypotensive rabbits, IV catheterization may not be possible. In these scenarios, the placement of an intraosseous (IO)

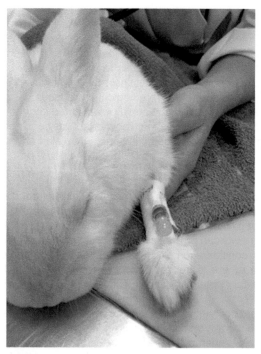

Fig. 1. Cephalic intravenous catheter placement. (*Courtesy of* Miranda Sadar, DVM, DACZM, Colorado State University.)

catheter may be appropriate.[25] Almost all products that can be administered IV can be given via the IO route including crystalloids, colloids including blood products, various medications, dextrose, and emergency drugs.[25] Common locations for placement of an IO catheter include the trochanteric fossa of the femur, the greater tubercle of the proximal humerus, the wing of the ilium, or the tibial tuberosity.[24] Details regarding the placement of IO catheters have been described elsewhere.[24]

BALANCED MULTIMODAL ANESTHESIA

Multimodal or "balanced" anesthesia is a concept that uses a combination of drugs in a sufficient amount to produce the desired effect of anesthesia at its optimum degree but minimizes the undesirable effects that can occur.[26] This technique targets the triad of narcosis, analgesia, and muscle relaxation by acting on each element individually to avoid deep levels of central brain depression.[26]

PREMEDICATION

As in small animals, premedication of rabbits is ideal. Anxiety and stress can induce dyspnea, and result in the release of endogenous catecholamines and cortisol, which can result in complications during anesthesia and result in a less stable patient.[27] In addition, effective premedication protocols facilitate IV access, decrease induction drug doses, and often decrease the minimum alveolar concentration (MAC) of inhalant anesthetics required for anesthetic maintenance.[28–32] There are many premedication protocols that have been successfully used in rabbits and the selection of the protocol will depend, in part, on the procedure to be performed. In addition, certain breeds and strains have demonstrated differing responses to sedation protocols, and there is little information evaluating the influence of age, sex, or health status on drug effects.[33] Given the lack of scientific data and the higher anesthetic risks, the preferential use of reversible drugs should be considered to allow for better control of the depth of anesthesia and expedite recovery times.

BENZODIAZEPINES

The most commonly used benzodiazepine in rabbits is midazolam. Midazolam is a short-acting benzodiazepine that is water soluble and can be administered either intramuscularly (IM) or subcutaneously (SC) for a premedication, or IV during induction.[34] Midazolam is often used as a sole sedative for minor, noninvasive, nonpainful procedures, but is also commonly used in combination with an opioid, ketamine, or an alpha-2 agonist for more extensive procedures in the preoperative setting. Midazolam alone administered at 2 mg/kg IM produces muscle relaxation, mild sedation lasting for 30 to 60 minutes, and minimal to no respiratory depression characterized by a decreased respiratory rate but no changes in Po_2 or Pco_2.[35] More profound and longer sedation is obtained when midazolam is combined with an opioid.[35] Flumazenil is the common reversal agent for benzodiazepines and can be titrated to effect.[34] Diazepam is typically avoided because of the presence of propylene glycol in the injectable formulations that can result in hypotension and thrombophlebitis.[36]

Partial Opioid Agonists and Agonist/Antagonists

Butorphanol is a μ antagonist to partial μ agonist and κ opioid agonist. It has less analgesic potency than μ-pure agonists, a ceiling effect at high doses, and minimal MAC-sparing effects.[37–39] Due to its unique pharmacologic profile, butorphanol administration is only appropriate to treat mild pain and is an excellent sedative for minor diagnostic procedures.[35] Butorphanol alone causes mild, short-term sedation in healthy rabbits with minimal cardiorespiratory depression.[35] More profound sedation, but also significant respiratory depression, can be seen when it is combined with other sedatives such as midazolam or alpha-2 agonists.[35,40,41] Butorphanol is often administered IM or IV, but it is also well absorbed when given intranasally.[42]

Buprenorphine is a μ-partial agonist and an effective analgesic to treat mild to moderate pain. Used alone, buprenorphine produces mild sedation, no cardiovascular side effects, and mild respiratory depression.[35,43] A study examining buprenorphine use in rabbits as a single dose demonstrated no adverse effects on gastrointestinal motility[44]; however, other multidose studies have demonstrated potential effects of buprenorphine on food intake and gastrointestinal motility.[45] The combination of midazolam and buprenorphine can result in marked sedation lasting 90 to 120 minutes.[35]

PURE μ AGONISTS

Pure agonists such as morphine, methadone, hydromorphone, and fentanyl are preferred as part of the premedication regimen when moderate to severe pain is present, or before an invasive procedure. Comparison of the sedative effects of morphine (2 mg/kg SC) and methadone (2 mg/kg SC) demonstrated more profound sedation with methadone compared to morphine, with a maximum sedation score achieved between 30 and 60 minutes postinjection.[46] Fentanyl is a short-acting potent opioid that is commonly administered as a constant rate infusion (CRI) to provide analgesia and MAC-reduction during surgery. At clinical doses, fentanyl has minimal cardiovascular side effects except for mild to moderate bradycardia.[47] In healthy rabbits anesthetized with propofol, repeated boluses of fentanyl (5 μg/kg IV) caused no changes in cardiac contractility but significant decreases in heart rate and mean arterial pressures (MAPs).[48] Therefore, high doses should be used with caution in ill patients or when used concomitantly with drugs that depress the sympathetic system. Pharmacokinetics of fentanyl in rabbits after IV and sublingual administration have been described elsewhere.[49]

Tapentadol is a novel, atypical opioid that behaves as an agonist at the μ-receptor and is also a norepinephrine reuptake inhibitor.[50] Although few studies evaluate the effectiveness of this drug in small mammals, tapentadol is reported to have similar analgesic activity to morphine in humans, but lower affinity for the μ-receptors.[50] In rabbits, 5 mg/kg IV was administered before sevoflurane induction to perform orchiectomy and demonstrated rapid distribution, elimination, and no evidence of apnea.[51] In addition, the pharmacodynamic evaluation of the drug demonstrated that tapentadol provided adequate postsurgery analgesia.[51]

ALPHA-2 AGONISTS

Commonly used alpha-2 adrenergic receptor agonists include xylazine, detomidine, medetomidine, and dexmedetomidine. These drugs are advantageous in premedication protocols because of their ability to provide excellent sedation and muscle relaxation, as well as commercially available reversal agents (yohimbine, atipamezole, tolazoline).[52] The cardiovascular effects can be significant and include vasoconstriction, decreased cardiac output, second-degree heart block, and bradyarrhythmias.[52] With cardiovascular compromise or concerns for cardiac disease, this class of drugs should typically be avoided.

N-METHYL-D-ASPARTATE (NMDA) ANTAGONISTS

Ketamine is a noncompetitive NMDA receptor antagonist that results in the prevention of central sensitization, provision of analgesia, and induction of dissociative anesthesia.[53] In healthy patients, ketamine is well tolerated and can be an excellent adjunct to a premedication or injectable anesthetic protocol for short procedures; however, ketamine can cause muscle rigidity and should be used with drugs that are potent muscle relaxants such as alpha-2 agonists or benzodiazepines. Ketamine also has sympathomimetic properties that can result in an increased heart rate, increased myocardial contractility, and increased peripheral vascular resistance.[53] Ketamine is commonly used to produce profound sedation, or as an induction agent combined with midazolam.

Reports of tiletamine-zolazepam in New Zealand white rabbits demonstrated nephrotoxicity at certain dosages but provides the advantage of smaller drug volumes compared to ketamine if given as an IM injection.[54,55] This drug should be used with caution.

ANTICHOLINERGICS

The most common indication for anticholinergics in a premedication protocol include minimization of salivary and bronchial secretions, and reduction of vagally-induced bradyarrhythmias[56]; however, their utility in these scenarios has been questioned in the human medical field, and controlled studies in rabbits have not been performed.[57] In addition, atropine is not recommended because of lack of efficacy and clinical effects. This has been traditionally explained by approximately 61% of rabbits having a high level of atropine esterase activity that rapidly hydrolyses atropine from the systemic circulation, with a higher prevalence in males.[50,58] Even rabbits with low levels of atropine esterase activity also metabolize atropine quickly, which results in doses up to 2 mg/kg having no effect on heart rate.[47] Glycopyrrolate has a longer duration of action than atropine.[56] In rabbits, 0.1 mg/kg IM of glycopyrrolate has been demonstrated to increase heart rate for a period of 60 minutes.[56] Owing to the lack of proven efficacy and the confirmed negative effects on gastrointestinal motility in hindgut fermenters,[59] the routine use of anticholinergics as part of the premedication protocol is not recommended. **Table 2** lists common premedication protocols and indications for each protocol.

LOCAL ANESTHETICS

Local anesthetics such as lidocaine and bupivacaine are commonly used in small animals to reversibly inhibit neural transmission.[60] Routes of administration of local anesthetics include topical, infiltration, intraarticularly, or as a regional nerve block.[60]

EPIDURAL ANESTHESIA

For abdominal surgeries or painful procedures of the caudal half of the body, epidural anesthesia and analgesia offer a useful adjunct to pain management. Epidural anesthesia offers many avenues for use, including management of surgical cases, obstetric pain, postsurgical pain, and chronic pain.[60] Epidural drugs allow for the achievement of analgesia without the concern for systemic effects compared to when the same drugs are given IM or IV.[60] In addition, epidurals have been shown to reduce recovery time and it could be assumed a similar advantage would be seen in rabbits.[61]

Epidurals also allow a decrease in the amount of gas anesthesia required during the procedure, allowing for a safer and more stable anesthesia.[62] The lumbosacral

Table 2
Injectable preanesthetic sedation and premedication protocols commonly used in rabbits with reversal agents

Drug	Dosage	Common Uses	Reversal Agents
Midazolam + butorphanol ± ketamine	Midazolam 0.5–2 mg/kg SC or IM + butorphanol 0.5–2 mg/kg SC or IM ± ketamine 3–5 mg/kg SC or IM	Excellent for sedation for nonpainful procedures such as radiographs, computed tomography scan, and catheter placement	Flumazenil 0.05–0.1 mg/kg IM or SC
Midazolam + hydromorphone ± ketamine	Midazolam 0.5–2 mg/kg SC or IM + hydromorphone 0.1–0.3 mg/kg SC or IM ± ketamine 3–5 mg/kg SC or IM	Excellent for sedation for potentially painful procedures or as a premedication before surgery	Flumazenil 0.05–0.1 mg/kg IM or SC + naloxone 0.01–0.04 mg/kg IM or SC
Midazolam + butorphanol + dexmedetomidine	Midazolam 0.5–2 mg/kg SC or IM + butorphanol 0.5–2 mg/kg SC or IM ± dexmedetomidine 0.01–0.05 mg/kg SC or IM	Useful in young healthy rabbits when moderate to profound sedation is necessary	Flumazenil 0.05–0.1 mg/kg IM or SC + atipamezole 0.1–0.5 mg/kg SC or IM (depending on the dose of dexmedetomidine)
Midazolam + hydromorphone + dexmedetomidine	Midazolam 0.5–2 mg/kg SC or IM + hydromorphone 0.1–0.3 mg/kg SC or IM ± dexmedetomidine 0.01–0.05 mg/kg SC or IM	Useful in young healthy rabbits when moderate to profound sedation is necessary with analgesia in addition	Flumazenil 0.05–0.1 mg/kg IM or SC + naloxone 0.01–0.04 mg/kg IM or SC + atipamezole 0.1–0.5 mg/kg SC or IM (depending on the dose of dexmedetomidine)

These are suggested dosages and protocols based on published information and the authors' clinical experience. Species and individual variation in response to a drug can be unpredictable and therefore, each dose should be selected with knowledge of clinical status and underlying health concerns.

junction site is the most commonly used location in rabbits, with a technique similar to dogs and cats. It is important to note that injection into the lumbosacral space may result in intrathecal administration of drugs because the dural sac in rabbits extends into the sacrum.[63] The use of a shielded needle and electrical stimulation has been described to allow for successful entry into the subarachnoid space.[64] Successful needle placement was described when a muscle contraction was noted at 0.3 mA.[64] In one study, an epidural consisting of lidocaine and morphine were both demonstrated to be effective adjunct analgesia when administered to rabbits undergoing pelvic limb orthopedic surgery.[65]

REGIONAL NERVE BLOCKS

A unique anatomic feature of rabbits is their elodont and hypsodont dentition that results in frequent presentations of dental disease in some form.[66,67] The pain associated with dental disease and surgical treatment of dental disease can be substantial. The use of locoregional dental blocks can help provide a multimodal analgesic approach, and various dental blocks have been described in the literature.[68–70]

Sciatic and femoral nerve blocks have been successfully described in rabbits with the use of a nerve stimulator and can provide intraoperative and postoperative analgesia after pelvic limb surgery.[71,72] Ultrasound-guided axillary brachial plexus nerve blocks have also been described in rabbits.[73]

Many other ultrasound-guided blocks have been described in small animals including paravertebral blocks, radial, ulnar, median, and musculocutaneous nerve blocks; erector spinae plane blocks; intercostal blocks; transversus abdominis plane blocks; and quadratus lumborum blocks.[74] The details of these blocks are beyond the scope of this article but are well described elsewhere (DiGeronimo PM, da Cunha A. Local and regional anesthesia in zoological companion animal practice. Vet Clin Exot Anim 2022;25:1: in press.].[74]

INDUCTION

Induction of anesthesia can be achieved through the use of injectable drugs or inhalant gases. Induction using an inhalant agent is common practice in rabbits, but whenever possible should be preceded by appropriate premedication. Premedication before gas induction shortens the excitatory phase and the dose of inhalant agent required. Preoxygenation via face mask can provide benefits before administration of the inhalant anesthetic by increasing oxygen stores and delaying arterial hemoglobin desaturation during apnea (**Fig. 2**).[75] The mask should be loose, but well-fitted with enough room to allow for escape of carbon dioxide and heat.[76] Oxygen flow rates greater than 100 mL/kg/min are needed with a mask that is well-fit.[76] If the mask is large and poorly fitted, higher oxygen flow rates (300 mL/kg/min) may be needed.[76] Benefits of preoxygenation can be achieved in less than 1 minute in a healthy patient, but may require greater than 5 minutes with compromised respiratory function.[17]

Induction with an appropriately sized mask allows for better depth control and monitoring and is preferred, but commercially available induction chambers can be advantageous in very stressed rabbits that are resistant to facemask induction.[77] As soon as the righting reflex is lost, the patient should be removed and placed on a face mask to allow for better control of anesthetic depth. A comparison of the advantages and disadvantages of face mask versus chamber induction is provided in **Table 3**. Given the many benefits of safe injectable drugs available, the use of injectable techniques is recommended, allowing for reduced anesthetic waste gas, readily available IV and airway access, and less cardiovascular depression due to easier drug titration.

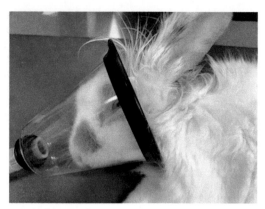

Fig. 2. Preoxygenation via face mask.

PROPOFOL

Propofol is a substituted isopropylphenol anesthetic. Its use as an injectable induction agent in rabbits is common because of its ability to provide a rapid, excitement-free induction and recovery.[78] The use of propofol requires IV or IO access, and the ability to rapidly intubate, as apnea is common after administration.[78] Propofol given as a bolus for induction causes a short-lived, dose-dependent vasodilation, and at supratherapeutic doses may decrease cardiac contractility.[79–81] These side effects are dose-related and may be exacerbated by rapid administration, and therefore, it is recommended to titrate propofol to effect. A calculated propofol induction dose can be given in one-quarter increments, administered over 30 to 60 seconds, to minimize side effects.[17] Propofol can also be used for anesthetic maintenance with doses of 24 to 36 mg/kg/h reported.[82] Pharmacokinetic data for propofol administered as a single bolus, and short and long infusion are available in the literature and appear to be affected by the time of the day with higher doses needed in the morning compared with the afternoon to reach the same anesthetic depth.[83–85]

ALFAXALONE

Alfaxalone is a neurosteroid anesthetic that is suitable as an induction agent through IV administration with a rapid onset and short duration of action.[86] Cardiovascular effects of the newest formulation of alfaxalone have not been well studied in rabbits but an older formulation of alfaxolone/alfadolone was demonstrated to produce dose-dependent cardiovascular depression similar to other general anesthetics.[87] This drug can also be administered IM or SC to provide sedation. Doses of 4 mg/kg and 6 mg/kg IM were reported to be well tolerated; however, one rabbit died following respiratory and cardiac arrest after a dose of 8 mg/kg was administered.[86] In one study, a combination of alfaxalone (6 mg/kg), dexmedetomidine (0.2 mg/kg), and butorphanol (0.3 mg/kg) IM produced anesthesia lasting approximately 1 hour with a recovery time of approximately two and a half hours.[88] An additional study examined a dose of 2 and 3 mg/kg IV for induction, and intubation was possible in all rabbits, although apnea was noted.[89] Therefore, as with propofol, preoxygenation and preparation for intubation is advised when alfaxalone is administered IM and IV.[89]

Table 3
Advantages and disadvantages to face mask and chamber induction methods in rabbits[17]

Method of Induction	Advantages	Disadvantages
Face mask	Rapid induction with a well-fitted mask	Waste gas high Staff exposure to anesthetic gases
Chamber induction	Waste gas lessened Short induction time	Staff exposure to anesthetic gases when patient is removed from chamber Inability to assess the depth of the patient Trauma during the excitement phase

ETOMIDATE

Etomidate is a potent, nonbarbiturate hypnotic agent with a short duration of action that is commonly used for induction and maintenance of anesthesia in animals and humans.[90] Similar to propofol and alfaxalone, etomidate does not possess analgesic properties.[90] Etomidate has been reported to cause hemolysis, thrombophlebitis, and pain on injection because of the formulation containing propylene glycol.[90] These side effects have been reduced with the creation of an aqueous formulation of the drug.[91] Although etomidate has been reported to have minimal cardiovascular side effects in other species, both formulations resulted in decreases in MAP and increases in HR when administered to rabbits.[91] Other common adverse effects include laryngeal reactivity and inhibition of cortisol secretion which preclude its use with adrenal insufficiency.[90]

Commonly used injectable induction protocols are listed in **Table 4**. **Table 5** describes reported combinations of drugs for premedication, induction, and maintenance of anesthesia.

AIRWAY ACCESS
Nasotracheal Intubation

Nasotracheal intubation can be a useful method of intubation in specific situations, including the emergency setting when respiration ceases or during dental procedures where an endotracheal tube can impede the ability to perform the procedure.[92,93] Commonly, nasotracheal intubation is used in cases where the oral cavity is the primary area of interest.[94] The tube should be directed ventrally and medially into the ventral nasal meatus.[93] Nasotracheal intubation uses the fact that rabbits are obligate nasal breathers.[93] The epiglottis is entrapped on the dorsal surface of the soft palate, and thus, facilitates the direct passage of air from the nasopharynx into the larynx and trachea.[93] Resultantly, a tube passed nasally should naturally traverse the pathway from the nasopharynx, to the larynx, to the trachea.[93] The flipped soft palate is one of the described difficulties with orotracheal intubation and is beneficial when performing nasotracheal intubation. Contraindications for the use of nasotracheal intubation include the presence of upper respiratory disease, preexisting edema of the nasal passages, and preexisting narrowing of the nasal passages, which may occur because of apical elongation from the teeth associated with dental disease.[93,95] Complications are usually associated with traumatic nasotracheal intubation where repeated attempts result in damage to the soft tissue structures and nasal turbinates which can result in swelling and nasal passageway obstruction.[94] Although there is little evidence to support introduction of bacteria into the lungs, in cases of known upper respiratory infection, it may be prudent to avoid the use of nasotracheal intubation.[93,95] In very small rabbits, this technique may not be feasible because of the small size of tube that would be required. Step-by-step directions on nasotracheal tube intubation are provided in **Box 1**.

Oral Endotracheal Intubation

Oral endotracheal intubation is the most common method of securing an airway in rabbits and allows for positive pressure ventilation to be performed throughout the anesthetic event. Orotracheal intubation presents challenges because of the narrow oral cavity lined by premolars and molars on both sides, the long tongue with a large base, decreased jaw opening ability, and potential for laryngospasm.[96] Many techniques have been described for intubation including the blind method, modified blind method, videoendoscopic methods, and direct visualization.[96] Complications with orotracheal intubation include difficult placement, trauma to the oropharyngeal soft tissue, laryngospasm, tube dislodgement, and postintubation oropharyngeal swelling after intubation.[96,97]

For intubation using the blind technique, visualization of airflow through the endotracheal tube, listening for respiration, or monitoring of end-tidal carbon dioxide (EtCO$_2$) followed by careful manipulation of the tube is required.[96] This technique is not useful in cases of respiratory arrest or prolonged apnea because of the absence of airflow and the necessity for breathing.[96] With inexperience, this technique can result in significant laryngospasm and laryngeal trauma.[96] Direct visualization of the larynx with a laryngoscope can also be attempted; however, this technique presents significant challenges, as often the laryngoscope blade is wider than the narrow oral cavity, premolars, and molars, preventing appropriate visualization and an inability to depress the tongue.[96] Other techniques include the use of a fiberoptic laryngoscope or an endoscope to visualize the larynx and guide placement of the endotracheal tube.[96]

The most common endotracheal tube sizes in rabbits range from 2.0 to 3.5 mm internal diameter.[98] The size selected should be the largest possible to reduce airflow resistance, and allow creation of a good seal to facilitate ventilation, but should also avoid iatrogenic trauma to the tracheal mucosa. Commercially available tubes are often too long and should be measured to the thoracic inlet and cut to ensure accidental bronchial intubation does not occur.

It is important to keep in mind that with small diameter tubes, risk of occlusion of the tube with saliva, or occlusion from kinking of the tube are significant risks and require close anesthetic monitoring.[99] Use of an EtCO$_2$ monitor can be useful to help correct tube placement and accidental detachments or obstructions.[99]

Confirmation of tube placement is similar to other species.[99] The rabbit may cough as the tube is passed, condensation may be seen on the inside of the endotracheal tube or on a glass slide placed at the end of the tube, air movement can be detected by listening for breath sounds, a wave form can be detected on the EtCO$_2$ monitor, or movement of the chest can be detected when a breath is provided with the rebreathing bag.[99]

Although complications of intubation are rare, reports of subtracheal injury, ulceration, and postintubation tracheal stricture following intubation with both cuffed and uncuffed endotracheal tubes have been documented.[100,101] The clinical presentation is typically dyspnea and upper respiratory tract obstruction signs, such as moist rales and cyanosis.[100,101] This highlights the importance of taking great care during the intubation process and the consideration for alternatives such as a face mask or laryngeal mask airway during very short procedures.[100,101] Other factors that have been

Table 4
Commonly used induction protocols and dosages used in rabbits

Drug	Dosage	Comments
Propofol	2–8 mg/kg IV	Apnea is common, especially when administered rapidly or at higher dosages Dose-dependent hypotension
Alfaxalone	1–4 mg/kg IV	Apnea is common, especially when administered rapidly or at higher doses Potential dose-dependent hypotension
Ketamine + midazolam	Ketamine 2.5–5 mg/kg IV + Midazolam 0.5 mg/kg IV	Apnea is uncommon Increases MAP and HR

These are suggested dosages and protocols based on published information and the authors' clinical experience. Species and individual variation in response to a drug can be unpredictable and therefore, each dose should be selected with knowledge of clinical status and underlying health concerns.

implicated in tracheal injury and stricture include ventilation technique and disinfection protocols for the endotracheal tubes.[100,101]

Laryngeal Mask Airway Devices and Supraglottic Airway Devices

The laryngeal mask was initially developed to serve as an alternative to mask ventilation for people and also for use in an emergency setting for the management of challenging airways.[102] The pediatric laryngeal mask airway (LMA) device has been used as an alternative to endotracheal tube placement in rabbits, and may result in easier placement than an endotracheal tube, especially in the emergency setting.[103] It is important to note that the LMA device results in more gas inhalant waste than when endotracheal intubation of the rabbit is performed.[103] In addition, as pediatric human devices have not been specifically designed for use in rabbits, complications such as lingual cyanosis, gastric tympany, and an incomplete airway seal have been documented with the use of these devices.[103–105]

More recently, a supraglottic airway device (SGAD), specifically designed to mirror the pharyngeal airway anatomic structures of the rabbit (v-gel ADVANCED, DocsInnovent Ltd, Hemel Hempstead, UK), has been created. This device allows for rapid management of the airway and when properly placed can also allow for the application of positive pressure ventilation (**Fig. 3**).[106] This SGAD is beneficial in certain scenarios because of its ease of placement by a novice clinician using $EtCO_2$ guidance combined with minimal to no airway trauma.[106] Placement time is rapid, ranging from 14 to 38 seconds.[106] In one study evaluating the placement of a v-gel compared to oral endotracheal intubation, the longest time for placement was 38 seconds compared to 171 seconds with an endotracheal tube.[106] The combination of the unique shape of the v-gel with the soft gel-like material allows for creation of a strong seal with minimal trauma to the airway.[106] In addition, it is suggested by the manufacturer that it does not result in narrowing of the airway which is seen with an endotracheal tube and thus, may resultantly decrease work of breathing.[107] The rabbit v-gel is available in a wide variety of weights (0.6 kg to 4.5+ kg).[107] When positive pressure ventilation is required, especially for an extended duration, placement of an endotracheal tube is a recommended safer option due to potential for complications such as

Table 5
Drug combination studies reported in rabbits for premedication, induction, and maintenance of anesthesia

Drug Protocol	Purpose of Protocol	Dosage	Comments
Ketamine + xylazine[149] Ketamine + xylazine + butorphanol[149]	Injectable anesthesia	K 35 mg/kg + X 5 mg/kg IM K 35 mg/kg + X 5 mg/kg + B 0.1 mg/kg IM	Addition of butorphanol to protocol resulted in a prolonged reflex loss (palpebral reflex, pedal reflex, righting reflex), as well as mild alterations in physiologic changes
Ketamine-propofol admixture[150]	Induction	K 1, 3, or 5 mg/kg + P 1 mg/kg	Time to loss of righting reflex shortest and duration of action longest with the highest dose of ketamine Mild to moderate sedation only achieved in the lowest dose ketamine group Hypoxemia observed at highest doses
Medetomidine + midazolam + atropine IM + propofol IV[82]	Induction + maintenance of anesthesia	Med 0.2 mg/kg IM + Mid 0.5 mg/kg IM + atropine 0.5 mg/kg IM + P to effect IV	Propofol at 0.5 mg/kg/min maintained general anesthesia with few side effects to the cardiopulmonary system apart from mild hypotension, hypercapnia, and respiratory acidosis Smooth recovery Two rabbits died within 24 h of the procedure
Ketamine + midazolam[151] Ketamine + medetomidine[151]	Induction	K 15 mg/kg + Mid 3 mg/kg IM K 15 mg/kg + Med 0.25 mg/kg IM	Time to loss of righting reflex was shorter with medetomidine Intubation was not possible with 3 rabbits in the medetomidine protocol and 4 rabbits in the midazolam protocol Mean heart rate, SPO$_2$, and vaporizer setting (isoflurane sparing) were lower in the medetomidine group Medetomidine rabbits were more prone to laryngospasm

Ketamine + midazolam[152] Ketamine + midazolam + tramadol[152]	Injectable anesthesia	K 25 mg/kg + Mid 2 mg/kg IM K 25 mg/kg + Mid 2 mg/kg + T 4 mg/kg IM	Faster time to loss of righting reflex and to standing with inclusion of tramadol Inclusion of tramadol did not provide additional analgesia in the protocol
Ketamine + medetomidine[153] Medetomidine + fentanyl + midazolam[153] Xylazine + ketamine[153]	Injectable anesthesia	K 35 mg/kg + Med 0.25 mg/kg Med 0.2 mg/kg + F 0.02 mg/kg + Mid 1 mg/kg X 4 mg/kg + K 50 mg/kg	Surgical anesthesia induced in most animals receiving medetomidine-based protocols Apnea was noted in the fentanyl protocol and endotracheal intubation is essential Supplemental oxygen needed for all protocols Quality of surgical anesthesia greatest with the medetomidine + ketamine protocol
Ketamine + medetomidine SC[154] Ketamine + medetomidine IM[154] Ketamine + medetomidine + butorphanol SC[154] Ketamine + medetomidine + butorphanol IM[154]	Injectable anesthesia	K 15 mg/kg + Med 0.25 mg/kg SC K 15 mg/kg + Med 0.25 mg/kg IM K 15 mg/kg + Med 0.5 mg/kg + B 0.4 mg/kg SC K 15 mg/kg + Med 0.25 mg/kg + B 0.4 mg/kg IM	All groups lost righting reflex and ear pinch response with time to loss of reflexes similar among all groups Higher dose of medetomidine and addition of butorphanol produced a greater duration of loss of ear pinch response Moderate hypoxemia and moderate bradycardia in all rabbits SC and IM administration were equivalent Addition of butorphanol increased the duration of anesthesia with a slight increase in the degree of respiratory depression

These are suggested dosages and protocols based on the published information. Species and individual variation in response to a drug can be unpredictable and therefore, each dose should be selected with knowledge of clinical status and underlying health concerns.

Box 1
Step-by-step instructions for the placement of a nasotracheal tube in the rabbit

To place a nasotracheal tube, adequate muscle relaxation and appropriate anesthetic depth are required. Supplemental oxygen via face mask or flow by should be provided over the duration of the procedure. A 2% lidocaine solution (1–2 mg/kg) can be infused into the nasal passages with a syringe or catheter 60 seconds before tube placement. Correct positioning is critical for successful intubation allowing for optimal alignment of the nasopharynx with the trachea. The rabbit is positioned in sternal recumbency with hyperextension of the head and neck. The diameter of the nasal passage, even in large individuals, is small, and therefore it is usually not possible to pass a tube larger than 2.0 to 2.5 mm. In small rabbits, it may not be feasible. Conservative application of sterile lubricant should be applied on the end of the tube before placement. Excessive lubricant can result in obstruction of the Murphy eye of the tube. The bevel of the endotracheal tube is inserted into the ventral nasal canal and directed in a ventromedial direction. A small degree of resistance is considered normal because of the nasal passageway anatomy, but if significant resistance or a "crunching" sound is encountered, it may be indicative of a tube that is too large or it is passing in the wrong direction through the nasal turbinates and requires redirection.[95] The rabbit often coughs when the tube enters the trachea.[95]

---

lingual edema and cyanosis, gastric tympany, and v-gel dislodgement.[108] A common challenge is dislodgement when the head is shifted. When performing surgical procedures, or an anesthetic event that may require substantial movement of the head, endotracheal intubation should be considered. A recent study demonstrated that the v-gel is a practical alternative to both endotracheal tubes and laryngeal masks.[109]

MAINTENANCE OF ANESTHESIA

Once the airway is secured, the maintenance stage of anesthesia begins. At this point, the most important considerations include monitoring the depth of anesthesia, providing supportive care to the rabbit as needed, and ensuring adequate monitoring is in place.

Active warming should occur after premedication and should continue until the rabbit is fully recovered, alert, and normothermic. Active warming options include warmed IV fluids, warmed anesthetic gases, warmed air beds, hot water bottles, circulating water blankets, or heat pads. In rabbits breathing a heated anesthetic mixture, the average body temperature was shown to be 1.01°C (1.8°F) higher than breathing a nonheated anesthetic mixture.[110] With any warming device, caution should always be used to ensure there is no direct contact that could result in thermal burns. Constant monitoring of temperature with either an esophageal probe or rectal thermometer is critical throughout the anesthesia.

In select situations (short-term procedure), maintenance of anesthesia with a face mask can be considered. Examples include a brief incisor trim or simple dental procedure, a biopsy for histopathological analysis, or endoscopic evaluation of the oral cavity; however, though face masks are easily placed, significant leakage occurs during controlled mechanical ventilation.[109]

ISOFLURANE, SEVOFLURANE, AND DESFLURANE

In most situations, maintenance of anesthesia is performed with an inhalant gas, either isoflurane, sevoflurane, or desflurane.[111] Sevoflurane has a less noxious smell and may be better tolerated for mask induction.[112] Very little of the anesthetic gases are metabolized, which reduces the impact on hepatic and renal function.[112]

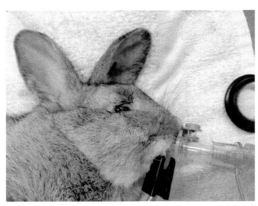

Fig. 3. Appropriate placement of a commercially available rabbit-specific supraglottic airway device.

Inhalant anesthetic can result in cardiovascular and respiratory depression. Most inhalants act in a dose-dependent manner to reduce systemic vascular resistance and cause decreases in stroke volume as a result of decreased myocardial contractility. Both these undesirable side effects result in dose-dependent hypotension.[111] Rabbits appear to be more sensitive to the vasodilatory effects of inhalant anesthetics than other species, with hypotension occurring at levels as low as 1 MAC and may be a contributing factor to the higher anesthetic mortality seen.[113,114] The underlying cause is unclear but a lower systemic vascular resistance and substantially lower arterial blood pressures have been reported at equipotent doses of inhalants.[115]

The negative effects of inhalant gases can be minimized by using a balanced anesthetic approach and the administration of sympathomimetics. Dopamine is commonly used to combat isoflurane-induced hypotension but has been ineffective in rabbits, where phenylephrine was only minimally effective at 2 μg/kg/min[114] Norepinephrine 0.5 to 1.0 μg/kg/min has been demonstrated as a potentially effective treatment to combat isoflurane-induced hypotension.[116]

Various drugs and drug combinations have been reported to reduce MACs, and should be considered (**Table 6**).

TOTAL AND PARTIAL INTRAVENOUS ANESTHESIA

Intravenous CRIs of anesthetic drugs have been used to provide total intravenous anesthesia (TIVA) in rabbits. These medications can be titrated to effect and support a balanced anesthetic approach by reducing other drug dosages. These techniques require IV or IO access. Studies examining propofol and fospropofol continuous IV infusion for anesthetic maintenance in rabbits demonstrated prolongation of recovery time with increasing infusion time for both drugs.[117] Fospropofol, the water-soluble prodrug of propofol, demonstrated greater prolongation of recovery time compared to propofol.[117] An additional study compared the physiologic effects of sufentanil-midazolam TIVA to sevoflurane for surgical anesthesia in premedicated rabbits.[118] This study demonstrated that both protocols provided similar quality of anesthesia and required mechanical ventilation.[118]

Table 6
Anesthetic drugs with clinically significant minimum alveolar concentration sparing effects in rabbits

Drug	Dose	Minimum Alveolar Concentration Reduction	Commonly Used Clinical Doses
Fentanyl[114]	Plasma concentration 2 ± 0.1 ng/mL to 36.8 ± 2.4 ng/mL	up to 63% (Isoflurane)	Loading dose: 3–10 μg/kg Intraoperative rate: 5–20 μg/kg/h Postoperative rate: 2–5.0 μg/kg/h
Ketamine[120]	1 mg/kg loading dose IV + 40 μg/kg/min IV	35% (Isoflurane)	Loading dose: 0.5–2 mg/kg Intraoperative rate: 0.5–3 mg/kg/h Postoperative rate: 0.25–1 mg/kg/h
Lidocaine[125]	50–100 μg/kg/min	10.5% to 21.7% (Isoflurane)	Loading dose:1–2 mg/kg Intraoperative rate: 50–100 μg/kg/min Postoperative rate: 10–50 μg/kg/min
Butorphanol[39]	0.4 mg/kg IV	2.30% to 2.33% (Isoflurane)	Significantly reduced MAC alone or in combination with meloxicam (more significant reduction with combination)

Both tramadol (4.4 mg/kg IV) and meloxicam (0.3 mg/kg IV, 1.5 mg/kg IV) have also been evaluated for MAC reduction in rabbits and did not show clinically significant effects.[39,155]

CRIs can be used to supplement inhalant anesthesia and provide analgesia. Ketamine as a CRI is useful for intraoperative analgesia, MAC reduction, and the benefit of minimal respiratory depression.[119] A ketamine CRI of 9 mg/kg/h resulted in a significant decrease in the MAC of isoflurane in rabbits.[120] μ-Receptor agonist opioids are also commonly used as CRIs during anesthetic maintenance, with fentanyl citrate being one of the more common. An IV fentanyl CRI resulted in a reduction of the MAC of isoflurane by up to 63% in rabbits, depending on the plasma concentrations that were evaluated.[121] In addition, the higher concentrations of fentanyl caused increases in blood pressure with no change in cardiac output.[122] Another study examined the use of sufentanil in combination with midazolam for use as TIVA, and demonstrated similar quality surgical anesthesia to sevoflurane anesthesia in ovariohysterectomized rabbits with both protocols requiring mechanical ventilation.[123]

Lidocaine as an IV infusion has the potential for multiple benefits including visceral analgesia, promotion of gastrointestinal motility, MAC reduction, and an increase in visceral perfusion.[124,125] In rabbits, lidocaine CRI (100 μg/kg/min for 2 days) decreased pain behavior; increased gastrointestinal motility, food intake, and fecal output, and decreased heart rate compared to buprenorphine (0.06 mg/kg IV q 8 h for 2 days) in the postoperative period following ovariohysterectomy.[126] Commonly used drugs for CRIs are listed in **Table 7**.

Table 7
Commonly used constant rate infusions in rabbits

Drug	Dose	Comments
Ketamine[17,120]	Loading dose: 2–5 mg/kg Perioperative rate: 1–2 mg/kg/h Postoperative rate: 0.25–1 mg/kg/h	Less respiratory depression was noted compared to opioids that are administered as a CRI
Fentanyl citrate[17,122]	Loading dose: 5–10 μg/kg Perioperative rate: 10–40 μg/kg/h Postoperative rate: 1.25–5.0 μg/kg h	Apnea is common and ventilation of the rabbit is often necessary
Lidocaine[126]	50–100 μg/kg/min	

These are suggested dosages and protocols based on the published information. Species and individual variation in response to a drug can be unpredictable and therefore, each dose should be selected with knowledge of clinical status and underlying health concerns.

MONITORING OF ANESTHESIA

Common anesthetic complications in rabbits include hypothermia, respiratory depression, hypotension, and bradycardia.

CARDIOVASCULAR SYSTEM

Thoracic auscultation should be performed throughout anesthesia to allow for evaluation of the heart rate, rhythm, and presence of abnormal cardiac sounds. The normal anatomy of the heart, including the differences from common domestic species has been well described.[127–129] Pulse strength can be evaluated with the femoral artery, the dorsal pedal artery, and the auricular artery.[130,131] Mucous membrane color and capillary refill time should be assessed as part of a thorough evaluation of the cardiovascular system throughout the anesthetic procedure.[132]

Doppler evaluation of the cardiovascular system is useful to evaluate the rate and rhythm of the heart.[130] The Doppler transducer can be placed directly on a superficial artery such as the carotid, radial carpal artery (medial aspect of forelimb), auricular, dorsal pedal (dorsal aspect of hindlimb), or femoral.[131,133–136]

Blood pressure measurement in rabbits can be challenging. Arterial blood pressure is evaluated as a function of heart rate, blood volume, stroke volume, and arterial compliance.[137] The evaluation of blood pressure should be used in conjunction with other diagnostics as part of the cardiovascular assessment and evaluation of tissue perfusion.[138] A low blood pressure can be indicative of reduced blood flow and impaired oxygenation of major organs.[138] Blood pressure can be measured directly or indirectly.[130] Direct arterial blood pressure monitoring can be reliable and accurate when an over-the-needle catheter is placed in the central auricular artery (**Fig. 4**).[134] In small rabbits, less than 2 kg, the arterial wave may be overdamped, making interpretation challenging, and are also at increased risk of thromboembolism.[139]

Indirect blood pressure measurement is more commonly used and is less invasive.[130] There are 2 main methods of indirect blood pressure: oscillometry and Doppler ultrasonic sphygmomanometry.[130] In other species, systolic arterial pressure is measured by the Doppler technique, although in cats, there is evidence that Doppler blood pressure may be more reflective of MAP.[140] Regardless, the cuff width to limb circumference ratio should be 30% to 40%.[141] Typically, Doppler is recommended over oscillometric monitoring in rabbits for several reasons. Oscillometric techniques

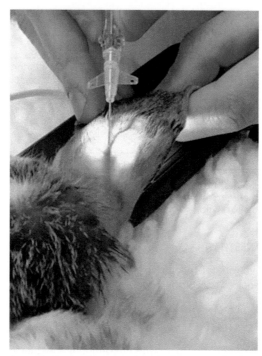

Fig. 4. Placement of a catheter in the central auricular artery for invasive blood pressure monitoring.

can fail to obtain accurate measurements in animals with rapid heart rates (>200 bpm), of small size, and with hypothermia.[133,134]

Attempts to validate noninvasive blood pressure monitors in rabbits have been made with mixed results. One study (n = 17) found good agreement between Doppler measurements at the dorsal carpal branch of the radial artery and those that directly obtain auricular systolic pressures; in addition, the same study found that Doppler measurements below 80 mm Hg were a reliable indicator of arterial hypotension.[133] On the contrary, a second study with a smaller sample size (n = 6) concluded that both oscillometric and Doppler blood pressure measurements were poor substitutes for carotid blood pressure measurement because of changing bias and large limits of agreement.[115]

When using oscillometric devices, the forelimb is preferred because measurements from the pelvic limb have a poor correlation with the abdominal aorta (criterion standard) readings, but measurements from the forelimb appear to correlate well at low and normal pressure ranges.[134]

Electrocardiograms

Cardiac muscle cells produce electrical activity and this can be monitored with the use of an electrocardiogram (ECG) tracing.[131] The ECG tracing is composed of 3 primary complexes, which includes the P wave, QRS complex, and T wave.[142] An ECG evaluation is useful when detection of arrhythmias occurs, which is common with acid-base and electrolyte abnormalities. Given that rabbits have rapid heart rates, low-voltage machines and fast recording speeds (up to 100 mm/s) are recommended.[136,143] Rabbits have very delicate skin and the standard alligator clips can tear it. It is preferred that the clips be attached to small-gauge hypodermic needles placed through the skin. Adhesive pads can be used but may tear the skin on removal. These pads do not work well on the feet of rabbits as they require the protective fur on the plantar and palmar aspect of the feet to be shaved, which can lead to severe pododermatitis because of a lack of protective foot pads.

Pulse Oximeter

Pulse oximetry is commonly used in rabbits, but with limited information available about its accuracy. Pulse oximetry measures oxygen saturation of the blood through illumination of the skin and detection of changes in light absorption between oxygenated blood (oxyhemoglobin) and deoxygenated blood (reduced hemoglobin).[144] The pulse oximeter determines the ratio of absorbance between these wavelengths with calibration against direct measurements of arterial oxygen saturation (SaO_2) to determine the measurement of arterial saturation (SpO_2) by the pulse oximeter.[144] In humans, the difference between SpO_2 and SaO_2 is less than 2% when the SaO_2 value is above 90%; however, the precision of the reading worsens when the SaO_2 is lower than 90%.[144] The use of pulse oximetry has been validated in rabbits, with accuracy at hemoglobin saturation values greater than 85%.[145] The pulse oximeter can be placed in various locations, working most effectively on unpigmented regions of the skin (toe, ear, perianal region). Pulse oximeters may also provide valuable information on heart rate.

Capnograph

Capnography is a useful tool in anesthetized rabbits that are intubated.[146] Capnometry measures the maximum value of carbon dioxide that is measured at the end of expiration, which in turn is a reflection of the amount of CO_2 that is present in the alveolar gas.[146] Measurement of the $EtCO_2$ has demonstrated utility in determining the arterial concentration of carbon dioxide ($Paco_2$).[146] Normocapnia in mammals is associated with an $EtCO_2$ of 35 to 45 mm Hg.[147] Values less than 35 mm Hg are hypocapnic, and values from 65 to 75 mm Hg are hypercapnic.[147] Both hypoventilation and hypercapnia are concerns for rabbits under general anesthesia.[146] The capnograph wave is useful for assessing the adequacy of ventilation and perfusion to the lungs as it has been well correlated with arterial CO_2.[146] Capnography has been demonstrated to provide useful estimations of the $Paco_2$ in rabbits.[148]

THE POSTANESTHETIC PERIOD

The recovery period following an anesthetic event requires equally intense monitoring as the preanesthetic and intra-anesthetic periods. As previously noted, many anesthetic deaths occur in the postanesthetic period.[3–5] If the endotracheal tube is removed too soon, there is risk of airway obstruction, hypoventilation, and hypoxemia. As a result, rabbits should be maintained on oxygen until spontaneous respiration and movement returns. Even after extubation, maintain the rabbit on a face mask or in an oxygen cage until they are fully alert and aware of their surroundings.

Following extubation, it is critical to continue close monitoring and provide any necessary supportive care. Once sufficiently recovered, the rabbit should be placed into a stress-free, warm, dark, recovery cage. Given that many anesthetic deaths occur in the postanesthesia recovery period, ongoing monitoring of body temperature, heart rate, respiratory rate, and comfort should be assessed on a regular basis, with issues addressed as needed.

Once the rabbit can stand and move confidently about the cage, provision of food and water is critical, to not only preserve energy requirements but also to ensure restoration of gastrointestinal motility. If hyporexia, anorexia, or reduced or lack of fecal output is noted, supplemental feeding and analgesia should be instituted.

SUMMARY

Rabbits are increasingly presented to their veterinarian for evaluation and treatment. Owners frequently expect high-level medical and surgical care, which often results in the need for intensive and thorough anesthetic management. Successful anesthetic management requires knowledge of general anesthetic principles, awareness of the limitations and risks of anesthesia, and knowledge of the current literature to all for continuation of provision of high standards of care.

REFERENCES

1. AVMA. In: AVMA pet ownership and demographics sourcebook. Schaumburg, IL: American Veterinary Medical Association; 2017.
2. Donnelly TM, Vella D. In: Quesenberry KE, Orcutt CJ, Mans C, et al, editors. Basic anatomy, physiology, and husbandry of rabbits. 4th edition. St. Louis, Missouri: Elsevier; 2020.
3. Brodbelt DC, Blissitt KJ, Hammond RA, et al. The risk of death: the confidential enquiry into perioperative small animal fatalities. Vet Anaesth Analg 2008;35: 365–73.
4. Lee HW, Machin H, Adami C. Peri-anaesthetic mortality and nonfatal gastrointestinal complications in pet rabbits: a retrospective study on 210 cases. Vet Anaesth Analg 2018;45:520–8.
5. Ishida T, Onuma M, Ono S, et al. Anesthesia-associated death in 160 rabbits. Jpn J Vet Anesth Surg 2014;45:7–12.
6. Brandão J, Graham J, Quesenberry KE. In: Quesenberry KE, Orcutt CJ, Mans C, et al, editors. Basic approach to veterinary care of rabbits. 4th edition. St. Louis, Missouri: Elsevier; 2020.
7. Carrero EJ, Fàbregas N. Thermoregulation and neuroanesthesia. Saudi J Anaesth 2012;6:5–7.
8. Brodbelt D, Flaherty D, Pettifer G. Anesthetic risk and informed consent. In: Grimm K, Lamont L, Tranquilli W, et al, editors. Lumb and Jones veterinary anesthesia and analgesia. 5th edition. Ames, Iowa: Wiley Blackwell; 2015. p. 11–22.
9. Clarke K, Trim C, Hall L, editors. Veterinary anesthesia. 11th edition. China: Elsevier; 2013.
10. Shimokawa M, Kitaguchi K, Kawaguchi M, et al. The influence of induced hypothermia for hemostatic function on temperature-adjusted measurements in rabbits. Anesth Analg 2003;96:1209–13.
11. Di Girolamo N, Toth G, Selleri P. Prognostic value of rectal temperature at hospital admission in client-owned rabbits. J Am Vet Med Assoc 2016;248:288–97.
12. Oparil KM, Gladden JN, Babyak JM, et al. Clinical characteristics and short-term outcomes for rabbits with signs of gastrointestinal tract dysfunction: 117 cases (2014-2016). J Am Vet Med Assoc 2019;255:837–45.
13. Nowland MH, Brammer DW, Garcia A, et al. Biology and diseases of rabbits. In: Laboratory animal medicine. 3rd edition. London: Academic Press, Elsevier; 2015. p. 411–61.
14. Harcourt-Brown FM, Harcourt-Brown S. Clinical value of blood glucose measurement in pet rabbits. Vet Rec 2012;170:674.

15. Sharma D, Hill AE, Christopher MM. Hypercholesterolemia and hypertriglyceridemia as biochemical markers of disease in companion rabbits. Vet Clin Pathol 2018;47:589–602.

16. Harcourt-Brown FM. Gastric dilation and intestinal obstruction in 76 rabbits. Vet Rec 2007;161:409–14.

17. Hawkins MG, Pascoe PJ. In: Quesenberry KE, Orcutt CJ, Mans C, et al, editors. Anesthesia, analgesia, and sedation of small mammals. 4th edition. St. Louis, Missouri: Elsevier; 2021.

18. Jang SJ, Kang SS, Son SJ, et al. Cortisol levels and gastrointestinal disorders after stressful surgery in rabbits. In Vivo (Brooklyn) 2017;31:637–40.

19. Lichtenberger M, Lennox A. Updates and advanced therapies for gastrointestinal stasis in rabbits. Vet Clin North Am Exot Anim Pract 2010;13:525–41.

20. Muir W. Rethinking your approach to preoperative fluid therapy. Vet Med 2013; 108:67–70.

21. Tschudin A, Clauss M, Codron D, et al. Water intake in domestic rabbits (Oryctolagus cuniculus) from open dishes and nipple drinkers under different water and feeding regimes. J Anim Physiol Anim Nutr (Berl) 2011;95:499–511.

22. Cizek L. Relationship between food and water ingestion in the rabbit. Am J Physiol 1961;201:557–66.

23. Keating SCJ, Thomas AA, Flecknell PA, et al. Evaluation of EMLA cream for preventing pain during tattooing of rabbits: changes in physiological, behavioural and facial expression responses. PLoS One 2012;7:e44437.

24. Paul-Murphy J. Critical care of the rabbit. Vet Clin North Am Exot Anim Pract 2007;10:437–61.

25. Petitpas F, Guenezan J, Vendeuvre T, et al. Use of intra-osseous access in adults: a systematic review. Crit Care 2016;20:102.

26. Mori K, Ohmura A, Toyooka H, et al. In: Mori K, Ohmura A, Toyooka H, et al, editors. New balanced anesthesia. Tokyo: Elsevier; 1998. p. 1–384.

27. Baias A, Bodnariu A, Nichita I, et al. Stress in laboratory juvenile rabbits: physiological indicators. Lucr tiinţifice - Zooteh i Biotehnol Univ tiinţe Agric i Med Vet A Banat Timişoara 2012;45:142–5.

28. Monteiro ER, Figueroa CDN, Choma JC, et al. Effects of methadone, alone or in combination with acepromazine or xylazine, on sedation and physiologic values in dogs. Vet Anaesth Analg 2008;35:519–27.

29. Monteiro ER, Coelho K, Bressan TF, et al. Effects of acepromazine-morphine and acepromazine-methadone premedication on the minimum alveolar concentration of isoflurane in dogs. Vet Anaesth Analg 2016;43:27–34.

30. Ko JCH, Weil AB, Inoue T. Effects of carprofen and morphine on the minimum alveolar concentration of isoflurane in dogs. J Am Anim Hosp Assoc 2009;45: 19–23.

31. Hellyer PW, Mama KR, Shafford HL, et al. Effects of diazepam and flumazenil on minimum alveolar concentrations for dogs anesthetized with isoflurane or a combination of isoflurane and fentanyl. Am J Vet Res 2001;62:555–60.

32. Credie RG, Teixeira Neto FF, Ferreira TH, et al. Effects of methadone on the minimum alveolar concentration of isoflurane in dogs. Vet Anaesth Analg 2010;37: 240–9.

33. Avsaroglu H, Versluis A, Hellebrekers LJ, et al. Strain differences in response to propofol, ketamine and medetomidine in rabbits. Vet Rec 2003;152:300.

34. Lingamchetty T, Alireza Hosseini S, Saadabadi A. Midazolam - StatPearls. In: NCBI bookshelf. Treasure Island, Fl: StatPearls Publishing LLC; 2020.

35. Schroeder CA, Smith LJ. Respiratory rates and arterial blood-gas tensions in healthy rabbits given buprenorphine, butorphanol, midazolam, or their combinations. J Am Assoc Lab Anim Sci 2011;50:205–11.

36. Korttila K, Aromaa U. Venous complications after intravenous injection of diazepam, flunitrazepam, thiopentone and etomidate. Acta Anaesthesiol Scand 1980;24:227–30.

37. Dyson DH. Update on butorphanol tartrate: use in small animals. Can Vet J 1990;31:120–1.

38. Bortolami E, Love EJ. Practical use of opioids in cats: a state-of-the-art, evidence-based review. J Feline Med Surg 2015;17:283–311.

39. Turner PV, Kerr CL, Healy AJ, et al. Effect of meloxicam and butorphanol on minimum alveolar concentration of isoflurane in rabbits. Am J Vet Res 2006;67:770–4.

40. Santangelo B, Micieli F, Marino F, et al. Plasma concentrations and sedative effects of a dexmedetomidine, midazolam, and butorphanol combination after transnasal administration in healthy rabbits. J Vet Pharmacol Ther 2016;39:408–11.

41. Kirihara Y, Takechi M, Kurosaki K, et al. Effects of an anesthetic mixture of medetomidine, midazolam, and butorphanol and antagonism by atipamezole in rabbits. Exp Anim 2019;68:443–52.

42. Santangelo B, Micieli F, Mozzillo T, et al. Transnasal administration of a combination of dexmedetomidine, midazolam and butorphanol produces deep sedation in New Zealand White rabbits. Vet Anaesth Analg 2016;43:209–14.

43. Shafford HL, Schadt JC. Respiratory and cardiovascular effects of buprenorphine in conscious rabbits. Vet Anaesth Analg 2008;35:326–32.

44. Deflers H, Gandar F, Bolen G, et al. Influence of a single dose of buprenorphine on rabbit (Oryctolagus cuniculus) gastrointestinal motility. Vet Anaesth Analg 2018;45:510–9.

45. Martin-Flores M, Singh B, Walsh CA, et al. Effects of buprenorphine, methylnaltrexone, and their combination on gastrointestinal transit in healthy New Zealand white rabbits. J Am Assoc Lab Anim Sci 2017;56:155–9.

46. Touzot-Jourde G, Nino V, Holopherne-Doran D. Comparison of methadone and morphine sedation and analgesia in the NZW rabbit. J Vet Pharmacol Ther 2015;38:70–1.

47. Bowery NG. Fentanyl. In: xPharm: the comprehensive pharmacology reference. London: Elsevier Inc; 2007. p. 1–5.

48. Baumgartner CM, Koenighaus H, Ebner JK, et al. Cardiovascular effects of fentanyl and propofol on hemodynamic function in rabbits. Am J Vet Res 2009;70:409–17.

49. Malkawi AH, Al-Ghananeem AM, Crooks PA. Development of a GC-MS assay for the determination of fentanyl pharmacokinetics in rabbit plasma after sublingual spray delivery. AAPS J 2008;10:261–7.

50. Hartrick CT, Rozek RJ. Tapentadol in pain management: a μ-Opioid receptor agonist and noradrenaline reuptake inhibitor. CNS Drugs 2011;25:359–70.

51. Giorgi M, Mills PC, Tayari H, et al. Plasma concentrations of Tapentadol and clinical evaluations of a combination of tapentadol plus sevoflurane for surgical anaesthesia and analgesia in Rabbits (Oryctolagus Cuniculus) undergoing orchiectomy. Isr J Vet Med 2013;68:141–8.

52. Nguyen V, Tiemann D, Park E, et al. Alpha-2 Agonists. Anesthesiol Clin 2017;35:233–45.

53. Sinner B, Graf BM. Ketamine. In: Schüttler J, Schwilden H, editors. Handbook of Experimental pharmacology, vol. 182. Berlin, Heidelberg: Springer Science and Business Media, LLC; 2008. p. 313–33.
54. Brammer DW, Doerning BJ, Chrisp CE, et al. Anesthetic and nephrotoxic effects of Telazol® in New Zealand white rabbits. Lab Anim Sci 1991;41:432–5.
55. Doerning BJ, Brammer DW, Chrisp CE, et al. Nephrotoxicity of tiletamine in New Zealand white rabbits. Lab Anim Sci 1992;42:267–9.
56. Olson ME, Vizzuti D, Morck DW, et al. The parasympatholytic effects of atropine sulfate and glycopyrrolate in rats and rabbits. Can J Vet Res 1994;58:254–8.
57. Cowl CT, Prakash UBS, Kruger BR. The role of anticholinergics in bronchoscopy: a randomized clinical trial. Chest 2000;118:188–92.
58. Liebenberg SP, Linn JM. Seasonal and sexual influences on rabbit atropinesterase. Lab Anim 1980;14:297–300.
59. Bachrach WH. Anticholinergic drugs - survey of the literature and some experimental observations. Am J Dig Dis 1958;3:743–99.
60. Barter LS. Rabbit analgesia. Vet Clin North Am Exot Anim Pract 2011;14:93–104.
61. Liu J, Cui F, Li S, et al. Nonintubated video-assisted thoracoscopic surgery under epidural anesthesia compared with conventional anesthetic option: a randomized control study. Surg Innov 2015;22:123–30.
62. Souza SS, Intelisano TR, De Biaggi CP, et al. Cardiopulmonary and isoflurane-sparing effects of epidural or intravenous infusion of dexmedetomidine in cats undergoing surgery with epidural lidocaine. Vet Anaesth Analg 2010;37:106–15.
63. Greenaway JB, Partlow GD, Gonsholt NL, et al. Anatomy of the lumbosacral spinal cord in rabbits. J Am Anim Hosp Assoc 2001;37:27–34.
64. Otero PE, Portela DA, Brinkyer JA, et al. Use of electrical stimulation to monitor lumbosacral epidural and intrathecal needle placement in rabbits. Am J Vet Res 2012;73:1137–41.
65. Antończyk A, Liszka B, Skrzypczak P, et al. Comparison of analgesia provided by lidocaine or morphine delivered epidurally in rabbits undergoing hindlimb orthopedic surgery. Pol J Vet Sci 2019;22:31–5.
66. Harcourt-Brown FM. The progressive syndrome of acquired dental disease in rabbits. J Exot Pet Med 2007;16:146–57.
67. Lennox AM. Diagnosis and treatment of dental disease in pet rabbits. J Exot Pet Med 2008;17:107–13.
68. Pena I, Campoy L, de Matos R. Investigation of a maxillary nerve block technique in healthy New Zealand white rabbits (Oryctolagus cuniculus). Am J Vet Res 2020;81:843–8.
69. Capello V. Diagnosis and treatment of dental disease in pet rodents. J Exot Pet Med 2008;17:114–23.
70. Lennox AM. Clinical technique: small exotic companion mammal dentistry-anesthetic considerations. J Exot Pet Med 2008;17:102–6.
71. D'Ovidio D, Rota S, Noviello E, et al. Nerve stimulator-guided sciatic-femoral block in pet rabbits (Oryctolagus cuniculus) undergoing hind limb surgery: a case series. J Exot Pet Med 2014;23:91–5.
72. Kluge K, Larenza Menzies MP, Kloeppel H, et al. Femoral and sciatic nerve blockades and incision site infiltration in rabbits undergoing stifle joint arthrotomy. Lab Anim 2017;51:54–64.
73. Fonseca C, Server A, Esteves M, et al. An ultrasound-guided technique for axillary brachial plexus nerve block in rabbits. Lab Anim (NY) 2015;44:179–84.
74. Otero P, Portela D. In: Otero P, Portela DA, editors. Manual of small animal regional anesthesia: illustrated anatomy for nerve stimulation and ultrasound-

guided nerve blocks. 2nd edition. Buenos Aires, Argentina: 5m Publishing; 2019.

75. Nimmagadda U, Salem MR, Crystal GJ. Preoxygenation: physiologic basis, benefits, and potential risks. Anesth Analg 2017;124:507–17.

76. Boysen SR, Mathews KA. Respiratory emergencies. In: Mathews KA, editor. Veterinary emergency and critical care manual. 3rd edition. Guelph, ON: Lifelearn, Inc; 2017. p. 37–84.

77. Schmid RD, Hodgson DS, McMurphy RM. Comparison of anesthetic induction in cats by use of isoflurane in an anesthetic chamber with a conventional vapor or liquid injection technique. J Am Vet Med Assoc 2008;233:262–6.

78. Bryson HM, Fulton BR, Faulds D. Propofol: an update of its use in anaesthesia and conscious sedation. Drugs 1995;50:513–59.

79. Baumgartner C, Bollerhey M, Henke J, et al. Effects of propofol on ultrasonic indicators of haemodynamic function in rabbits. Vet Anaesth Analg 2008;35: 100–12.

80. Royse CF, Liew DFL, Wright CE, et al. Persistent depression of contractility and vasodilation with propofol but not with sevoflurane or desflurane in rabbits. Anesthesiology 2008;108:87–93.

81. Ouattara A, Langeron O, Souktani R, et al. Myocardial and coronary effects of propofol in rabbits with compensated cardiac hypertrophy. Anesthesiology 2001;95:699–707.

82. Rozanska D. Evaluation of medetomidine-midazolam-atropine (MeMiA) anesthesia maintained with propofol infusion in New Zealand White rabbits. Pol J Vet Sci 2009;12:209–16.

83. Cockshott ID, Douglas EJ, Plummer GF, et al. The pharmacokinetics of propofol in laboratory animals. Xenobiotica 1992;22:369–75.

84. Campos S, Monteiro J, Valenzuela B, et al. Evidence of different propofol pharmacokinetics under short and prolonged infusion times in rabbits. Basic Clin Pharmacol Toxicol 2016;118:421–31.

85. Bienert A, Płotek W, Zawidzka I, et al. Influence of time of day on propofol pharmacokinetics and pharmacodynamics in rabbits. Chronobiol Int 2011;28: 318–29.

86. Huynh M, Poumeyrol S, Pignon C, et al. Intramuscular administration of alfaxalone for sedation in rabbits. Vet Rec 2015;176:255.

87. McGrath JC, Mackenzie JE. The effects of intravenous anaesthetics on the cardiovascular system of the rabbit. Br J Pharmacol 1977;61:199–212.

88. Bradley MP, Doerning CM, Nowland MH, et al. Intramuscular administration of alfaxalone alone and in combination for sedation and anesthesia of rabbits (Oryctolagus cuniculus). J Am Assoc Lab Anim Sci 2019;58:216–22.

89. Grint NJ, Smith HE, Senior JM. Clinical evaluation of alfaxalone in cyclodextrin for the induction of anaesthesia in rabbits. Vet Rec 2008;163:395–6.

90. Williams L, Boyd K, Fitzgerald B. Etomidate. In: StatPearls. Treasure Island, FL: StatPearls Publishing; 2020.

91. McIntosh MP, Narita H, Kameyama Y, et al. Evaluation of mean arterial blood pressure, heart rate, and sympathetic nerve activity in rabbits after administration of two formulations of etomidate. Vet Anaesth Analg 2007;34:149–56.

92. Roppolo LP, Vilke GM, Chan TC, et al. Nasotracheal intubation in the Emergency Department, revisited. J Emerg Med 1999;17:791–9.

93. Devalle JMS. Successful management of rabbit anesthesia through the use of nasotracheal intubation. J Am Assoc Lab Anim Sci 2009;48:166–70.

94. Prasanna D, Bhat S. Nasotracheal intubation: an overview. J Maxillofac Oral Surg 2014;13:366–72.

95. Varga M. Airway management in the rabbit. J Exot Pet Med 2017;26:29–35.

96. Thompson KL, Meier TR, Scholz JA. Endotracheal intubation of rabbits using a polypropylene guide catheter. J Vis Exp 2017;2017:56369.

97. Lee LY, Lee D, Ryu H, et al. Capnography-guided endotracheal intubation as an alternative to existing intubation methods in rabbits. J Am Assoc Lab Anim Sci 2019;58:240–5.

98. Dehn S. Intubation of select exotic species for the veterinary technician. In: NAVC conference. 2009. p. 36. Orlando, FL.

99. Johnson DH. Endoscopic intubation of exotic companion mammals. Vet Clin North Am Exot Anim Pract 2010;13:273–89.

100. Grint NJ, Sayers IR, Cecchi R, et al. Postanaesthetic tracheal strictures in three rabbits. Lab Anim 2006;40:301–8.

101. Phaneuf LR, Barker S, Groleau MA, et al. Tracheal injury after endotracheal intubation and anesthesia in rabbits. J Am Assoc Lab Anim Sci 2006;45:67–72.

102. Verghese C, Mena G, Ferson DZ, et al. Laryngeal mask airway. In: Hagberg CA, editor. Benumof and Hagberg's airway management. 4th edition. Philadelphia, PA: Elsevier; 2013. p. 443–65.

103. Smith JC, Robertson LD, Auhll A, et al. Endotracheal tubes versus laryngeal mask airways in rabbit inhalation anesthesia: ease of use and waste gas emissions. Contemp Top Lab Anim Sci 2004;43:22–5.

104. Bateman L, Ludders JW, Gleed RD, et al. Comparison between facemask and laryngeal mask airway in rabbits during isoflurane anesthesia. Vet Anaesth Analg 2005;32:280–8.

105. Kazakos GM, Anagnostou T, Savvas I, et al. Use of the laryngeal mask airway in rabbits: Placement and efficacy. Lab Anim (NY) 2007;36:29–34.

106. Engbers S, Larkin A, Rousset N, et al. Comparison of a supraglottic airway device (v-gel®) with blind orotracheal intubation in rabbits. Front Vet Sci 2017; 4:49.

107. Anon. Docsinnovent. Available at: https://docsinnovent.com/products/product/rabbit-v-gel. Accessed November 16, 2019.

108. Crotaz IR. An observational clinical study in cats and rabbits of an anatomically designed supraglottic airway device for use in companion animal veterinary anaesthesia. Vet Rec 2013;172:606.

109. Wenger S, Müllhaupt D, Ohlerth S, et al. Experimental evaluation of four airway devices in anaesthetized New Zealand White rabbits. Vet Anaesth Analg 2017; 44:529–37.

110. Nogradi AL, Battay M, Cope I. Effects on intraoperative body temperature in rabbits (Oryctolagus cuniculus) and guinea pigs (Cavia porcellus) by heating the inhalational gas mixture. Magy Állatorvosok Lapja 2019;141:93–100.

111. Lopez LA, Hofmeister EH, Pavez JC, et al. Comparison of recovery from anesthesia with isoflurane, sevoflurane, or desflurane in healthy dogs. Am J Vet Res 2009;70:1339–44.

112. Behne M, Wilke HJ, Harder S. Clinical pharmacokinetics of sevoflurane. Clin Pharmacokinet 1999;36:13–26.

113. Imai A, Steffey E, Ilkiw J, et al. Comparison of clinical signs and hemodynamic variables used to monitor rabbits during halothane- and isoflurane-induced anesthesia. Am J Vet Res 1999;60:1189–95.

114. Gosliga JM, Barter LS. Cardiovascular effects of dopamine hydrochloride and phenylephrine hydrochloride in healthy isofluraneanesthetized New Zealand White rabbits (Oryctolagus cuniculus). Am J Vet Res 2015;76:116–21.

115. Barter LS, Epstein SE. Comparison of Doppler, oscillometric, auricular and carotid arterial blood pressure measurements in isoflurane anesthetized New Zealand white rabbits. Vet Anaesth Analg 2014;41:393–7.

116. Uccello O, Sanchez A, Valverde A, et al. Cardiovascular effects of increasing dosages of norepinephrine in healthy isoflurane-anesthetized New Zealand White rabbits. Vet Anaesth Analg 2020;47:781–8.

117. Li R, Zhang WS, Liu J, et al. Minimum infusion rates and recovery times from different durations of continuous infusion of fospropofol, a prodrug of propofol, in rabbits: a comparison with propofol emulsion. Vet Anaesth Analg 2012;39: 373–84.

118. Hedenqvist P, Jensen-Waern M, Fahlman Å, et al. Intravenous sufentanil-midazolam versus sevoflurane anaesthesia in medetomidine pre-medicated Himalayan rabbits undergoing ovariohysterectomy. Vet Anaesth Analg 2015;42: 377–85.

119. Tobias JD, Leder M. Procedural sedation: a review of sedative agents, monitoring, and management of complications. Saudi J Anaesth 2011;5:395–410.

120. Gianotti G, Valverde A, Sinclair M, et al. Prior determination of baseline minimum alveolar concentration (MAC) of isoflurane does not influence the effect of ketamine on MAC in rabbits. Can J Vet Res 2012;76:261–7.

121. Barter LS, Hawkins MG, Pypendop BH. Effects of fentanyl on isoflurane minimum alveolar concentration in New Zealand White rabbits (Oryctolagus cuniculus). Am J Vet Res 2015;76:111–5.

122. Tearney CC, Barter LS, Pypendop BH. Cardiovascular effects of equipotent doses of isoflurane alone and isoflurane plus fentanyl in New Zealand white rabbits (Oryctolagus cuniculus). Am J Vet Res 2015;76:591–8.

123. Hedenqvist P, Edner A, Fahlman Å, et al. Continuous intravenous anaesthesia with sufentanil and midazolam in medetomidine premedicated New Zealand White rabbits. BMC Vet Res 2013;9:21.

124. Eipe N, Gupta S, Penning J. Intravenous lidocaine for acute pain: an evidence-based clinical update. BJA Educ 2016;16:292–8.

125. Schnellbacher RW, Carpenter JW, Mason DE, et al. Effects of lidocaine administration via continuous rate infusion on the minimum alveolar concentration of isoflurane in New Zealand White rabbits (Oryctolagus cuniculus). Am J Vet Res 2013;74:1377–84.

126. Schnellbacher RW, Divers SJ, Comolli JR, et al. Effects of intravenous administration of lidocaine and buprenorphine on gastrointestinal tract motility and signs of pain in New Zealand white rabbits after ovariohysterectomy. Am J Vet Res 2017;78:1359–71.

127. Heatley JJ. Cardiovascular anatomy, physiology, and disease of rodents and small exotic mammals. Vet Clin North Am Exot Anim Pract 2009;12:99–113.

128. Truex RC, Belej R, Ginsberg LM, et al. Anatomy of the ferret heart: an animal model for cardiac research. Anat Rec 1974;179:411–22.

129. Pariaut R. Cardiovascular physiology and diseases of the rabbit. Vet Clin North Am Exot Anim Pract 2009;12:135–44.

130. Flecknell P. Managing and monitoring anaesthesia. In: Flecknell P, editor. Laboratory animal anaesthesia. 4th edition. Boston: Elsevier; 2015. p. 77–108.

131. Ozeki L, Caulkett N. Monitoring. In: West G, Heard D, Caulkett N, editors. Zoo animal and wildlife immobilization and anesthesia. 2nd edition. Ames, Iowa: Wiley-Blackwell; 2015. p. 149–65.
132. Reineke EL. Evaluation and triage of the critically ill patient. 2nd edition. Elsevier Inc; 2014.
133. Harvey L, Knowles T, Murison PJ. Comparison of direct and Doppler arterial blood pressure measurements in rabbits during isoflurane anaesthesia. Vet Anaesth Analg 2012;39:174–84.
134. Ypsilantis P, Didilis VN, Politou M, et al. A comparative study of invasive and oscillometric methods of arterial blood pressure measurement in the anesthetized rabbit. Res Vet Sci 2005;78:269–75.
135. Kuwahara M, Yagi Y, Birumachi JI, et al. Non-invasive measurement of systemic arterial pressure in guinea pigs by an automatic oscillometric device. Blood Press Monit 1996;1:433–7.
136. Heard D. Lagomorphs (Rabbits, hares, and pikas). In: West G, Heard D, Caulkett N, editors. Zoo animal and wildlife immobilization and anesthesia. 2nd edition. Ames, Iowa: Wiley-Blackwell; 2015. p. 1558–9.
137. Shahoud JS, Aeddula NR. Physiology, arterial pressure regulation. Treasure Island, Fl: StatPearls Publishing LLC; 2019.
138. Cooper E. Hypotension. In: Silverstein DC, Hopper K, editors. Small animal critical care medicine. 2nd edition. Elsevier Health Sciences; 2015. p. 46–50.
139. Heard D. Anesthesia. In: Speer B, editor. Current therapy in avian medicine and surgery. St. Louis, Missouri: Elsevier Inc; 2016. p. 612.
140. Caulkett NA, Cantwell SL, Houston DM. A comparison of indirect blood pressure monitoring techniques in the anesthetized cat. Vet Surg 1998;27:370–7.
141. Acierno MJ, Brown S, Coleman AE, et al. ACVIM consensus statement: Guidelines for the identification, evaluation, and management of systemic hypertension in dogs and cats. J Vet Intern Med 2018;32:1803–22.
142. Hancock EW, Deal BJ, Mirvis DM, et al. AHA/ACCF/HRS recommendations for the standardization and interpretation of the electrocardiogram. Part V: electrocardiogram changes associated with cardiac chamber hypertrophy a scientific statement from the American Heart Association electrocardiography. J Am Coll Cardiol 2009;53:992–1002.
143. Heard D. Rodents. In: West G, Heard D, Caulkett N, editors. Zoo animal and wildlife immobilization and anesthesia. 2nd edition. Ames, Iowa: Wiley-Blackwell; 2014. p. 893–903.
144. Jubran A. Pulse oximetry: review. Crit Care 2015;19:272.
145. Vegfords M, Sjöberg F, Lindberg LG, et al. Basic studies of pulse oximetry in a rabbit model. Acta Anaesthesiol Scand 1991;35:596–9.
146. Stanford M. Practical use of capnography in exotic animal anesthesia. ExoticDVM 2004;6:57–60.
147. Beck C, Barthel F, Hahn AM, et al. Evaluation of a new side-stream, low dead space, end-tidal carbon dioxide monitoring system in rats. Lab Anim 2014;48:1–5.
148. Evans JM, Hogg MIJ, Rosen M. Correlation of alveolar PCO 2 estimated by infrared analysis and arterial PCO 2 in the human neonate and the rabbit. Br J Anaesth 1977;49:761–4.
149. Marini RP, Avison DL, Corning BF, et al. Ketamine/xylazine/butorphanol: a new anesthetic combination for rabbits. Lab Anim Sci 1992;42:57–62.
150. Santos M, Viñuela A, Vela AA, et al. Single-syringe ketamine–propofol for induction of anaesthesia in rabbits. Vet Anaesth Analg 2016;43:561–5.

151. Grint NJ, Murison PJ. A comparison of ketamine-midazolam and ketamine-medetomidine combinations for induction of anaesthesia in rabbits. Vet Anaesth Analg 2008;35:113–21.

152. Oguntoye CO, Oyewande OA, Afolabi OO. Evaluation of tramadol-midazolam-ketamine anaesthesia in rabbits. Niger J Physiol Sci 2018;33:145–9.

153. Henke J, Astner S, Brill T, et al. Comparative study of three intramuscular anaesthetic combinations (medetomidine/ketamine, medetomidine/fentanyl/midazolam and xylazine/ketamine) in rabbits. Vet Anaesth Analg 2005;32:261–70.

154. Hedenqvist P, Orr HE, Roughan JV, et al. Anaesthesia with ketamine/medetomidine in the rabbit: Influence of route of administration and the effect of combination with butorphanol. Vet Anaesth Analg 2002;29:14–9.

155. Egger CM, Souza MJ, Greenacre CB, et al. Effect of intravenous administration of tramadol hydrochloride on the minimum alveolar concentration of isoflurane in rabbits. Am J Vet Res 2009;70:945–9.

Sedation and Anesthesia in Rodents

Katarina Bennett, DVM, DABVP-ECM[a],*, Kerrie Lewis, DVM, DACVAA[b,1]

KEYWORDS

- Rodent • Myomorpha • Caviomorpha • Sciuromorpha • Anesthesia • Sedation
- Premedication • Monitoring

KEY POINTS

- Knowledge of basic as well as species-specific anatomy and physiology is important for clinician success.
- Additional risk factors for rodents include high metabolism, low tolerance of hypoxemia, and low glycogen reserves.
- Specialty equipment is available to decrease dead space and facilitate patient monitoring.

INTRODUCTION

The order Rodentia is extraordinarily varied and diverse, with extensive ranges in morphology, diet, activity, metabolism, and anatomy among its members. The order boasts 29 families and more than 2000 species, which have adapted to habitats in most areas of the globe. This remarkable adaptation (and accelerated life cycle) has resulted in rodents becoming the predominant animal used in laboratories, and they are rising in popularity an interactive pets.[1] Owners consider their pets to be family members[1] and continue to demand a high level of care regardless of the species. Due to their nature as high-stress prey animals, much of what can be achieved in the conscious patient is through a distant examination or brief handling period. This article details considerations for sedation and anesthesia in the individual rodent patient and outlines methods, delivery, monitoring, recovery, and a review of recommended doses.

The authors do not have any commercial or financial conflicts of interest or funding sources to disclose.

[a] Avian & Exotics Service, Bluepearl Emergency and Specialty Hospital, 7414 S Tamiami Trl. Sarasota, FL 34231, USA; [b] Pebble Creek Animal Hospital, 19440 Bruce B Downs Boulevard, Tampa, FL 33647, USA
[1] Present address: 526 Suwanee Circle, Tampa FL 33606.
* Corresponding author. 2568 Floyd Street, Sarasota, FL 34239.
E-mail address: zcavetbennett@gmail.com

GENERAL REMARKS

Prior to pursuing sedation or anesthesia, a physical examination and thorough history should be obtained. Knowledge of species-specific anatomy and vital parameters is essential in determining the health of the rodent prior to applying chemical restraint. See **Table 1** for vital parameters. It is equally important to investigate the husbandry set-up, including ambient temperature and hygiene practices. These animals spend most of their time in their enclosures, and poor conditions have a marked effect on immune defenses and stress levels.

Anesthetic risk is higher in rodents than in larger mammals, such as cats and dogs.[4,5] A prospective study on perianesthetic mortality rates of healthy guinea pigs (*Cavia porcellus*) reported 3.8%, a figure approximately 10 times higher than cat and dog mortalities.[6] There are many reasons for this, including a higher metabolism and, therefore, oxygen and glucose demands, which means they have an extremely low tolerance to even brief hypoxemia. Irreversible central nervous system (CNS) injury occurs within 30 seconds of respiratory arrest.[7] Lower glycogen reserves predispose rodents to hypoglycemia and a higher surface area–to–volume ratio allows for rapid loss of heat, predisposing to hypothermia. The aforementioned rapid metabolism increases the speed of elimination of drugs, so rodents typically require higher doses and more frequent administration.[7] Elevated respiratory rates (RRs) increase alveolar ventilation, resulting in more rapid anesthetic uptake and excretion. There can be time-consuming and technical difficulties securing access to vascular and respiratory systems. Finally, rodents typically exhibit higher circulating catecholamine levels. Catecholamines (dopamine, norepinephrine, and epinephrine) are released in response to sympathetic nervous system activity and result in vasoconstriction, hypertension, tachycardia, elevated blood glucose, and dysrhythmias at high circulating levels.

SPECIES-SPECIFIC ANATOMIC AND PHYSIOLOGIC ATTRIBUTES

All rodents are obligate nasal breathers due to the dorsal location of the larynx in close association with the nasopharynx. The order Rodentia can be divided into 3 suborders to allow for simpler discussion of anatomic variations. The Caviomorpha (guinea pigs, chinchillas, and degus), the Myomorpha (rats, mice, hamsters, and gerbils), and the Sciuromorpha (prairie dogs, squirrels, and ground squirrels).

Caviomorpha

Members of Caviomorpha have a long and narrow oral cavity, with a soft palate that extends to the base of the large, elongated tongue and offers only 1 connection to the pharynx.[8] This small aperture between the oropharynx and pharynx is referred to as the palatal ostium and typically is 2 mm to 3 mm in width.[9] The palatal tissue around the ostium is called the velopharyngeal recess. It is highly vascular and vulnerable to injury, hemorrhage, and inflammation with manipulation.[9] Healthy guinea pigs and chinchillas (*Chinchilla lanigera*) retain food in the oropharynx normally. Degus (*Octodon degus*) are prone to development of elodontomas, which can cause partial obstruction of the nasal passage and predispose to respiratory infections. In a retrospective study conducted of degus, aerophagia due to nasal obstruction was a predisposing factor for development of gastrointestinal stasis.[10] As obligate nasal breathers, disease processes affecting the nasal passage must be considered during planning.

Auscultation of the guinea pig heart consists of the standard lub-dub sounds but normally may be preceded by a fourth heart sound that corresponds to atrial contraction.[11] Guinea pigs have 2 pericardial layers: a fibrous outer and serous inner layer.

Table 1
Vital parameters for selected rodent species[2,3]

Parameter	Mouse	Rat	Guinea Pig	Hamster	Gerbil	Chinchilla	Ground Squirrel	Prairie Dog
Body weight (g)	25–40	300–500	700–1200	85–150	85–150	400–600	—	—
Temperature (°C)	37.5	38	38	37.4	39	37–38	34–38	34.4–38.2
RR (per min)	80–200	70–115	50–140	80–135	90	20–80	100–200	40–60
HR (per min)	350–600 310–840	250–350	150–250 230–380	250–500	260–300	100–150 137–201	200–300	83–318

Coronary vascular supply in guinea pigs is heavily collateralized, making myocardial infarction unlikely.[11] In chinchillas, the right coronary artery is absent.[11] Heart murmurs are prevalent in chinchillas (23%) but often benign if low grade. Heart murmurs of grade 3/6 or higher correspond with a 29-times higher instance of echocardiographic abnormalities; therefore, an echocardiogram is recommended prior to anesthesia.[12,13]

Passive regurgitation has been noted anecdotally in Caviomorpha during the sedation/anesthetic period. These species do not engage in emesis due to reduced muscularity of the diaphragm, long abdominal esophagus length, small abdominal esophagus circumference, and medial position of the esophagus in the stomach, which consequently does not form a cone shape as in emetic species.[14] Caviomorpha also lack the coordinated brainstem response to complete a full emetic episode, which includes phrenic nerve activity, intercostal and esophageal movements, and diaphragmatic and abdominal muscle contractions. Individual or episodic retches or heaves have been identified in some caviomorphs, which consists only of abdominal and crural/costal diaphragmatic contractions. This results in a net increase in intra-abdominal pressure, which could result in movement of ingesta toward the esophagus.[14] Evidence of nausea has been identified in rodents, including guinea pigs, exhibited as increased salivation when administered drugs with known emetic properties, such as apomorphine.[14]

The lung fields are small due to a combination of comparatively large hearts and profuse gastrointestinal volume,[4,8] and they exhibit high chest wall compliance with low functional residual capacity.[15] This allows them to capitalize on oxygen intake and compensate for high oxygen demand without having an increased lung field.[15] Rodents have more alveoli with thinner diameters to maximize oxygen exchange. Bony spicules composed of dense lamellar bone may appear radiographically in the lungs of guinea pigs.[8] If misinterpreted, this normal finding could lead to a misdiagnosis of inhaled foreign body or osseous metaplasia.

Myomorpha

Mongolian gerbils (Meriones unguiculatus) lack a complete circle of Willis (anastomosis of arteries at the base of brain), which makes them susceptible to cerebral ischemia upon ligation of the common carotid artery.[15] Idiopathic epilepsy has been reported in certain gerbil strains, so contraindications exist for sedatives that may lower the seizure threshold.[4] Chinese hamsters (Cricetulus griseus) may exhibit hereditary diabetes.[4]

Hamsters (Cricetidae) have cheek pouches with orifices located near the angle of the mouth. This can be a source of aspirated food material if not addressed prior to anesthesia.[7] In mice (Mus musculus) and rats (Rattus norvegicus), the esophagus enters the stomach in the middle of the lesser curvature, and the limiting ridge terminates in this region. This anatomic combination prevents emesis.[14] In hamsters, vomiting is prohibited by the location of the cardia extremely close to the pylorus with little presence of a lesser curvature.[14]

Tracheal diameter of the adult rat is approximately 1.6 mm to 1.7 mm, and extension of the neck can increase the length by 50% with no change in lumen diameter.[15] Myomorpha have high chest wall compliance, low residual capacity, and a robust Bohr effect, and small changes in pH have a stronger effect on hemoglobin's affinity for oxygen. Hamsters in torpor or hibernating become mildly acidotic. The left lung is not separated into lobes in Myomorpha, whereas the right is separated into 4 or 5 lobes.[8] Cardiac striated muscle in the rat and hamster extends along the pulmonary vessel walls and into the lung tissue, making them susceptible to spread of infectious agents between these structures.[11] Blood supply of the rat heart is largely extracoronary from branches of the mammary and subclavian arteries.

Sciuromorpha

Most members have pouch-like paraoral structures that commonly are used to store food. As discussed previously, these should be examined prior to induction. Prairie dogs (*Cynomys* sp) have a large, fleshy tongue and an oropharyngeal ostium similar to that of Caviomorpha, making endotracheal intubation challenging. Odontogenic tumors have been reported frequently in prairie dogs between 2 years and 6 years old. The apex and reserve crown of the maxillary incisors are affected most commonly, and the resulting obstruction of the nasal passage can have severe consequences on patient stability.[16]

Black-tailed prairie dogs (*Cynomys ludivicianus*) are a primitive sciurid and have a unilobate left lung as in Myomorpha.[8] Heart disease is diagnosed in a high percentage of pet prairie dogs over 2 years to 3 years of age, so thorough auscultation is warranted. Illnesses or ambient cold temperatures in prairie dogs can trigger dormancy, which may respond dramatically to warmth and rehydration. Reassessment after 24 hours of supportive care is indicated.[17] A recent study in 13-lined ground squirrels (*Ictidomys tridecemlineatus*) showed they are resistant to cardiac ischemia and exhibit hypocoagulation during torpor and hibernation.[18]

PRESCREENING AND PREPARATION

Preparation for sedation or anesthesia begins prior to arrival of the patient to the hospital. Stress levels in rabbits are elevated by the period of travel from their home,[19] a finding that has not been studied in rodents but is likely a shared stressor. It is recommended to allow rodents an hour in the hospital environment to acclimate in a dark, quiet, and safe area before pursuing anesthesia, as a means of reducing morbidity. To reduce stress and maximize efficiency, it is recommended to plan and organize all machinery, medications, and supplies before the patient is handled. Lists can help maintain organization and ensure handling and sedation time is not prolonged due to missing items (**Fig. 1**).

Ideally, baseline bloodwork, including a complete blood cell count and biochemistry, should be performed. This provides the clinician more assurance of patient anesthetic stability and ability to metabolize sedative and narcotic drugs prior to immobilization. In several rodent species, however, sedation is required to facilitate venipuncture. Additionally, blood volume must be considered. The total blood volume should be calculated in each patient and a threshold for fatal blood loss (>20% blood volume) established. Blood volume for rodents is calculated as 60 mL/kg to 80 mL/kg of body weight, or 6% to 8% of the body weight. Recommended maximum for collection is 10% of blood volume. Many clinicians alternatively calculate for 1% body weight. If anticipated blood loss of a surgical procedure is greater than 10%, preoperative bloodwork may not be a viable option. In rodents where the allowable blood volume is not enough for a full panel, useful information can be gathered from preparation of a blood smear, packed cell volume, total protein/total solids, blood glucose, blood urea nitrogen, and lactate in some cases.

In patients exhibiting evidence of systemic instability, anemia, or dehydration, it is indicated to delay anesthesia until fluid deficits have been corrected and minimum database bloodwork has been performed. Severe anemia with a hematocrit of less than 20% should be corrected if possible, because anesthetized patients may be unable to compensate for decreased oxygen delivery.[4] Assessment of patient stability

Checklist for Biopsy Procedure

Monitoring
- ☐ Premedications
- ☐ Reversals (if applicable)
- ☐ Monitoring equipment (doppler, sphygmomanometer, ECG, pulse oximeter)
- ☐ Warming device
- ☐ Oxygen for mask or flow-by
- ☐ Anesthesia machine
- ☐ Nose mask - small
- ☐ Thermometer

Procedure
- ☐ Sterile scrub
- ☐ Sterile gloves
- ☐ Scalpel
- ☐ Formalin jar – small
- ☐ Minor surgical pack or closing pack
- ☐ Skin punch biopsy (if applicable)
- ☐ Cautery +/- gelfoam
- ☐ Suture package
- ☐ Recovery cage

Fig. 1. Example of an anesthesia checklist for a minor procedure.

should be performed with the intention of assigning a physical status (from I to V), as outlined by the American Society of Anesthesiologists (**Table 2**).

FASTING

Fasting of rodents prior to anesthesia is controversial and without clear guidelines. Overall, fasting is not recommended for small rodents because they are not capable of vomiting, and hypoglycemia due to exhaustion of glycogen reserves is a potential consequence.[20] A study in rats showed a decrease in gastric volume by 27% after a 4-hour fast, which could reduce pressure on small lung fields.[21] In guinea pigs and chinchillas, there are variable recommended fasting times, ranging from 0 to 8 hours for food and 0 to 2 hours for water.[5,9,17,20] The postulated reason for fasting caviomorphs is to reduce or eliminate food material in the oropharynx, reduce incidence of passive regurgitation, and potentially reduce gastrointestinal volume. The large size of the cecum in guinea pigs and chinchillas likely negates significant reduction in overall volume. Consequences of fasting in these species may include gastrointestinal stasis and hypoglycemia.

Table 2
Patient physical status as defined by the American Society of Anesthesiologists

Physical Status	Criteria	Examples
ASA I	Healthy patient, elective procedure	Spay, neuter
ASA II	Mild/localized systemic disease	Tooth trim, broken tail
ASA III	Systemic disease without immediate risk to life	Gastrointestinal stasis
ASA IV	Systemic disease with immediate risk to life	Foreign body, ketosis
ASA V	Will die with 24 h without intervention	Gastric dilatation and volvulus

Abbreviation: ASA, American Society of Anesthesiologists physical status classification system score.

To the authors' knowledge, there have been no studies to support the various recommendations, and most are based on individual clinician experience. These recommendations are used in the authors' clinics and have been recognized by other specialists.[22] Rinse the oral cavity of guinea pigs, chinchillas, degus, and prairie dogs using 2 mL to 5 mL of water and thoroughly clear the mouth of food material using cotton-tipped applicators 30 minutes to 60 minutes prior to anesthetic events. Food should be removed at the same time. Sedation or premedication can be administered any time after rinsing the oral cavity.

SEDATION AND PREMEDICATION

Sedation is defined as a drug-induced, reversible state of decreasing consciousness, including anxiolysis and reduced responses to external stimuli. In high-stress rodent species, sedation is indicated for minimally invasive procedures, such as imaging or venipuncture. Depending on the protocol and depth of sedation, some moderately invasive procedures, such as lancing of an abscess or biopsy can be accomplished, negating the need for general anesthesia. Addition of local anesthetics (eg, lidocaine and bupivacaine) can increase the effectiveness of sedation for moderately invasive procedures greatly.

Premedication is a method of using sedation to facilitate induction to anesthesia and to reduce the amount of anesthetic required to maintain a surgical plane of anesthesia. Drug protocols and routes of administration are similar to sedation alone and are discussed together. The sedative drugs used in rodents are like those used in other mammal species. In most cases, the dose requirements are higher, reflecting their metabolic rate. A discussion of the drug class, method of action, and physiologic effects is summarized in **Table 3**. The bulk of research performed on rodents is in a laboratory setting, and the established dose ranges presented in the literature can be higher than would be used in a clinical setting. The authors use half of the suggested lower dose range from laboratory animal references when using a protocol for the first time. It is easier to add more sedative than to try to reverse an overdose. The current dose ranges and recent studies assessing sedation protocols are presented in **Table 4**.[4,17,24,29–49]

A sedation scale has been published to assess depth of sedation for 2 protocols in rats.[23] After intramuscular (IM) sedation, assessments were made using criteria in the scale every 5 minutes until 20 minutes postinjection. This allowed for a determination of time to maximal sedation between the 2 protocols. As described in the study, frequent assessment of the patient is imperative, not only to identify negative reactions

Table 3
Premedication drug classification and effects

Premedication Drugs	Class	Method of Action, Metabolism, and Excretion	Physiologic Effects	Adverse Effects and Comments
Glycopyrrolate	Parasympatholytic, anticholinergic	Synthetic antimuscarinic agent. Competitively inhibits acetylcholine at postganglionic parasympathetic neuroeffector sites • Majority is eliminated unchanged in the feces and urine[24]	Reduces salivary and bronchial secretions Increases HR, minimizes vagally induced bradyarrhythmias[24]	Increases secretion viscosity, alters gastrointestinal motility at higher doses. Longer duration of activity compared with atropine (240 min in rats) Increases myocardial oxygen consumption. Urine retention Poor lipid solubility—does not cross appreciably the blood-brain and blood-placenta barriers[24]
Atropine	Parasympatholytic, anticholinergic	Competitively inhibits acetylcholine at postganglionic parasympathetic neuroeffector sites • Atropine is metabolized in the liver and excreted into the urine (30%–50% excreted unchanged)[24]	Reduces salivary and bronchial secretions Increases HR, minimizes vagally induced bradyarrhythmias[24]	Increase secretion viscosity; may decrease gut motility and induce colic in susceptible animals[24] Readily crosses brain and blood-placenta barriers.Increases myocardial oxygen consumption.
Midazolam	Benzodiazepine	Causes depression of subcortical levels (primarily limbic, thalamic, and hypothalamic) of the CNS The mechanism of action includes antagonism of	No significant cardiovascular or respiratory effects Anxiolytic, sedative, skeletal muscle relaxant, and anticonvulsant effects	No analgesic properties Paradoxic sedation, dysphoria, or excitement is seen in some species. Three times as potent as diazepam Reduced bioavailability

Drug	Class	Mechanism	Effects	Notes
		serotonin, increased γ-aminobutyric acid activity, and diminished release or turnover of acetylcholine in the CNS. • Hydroxylated into active metabolites in the liver • Eliminated by renal mechanisms[24]		when given PO due to first-pass effect[24] Reversal = flumazenil
Diazepam	Benzodiazepine	Binds to GABA$_A$ receptors and increases the affinity of the receptor for γ-aminobutyric acid. Results in increased chloride conductance and hyperpolarization of the postsynaptic cell membrane[24]	No significant cardiovascular or respiratory effects Anxiolytic, sedative, skeletal muscle relaxant, and anticonvulsant effects	Erratic efficacy with SC or IM use due to osmolality Hypotension if given rapidly IV due to propylene glycol vehicle Transient lameness with IM injection. No analgesic properties May be preferred in status epilepticus over midazolam because it is longer acting[24] Reversal = flumazenil
Acepromazine	Phenothiazine sedative/tranquilizer	Blocks postsynaptic dopamine receptors in the CNS and may inhibit the release of dopamine Depresses portions of the reticular activating system that assist in the control of body temperature, basal metabolic rate, emesis, vasomotor tone[24]	Minimal effect on respiratory function[24] Lower arterial blood pressure in dogs, causes increases in central venous pressure, a vagally induced bradycardic effect, and transient sinoatrial arrest[24] Peripheral vasodilation	Dose-dependent reduction of seizure threshold in gerbils. May allow for successful venipuncture due to vasodilation[4] Negligible analgesic effects, may potentiate analgesics[24] In some species, hematocrit reduction appreciated

(continued on next page)

Table 3
(continued)

Premedication Drugs	Class	Method of Action, Metabolism, and Excretion	Physiologic Effects	Adverse Effects and Comments
			even at low doses Decreases tear production[4]	associated with splenic sequestration[24]
Dexmedetomidine	α_2-Adrenergic agonist	Stimulates α_2-receptors in arterioles Depression of CNS, gastrointestinal, and endocrine functions[24] • Primarily metabolized in the liver via hydroxylation; metabolism depends on hepatic blood flow • Nonactive metabolites. Eliminated primarily in the urine and some elimination in the feces[24]	Negative chronotropic and inotropic effects Peripheral and cardiac vasoconstriction Dose-dependent respiratory depression Some somatic and visceral analgesia Bradycardia, cardiac output decrease in peripheral resistance[7] Sedation, anxiolysis, reduced intestinal smooth muscle tone[24]	Hyperglycemia may be transiently observed due to reduction of insulin release. Not recommended for use in patients that are measuring glucose curves Reversal = atipamezole
Medetomidine	α_2-Adrenergic agonist	Stimulates α_2-receptors in arterioles Exerts inhibitory feedback role on the release of subsequent norepinephrine; results in decreased sympathetic nervous system efferent activity[7]	Hypothermia, bradycardia[25] Vasoconstriction and increased peripheral resistance Muscle relaxation, sedative	Variable sedation alone but potentiates the effects of other sedatives Reversal = atipamezole
Xylazine	α_2-Adrenergic agonist	Stimulates α_2-receptors in arterioles. Depression of CNS, gastrointestinal,	Sedative, muscle relaxation, and analgesic properties Increases blood pressure,	Variable sedation alone but potentiates the effects of other sedatives[20]

	and endocrine functions Causes skeletal muscle relaxation through inhibition of central mediated pathways[24]	decreases HR, decreases cardiac output[20] Initial increase in blood pressure followed by longer period of hypotension[24] Insignificant effect on respiratory system May cause arrhythmias, reduce cardiac output, and increase risk for general anesthesia-related death[24]	In rats and mice, acute reversible lens opacity has been observed with xylazine and xylazine/ketamine combination Less selective for α_2-receptors than other agonists. Visceral analgesia has been demonstrated in horses and other ruminants.[24] When given in combination with ketamine over multiple anesthetic episodes, has been associated with myocardial necrosis and fibrosis in rabbits[4] Not recommended in animals with cardiopulmonary compromise[4] Reversals = yohimbine, tolazoline[7] Atipamezole, 1 mg/kg SC, IM, IO, or IV, can be used to reverse xylazine.[26]
Alfaxalone (alfaxalone-2-hydroxypropyl-β-cyclodextrin)	Neurosteroidal anesthetic acting on the $GABA_A$ receptor, sharing a common mechanism with propofol and the barbiturates[23]	Sedation at lower doses, anesthesia at higher doses Respiratory depression or apnea when administered IV	Used as an induction agent when given IV Negligible analgesic effects Dose-dependent respiratory depression. Should not be mixed with

(continued on next page)

Table 3
(continued)

Premedication Drugs	Class	Method of Action, Metabolism, and Excretion	Physiologic Effects	Adverse Effects and Comments
		Neuroactive steroid compounds inhibit action potential propagation and decrease activation of pathways related to awareness and arousal.[26] • Rapidly metabolized by the liver, minimal cumulative effects[20,26] • Eliminated by hepatic/fecal and renal routes[24]	Limited effect on cardiovascular system	other induction or sedative agents prior to administration[24,26] In human medicine, neurosteroid agents are considered to have a positive neurologic profile by decreasing cerebral metabolic demands, blood flow, and intracranial pressure. Violent recovery (paddling muscle twitching) if used alone[26] Ataxia, muscular tremors, and opisthotonus-like posture can be observed after IM and IV administration.[24]
Ketamine	Dissociative	Noncompetitive N-methyl-D-aspartate receptor antagonist. Depresses the thalamo-neocortical system while activating the limbic system. Inhibits the binding of γ-aminobutyric acid and also may block serotonin,	Sympathomimetic properties—increases HR, myocardial contractility, and peripheral vascular resistance. Increases myocardial oxygen demand[20] Negative inotrope Increased salivation, apneustic ventilation[7,27]	May be used as an induction agent Renal impairment causes prolonged recovery. Muscle rigidity regardless of dose makes this drug less appropriate for use alone. Synergistic with use of α₂-agonist or benzodiazepine. Acid pH

		norepinephrine, and dopamine in the CNS[27] Prevents central sensitization • Hepatic biotransformation to norketamine (M1) and dehydronorketamine (M2) is the major route of metabolism.[7] • Renal elimination	Depresses respiration, increasing $Paco_2$ Increases intracranial pressure[7] Moderate analgesic	may cause pain at injection site.[27] Causes cutaneous irritation and possible muscle necrosis when administered SC or IM.[28] Causes eyes to remain open during sedative period[20] Due to increase in intracranial pressure, not recommended for use in head trauma patients[7]
Tiletamine/zolazepam	Dissociative/tranquilizer	Combination of equal parts tiletamine hydrochloride, a dissociative anesthetic, and zolazepam hydrochloride, a benzodiazepine having minor tranquilizing properties[7] • Metabolized in liver, excreted in urine	Apnea may occur at higher doses.[24] Transient hypotension Tachycardia Cardiac output unchanged[24]	Dose-dependent nephrotoxicity in New Zealand white rabbits[29] Poor analgesia The duration of effect of the zolazepam component is longer than that of the tiletamine. Involuntary muscle twitching, athetoid movements, rough recovery[24]
Butorphanol Buprenorphine Fentanyl hydromorphone Morphine Methadone Oxymorphone	Opiods • Kappa • Mu • Delta	Interact with specific opioid receptors and mimic naturally occurring molecules, known as endogenous opioid peptides Binds to receptor, inhibits cyclic adenosine	Minimal cardiovascular effect Dose-dependent respiratory depression or apnea[7]	CNS depression or arousal may be exhibited. Hyperthermia or hypothermia potential, particularly when administered postoperatively Nausea and vomiting due

(continued on next page)

Table 3
(continued)

Premedication Drugs	Class	Method of Action, Metabolism, and Excretion	Physiologic Effects	Adverse Effects and Comments
		monophosphate activity, decreases Ca2+ influx. Reduced release of substance P from primary afferent fibers in the spinal cord dorsal horn, inhibiting synaptic transmission of nociceptive input[7] • Metabolized by conjugation in the liver with glucuronic acid forming M1 and M2 • Excretion through glomerular filtration[24]		to direct stimulation of the chemoreceptor trigger zone Rapid IV administration of morphine may result in histamine release.[7] Spasm of gastrointestinal smooth muscle may predispose to ileus. Reversals = naloxone, naltrexone

Abbreviations: GI, gastrointestinal; Hct, Hematocrit.

Table 4
Premedication drug combinations, reports, and duration of effect

Premedication Drugs and Combinations	Dosing Recommendations for Premedication and/or Sedation	Time to Effect	Duration of Action	Comments
Glycopyrrolate	HAMSTER 0.5 mg/kg IM[4] MOUSE 0.02–0.5 mg/kg SC, IM[4] RAT 0.02–0.05 SC, IM, IV[4] GENERAL RODENT 0.01–0.02 mg/kg SC or IM.[24,31]		240 min in rats	• After IM or SC administration, peak effects occur approximately 30–45 min postinjection (in dogs)[24] • The vagolytic effects persist for 2–3 h and the antisialagogue effects persist for up to 7 h in dogs.[24]
Atropine	HAMSTER 0.04–0.4 mg/kg SC, IM[31] GERBIL 0.04–0.4 mg/kg SC, IM[31] MOUSE 0.04–0.4 mg/kg SC, IM[31] RAT 0.04–0.4 mg/kg SC, IM, IV, IP[4,31] CHINCHILLA 0.05–0.2 mg/kg SC, IM, IV[4,31] 0.1–0.2 mg/kg SC, IM[31] GUINEA PIG 0.05–0.2 mg/kg SC, IM, IV[4,31] 0.1–0.2 mg/kg SC, IM[31]			• After IV administration, peak effects in HRs occur within 3–4 min—most species.[24] • Absorbed readily PO, endotracheal • Higher doses required in some rats that express serum atropinesterase • Short duration of activity in rats
Midazolam	HAMSTER 5 mg/kg IP[4] GERBIL 2–3 mg/kg IM[31] 5 mg/kg IM, IP[4]			• Reversal is possible with flumazenil, 0.02–0.05 mg/kg IV/SC/IM, but it may precipitate seizures in susceptible patients.

(continued on next page)

Table 4
(continued)

Premedication Drugs and Combinations	Dosing Recommendations for Premedication and/or Sedation	Time to Effect	Duration of Action	Comments
	MOUSE 2–3 mg/kg IM[31] 1–5 mg/kg SC, IM, IV[4] RAT 2–3 mg/kg IM[31] 1–2.5 mg/kg SC, IM, IV[4] 5 mg/kg IP[4] CHINCHILLA 0.4–2 mg/kg IM[31] 1–2 mg/kg SC, IM, IV[4] GUINEA PIG 0.4–2 mg/kg IM[31] GENERAL RODENT 1–2 mg/kg IM[24,31] 3–5 mg/kg IM, IV[24]			
Midazolam + butorphanol	RAT [Mi] 2.5 mg/kg + [B] 2 mg/kg IP[32] DEGU [Mi] 0.2–0.8 mg/kg + [B] 0.3–0.5 mg/kg IM[31]			• Completely reversible protocol • When administered intraperitoneal prior to gas anesthetic induction, attenuates the respiratory depression of isoflurane in rats[32]
Midazolam + dexmedetomidine	RAT [Mi] 15 mg/kg + [D] 0.09 mg/kg IP[33] [Mi] 20 mg/kg + [D] 0.12 mg/kg IP[33]	1–3 min[33]	>60 min[33]	• It was demonstrated that midazolam potentiates the analgesic effects of dexmedetomidine in rats. Onset of profound analgesia was reached within 5–10 min.[33]

				Comments
Midazolam + medetomidine + butorphanol	MOUSE [Mi] 4 mg/kg + [Me] 0.3 mg/kg + [B] 5 mg/kg SC[34] [Mi] 4 mg/kg + [Me] 0.3 mg/kg + [B] 5 mg/kg IP[35] RAT [Mi] 2 mg/kg + [Me] 0.15 mg/kg + [B] 2.5 mg/kg IP[31,36] [Mi] 3 mg/kg + [Me] 0.23 mg/kg + [B] 3.75 mg/kg IP[36] [Mi] 1 mg/kg + [Me] 0.05 mg/kg + [B] 2 rr g/kg IP[37]	5 min[36] 4.5 min[36]	45 min[34] 52 ± 14 min of immobilization[35] 40 min of immobilization[36] 68 ± 40 min of immobilization[36] 25 min[37]	• Completely reversible protocol • Intraperitoneal route was determined to be ineffective in 1 experiment.[34] • Effect of anesthetic agent may vary by murine strain.[35] • Marked cardiorespiratory depression observed in rats as well as individual variation in efficacy Intraperitoneal administration of medetomidine and midazolam are subject to first-pass metabolism by liver via absorption through the portal vein.[36]
Midazolam + medetomidine + fentanyl	HAMSTER [Mi] 3.3 mg/kg + [Me] 0.33 mg/kg + [F] 0.033 mg/kg SC[31] RAT [Mi] 2 mg/kg + [Me] 0.15 mg/kg + [F] 0.005 mg/kg IM[38] CHINCHILLA [Mi] 1 mg/kg + [Me] 0.05 mg/kg + [F] 0.02 mg/kg IM[4,31] GUINEA PIG [Mi] 2 mg/kg + [Me] 0.2 mg/kg + [F] 0.025–0.05 mg/kg IM[31]		90 min[4]	• Completely reversible protocol using flumazenil (0.1 mg/kg), atipamezole (0.5–1 mg/kg), and naloxone (0.12–0.05 mg/kg)[31] • Marked hypertension and bradycardia seen in rats using telemetry measurements when compared with ketamine-xylazine or isoflurane[38] • Chinchillas had less respiratory and cardiovascular depression and swifter recovery than medetomidine/ketamine.[4]
Diazepam	HAMSTER 2.5–5 mg/kg IM, IP[4,31] GERBIL 2.5–5 mg/kg IM[31]			• Significant irritation when given IM

(continued on next page)

Table 4
(continued)

Premedication Drugs and Combinations	Dosing Recommendations for Premedication and/or Sedation	Time to Effect	Duration of Action	Comments
	MOUSE 2.5–5 mg/kg IM[31] 3–5 mg/kg PO, IP[4] RAT 2.5–5 mg/kg IM, IV, IP[4,31] CHINCHILLA 2.5–5 mg/kg IM[31] 0.5–3 mg/kg IV[4] GUINEA PIG 0.5–5 mg/kg IM[31] 0.5–3 mg/kg IV[4]			
Acepromazine	HAMSTER 0.5–5 mg/kg IM, SC, PO[31] GERBIL 3 mg/kg IM[4] MOUSE 0.5–5 mg/kg IM, SC, PO[31] 2–5 mg/kg IM, SC, IP[4] RAT 0.5–2.5 mg/kg IM, SC, PO[31] CHINCHILLA 0.5–1 mg/kg IM, SC[4] GUINEA PIG 0.5–5 mg/kg IM, SC, PO[31] 0.5–1 mg/kg IM, SC[4] GENERAL RODENT 0.5–1 mg/kg IM[31]	Peak effect at 30–40 min in most species[24]		• Higher doses should be given only PO for hamster/gerbil/mice.[31] • May induce seizures in gerbils[4]

Drug	Dose	Onset	Duration	Comments
Acepromazine + ketamine	MOUSE [A] 2.5–5 mg/kg + [K] 50–150 mg/kg IM[31] RAT [A] 2.5–5 mg/kg + [K] 50–150 mg/kg IM[31] CHINCHILLA [A] 0.5 mg/kg + [K] 40 mg/kg IM[31] PRAIRIE DOG [A] 0.4 mg/kg + [K] 40 mg/kg IM[17]		20–30 min[17]	• Prolonged recovery reported in Chinchillas[31] • Wide margin of safety in chinchillas[30]
Dexmedetomidine	MOUSE 0.015–0.5 mg/kg SC, IP[4] RAT 0.015–0.5 mg/kg SC, IP[4] CHINCHILLA 0.05 mg/kg SC[4] GUINEA PIG 0.05 mg/kg SC[4]			• Typically used in combination with other sedatives. See combinations. • Reversable using atipamezole In most cases, dosing for dexmedetomidine is comparable to half the dose of medetomidine.
Dexmedetomidine + ketamine	MOUSE [D] 0.5 mg/kg + [K] 75 mg/kg IP[31] RAT [D] 0.5 mg/kg + [K] 75 mg/kg IP[31] CHINCHILLA [D] 0.015 mg/kg + [K] 4 mg/kg IM[40–42] GUINEA PIG [D] 0.05 mg/kg + [K] 3.5 mg/kg SC, IM[31] GENERAL RODENT [D] 0.25 mg/kg + [K] 2–4 mg/kg IM[31]	5 min[40] 2–3 min[41]	45 min[40,41]	• Partially reversable using atipamezole • Dose-dependent depression in core and surface body temperature in rats[39] • Resulted in improved quality and length of sedation compared with alfaxalone-butorphanol and also reduced postanesthetic gastrointestinal effects in chinchillas[40] • Comparable depressant effect to isoflurane on echocardiographic parameters (reduced cardiac output,

(continued on next page)

Table 4
(continued)

Premedication Drugs and Combinations	Dosing Recommendations for Premedication and/or Sedation	Time to Effect	Duration of Action	Comments
				fractional shortening, flow velocity) in chinchillas[41] • Reduced Spo_2 during sedative period compared with isoflurane anesthesia. Reduced food intake and fecal output in chinchillas compared with isoflurane anesthesia[42]
Medetomidine	**HAMSTER** 0.1 mg/kg SC[31] 0.2–0.3 mg/kg SC[31] 0.03–0.1 mg/kg SC, IP[4] **GERBIL** 0.1–0.2 mg/kg SC[4,31] **MOUSE** 0.03–0.1 mg/kg SC, IP[4] **RAT** 0.15 mg/kg IM[37] 0.15–0.25 mg/kg IM[31] 0.03–0.1 mg/kg SC, IP[4] **CHINCHILLA** 0.1 mg/kg SC[4] **GUINEA PIG** 0.1 mg/kg SC[4]		25 min[37]	• Typically used in combination with other sedatives. See combinations. • Reversable using atipamezole
Medetomidine + butorphanol	**RAT** [Me] 0.1 mg/kg + [B] 2 mg/kg IM[37]		25 min[37]	

Drug	Dose	Onset	Duration	Comments
Xylazine	HAMSTER 1–5 mg/kg IM. IP[4] GERBIL 2 mg/kg IM[4] MOUSE 5–10 mg/kg IP[4] RAT 1–5 mg/kg IM, IV, IP[4] CHINCHILLA 2–10 mg/kg IM, IV[4] GUINEA PIG 2–10 mg/kg IM, IV[4] GENERAL RODENT 5–10 mg/kg SC, IM, IP[24]	IM or SC dose = 10–15 min IV dose = 3–5 min[24]	45–60 min[24]	• Reversable using yohimbine (0.5–1 mg/kg IV, IP)[31]
Alfaxalone	MOUSE 100 mg/kg SC, IP[34] 80 mg/kg IP[43] RAT 2–5 mg/kg IV[31] 20 mg/kg IP[44] CHINCHILLA 5–10 mg/kg SC, IM[40] GUINEA PIG 40 mg/kg IM, IP[31] 20 mg/kg[29]	2.2 min[43] 3–6 min[44] 6.8–8 min[29]	60 min[43] <15 min[31] 20–60 min[44] 73 ± 20 min[29]	• High doses often required, so IM administration may not be feasible in some cases. • Alfaxalone alone resulted in incomplete level of anesthesia in chinchillas. SC route not recommended in chinchillas due to limited effect at 10 mg/kg.[40] • No apnea when given intraperitoneal in rats compared with IV administration. Effective for surgical anesthesia in 7/10 rats[44] • Surgical anesthesia not induced at 100 mg/kg SC in mice[34] • Responses to intraperitoneal alfaxalone used alone in mice included limb-jerking, intense pruritis of the face,

(continued on next page)

Table 4
(continued)

Premedication Drugs and Combinations	Dosing Recommendations for Premedication and/or Sedation	Time to Effect	Duration of Action	Comments
				hyperresponsiveness to noise, and popcorn body movements in 10 of 14 subjects. Not recommended for use alone[43] • Twitching or bruxism appreciated sporadically with alfaxalone used alone in guinea pigs[29]
Alfaxalone + butorphanol	CHINCHILLA [A] 5 mg/kg + [B] 0.5 mg/kg IM[40]	5–15 min[40]	5–20 min[40]	• Less consistent anesthesia and higher impact on gastrointestinal intake and output postanesthetic compared with dexketamine in chinchillas[40]
Alfaxalone + butorphanol + midazolam	SQUIRREL [A] 8 mg/kg + [B] 1 mg/kg + [M] 1 mg/kg IM[45]	15 s[45]	40 min[45]	• Five-striped palm squirrel (*Funambulus pennantii*) anesthetic protocol.[45] • Partially reversible protocol
Alfaxalone + medetomidine + butorphanol	MOUSE [A] 40–80 mg/kg + [M] 0.3 mg/kg + [B] 5 mg/kg SC[34]	5–10 min[34]	35–85 min[34]	• Duration of anesthesia is dependent on dose of alfaxalone.[34]
Alfaxalone + dexmedetomidine + buprenorphine	GUINEA PIG [A] 15–20 mg/kg + [D] 0.25 mg/kg + [B] 0.05 mg/kg SC[29]	6–8 min[29]	90 min[29]	• Surgical plane of anesthesia was not achieved; appropriate for nonpainful procedures[29]
Alfaxalone + xylazine	MOUSE [A] 80 mg/kg + [X] 10 mg/kg IP[43]	2.3 min[43]	70–90 min[43]	

Agent	Species and Dose	Onset	Duration	Notes
Alfaxalone + ketamine	SQUIRREL [A] 6 mg/kg + [K] 40 mg/kg IM[45]	50 s[45]	62 min[45]	• Five-striped palm squirrel (*Funambulus pennantii*) anesthetic protocol[45] • All animals showed twitching and abnormal vocalization during recovery.[45]
Alfaxalone + ketamine + dexmedetomidine	SQUIRREL [A] 6 mg/kg + [K] 20 mg/kg + [D] 0.1 mg/kg IM[45]	60 s[45]	40 min[45]	• Five-striped palm squirrel (*Funambulus pennantii*) anesthetic protocol[45] • Partially reversible protocol
Ketamine	HAMSTER 20–40 mg/kg IM[31] GERBIL 40–60 mg/kg IM[43] MOUSE 80 mg/kg IP[43] 22–44 mg/kg IM[31] 150 mg/kg IP[46] RAT 22–40 mg/kg IM[31] CHINCHILLA 20–40 mg/kg IV[31] GUINEA PIG 22–44 mg/kg IM	8–10 min in most species[24] 5 min[43]	7 min[43]	• Provided only sedative effects in mice. Combination with xylazine provided reliable anesthesia IP[43] • Higher doses provide heavier sedation compared with lower doses • Marked individual variation among responses in gerbil[31] • In a study on echocardiogram performance in mice, ketamine alone exerted the least depressant effects on left ventricular function and HR compared with isoflurane and ketamine-xylazine combination.[46]
Ketamine + xylazine	HAMSTER [K] 200 mg/kg + [X] 10 mg/kg IP[24] [K] 80 mg/kg + [X] 5 mg/kg IM, IP[31] [K] 100 mg/kg + [X] 10 mg/kg IM[47] GERBIL [K] 50 mg/kg + [X] 2 mg/kg IP[24,31]	4 min[43] 2.5 min to loss of righting reflex[35] 2.5 min to loss of righting	37 ± 8 min[43] <40 min[31] <30 min[31] 27 min immobilization[35] 40 min immobilization[35] 35 min[36]	• Marked cardiorespiratory depression seen with high doses in rats when compared with isoflurane[36] • Prolonged recovery period compared with isoflurane or

(continued on next page)

Table 4
(continued)

Premedication Drugs and Combinations	Dosing Recommendations for Premedication and/or Sedation	Time to Effect	Duration of Action	Comments
	MOUSE [K] 80 mg/kg + [X] 10 mg/kg IP[43] [K] 60 mg/kg + [X] 6 mg/kg IP[31,35] [K] 80 mg/kg + [X] 8 mg/kg IP[31,35] RAT [K] 75 mg/kg + [X] 10 mg/kg IP[81] [K] 80 mg/kg + [X] 10 mg/kg IP[36] [K] 100 mg/kg + [X] 5 mg/kg IM, IP[38] CHINCHILLA [K] 40 mg/kg + [X] 2 mg/kg IM[31] GUINEA PIG [K] 40 mg/kg + [X] 5 mg/kg IP[81] [K] 20–40 mg/kg + [X] 2 mg/kg IM[31] SQUIRREL [K] 85 mg/kg + [X] 10 mg/kg IM, SC[48]	reflex[35] 6 min[36]	301 min[38] 20–30 min[48]	medetomidine-midazolam-fentanyl. Fewer cardiovascular effects than midazolam-fentanyl but more than isoflurane alone[38] • Reduced cardiovascular depression (left ventricular ejection fraction) seen on echocardiogram when compared with isoflurane or thiopental in hamsters[47] • Dose-dependent depression in core and surface body temperature in rats[39] • Surgical plane of anesthesia achieved in Richardson's ground squirrels (*Urocitellus richardsonii*)[48]
Ketamine + diazepam	CHINCHILLA [K] 20–40 mg/kg + [D] 1–2 mg/kg IM[31] GUINEA PIG [K] 20–30 mg/kg + [D] 1–2 mg/kg IM[31]			
Ketamine + medetomidine	HAMSTER [K] 100–200 mg/kg + [Me] 0.25 mg/kg SC, IP[31] GERBIL		20–30 min[31] 20–30 min[31] 20–30 min[31]	• Female mice may require a higher dose of ketamine.[31]

	[K] 75–90 mg/kg + [Me] 0.5 mg/kg IM, IP[31]	
	MOUSE	
	[K] 40–75 mg/<g + [Me] 1 mg/kg IP[31]	
	RAT	
	[K] 75–90 mg/kg + [Me] 0.5 mg/kg IM, IP[31]	
	DEGU	
	[K] 5–10 mg/kg + [Me] 0.02–0.04 mg/kg IM[31]	
	CHINCHILLA	
	[K] 4–5 mg/kg + [Me] 0.03 mg/kg IM	
	[K] 5 mg/kg + [Me] 0.06 mg/kg IM	
	GUINEA PIG	
	[K] 3–5 mg/kg + [Me] 0.1 mg/kg SC, IM[31]	
	[K] 40 mg/kg + [Me] 0.5 mg/kg IM, IP[31]	
	GENERAL RODENT	
	[K] 2–4 mg/kg + [Me] 0.05 mg/kg IM	
Ketamine + medetomidine + buprenorphine	GUINEA PIG [K] 3–5 mg/kg + [Me] 0.1 mg/kg + [B] 0.03 mg/kg IM[49]	• Used as premedication prior to fracture repair[49]
Ketamine + midazolam	RAT [K] 40 mg/kg + [Mi] 1–2 mg/kg IM, SC, IP[31]	
	CHINCHILLA [K] 5–10 mg/kg + [Mi] 0.5–1 mg/kg IM[31]	
	GUINEA PIG	

(continued on next page)

Table 4
(continued)

Premedication Drugs and Combinations	Dosing Recommendations for Premedication and/or Sedation	Time to Effect	Duration of Action	Comments
	[K] 5–10 mg/kg + [Mi] 0.5–1 mg/kg IM[31] PRAIRIE DOG [K] 5–10 mg/kg + [Mi] 0.5–1 mg/kg IM[31]			
Ketamine + midazolam + butorphanol	DEGU [K] 5–10 mg/kg + [Mi] 0.2–0.4 mg/kg IM + [B] 0.3–0.5 mg/kg IM[31]			
Tiletamine/zolazepam	HAMSTER 30 mg/kg IM, IP MOUSE 50–80 mg/kg IM RAT 50–80 mg/kg IM 20–40 mg/kg IM CHINCHILLA 20–40 mg/kg IM	IM injection averages 7.5 min[24]	IV: 15–20 min IM: 30–45 min[24]	
Tiletamine/zolazepam + xylazine	HAMSTER [T] 30 mg/kg + [X] 10 mg/kg IM, IP[31] GERBIL [T] 20 mg/kg + [X] 10 mg/kg IP[31]			

Abbreviations: [A], acepromazine; [B], butorphanol; [D], dexmedetomidine; [F], fentanyl; [K], ketamine; [Me, Medetomidine; [Mi], Midazolam; [T], tiletamine/zolazepam; [X], xylazine.

early but also to identify when maximal sedation has been achieved.[23] The authors reported that this scale exhibited good reproducibility. With consistent use of a sedation scale, dosing protocols can be developed in the individual clinic based on length and invasiveness of the procedure.

EQUIPMENT

Due to the small size and diversity of rodents, there are limitations to the ability to perform criterion standard maintenance and monitoring. Equipment used on small animals can be modified to assist with safe anesthesia. Laboratory specialty equipment has been designed for rodents but may not be price efficient for practices serving multiple species.

Anesthesia Machine

Delivery systems
Most machines made for anesthetic delivery used on small animals can be used. The limitation of these standard pieces of equipment is the vaporizer output accuracy at low fresh gas flow rates.[2] As a rule, 2 times the minute volume (MV) should be used as a flow rate, where MV equals tidal volume (TV) times RR: $MV = TV \times RR$. A minimum of 0.5 L/min should be used to provide adequate oxygen to the patient as well as most accurate vaporizer output. Higher fresh gas flow leads to decreased patient temperatures. Newer digital systems that allow injection of volatile gases with low flow oxygen are being developed for rats and mice.[60]

Anesthesia circuits
Because of patient size, selection should be weighted toward non-rebreathing circuits. Non-rebreathing circuits provide low resistance to accommodate for small TVs. Rebreathing circuits, because of the valves required to produce flow through the circuit, are higher in resistance and consequently increase the work of breathing. The increased resistance can be overcome with a mechanical ventilator. **Table 5** contains details about common circuits.

Ventilators

Breaths can be administered by using the rebreathing bag. TV can be calculated by multiplying weight (in kilograms) by 10 to 15. In general, 20 cm H_2O to 25 cm H_2O should not be exceeded because a breath or damage to alveoli may occur.[51] Lungs require approximately 5 cm H_2O to 8 cm H_2O of positive pressure to expand the alveoli for effective ventilation.[51]

Mechanical ventilators are a significant help during anesthesia. These devices allow control of respirations, maintain a more consistent depth of anesthesia, overcome respiratory depression from anesthetic drugs, and prevent atelectasis. The downsides of mechanical ventilation include increased thoracic pressure resulting in decreased cardiac output that can have an impact on systemic blood pressures and an increased risk of pulmonary trauma from over-ventilation. There also is evidence that mechanical ventilation longer than 4 hours suppressed peripheral immune function in rats.[52]

Standard small animal ventilators do not meet the delicate needs of ventilation for rodents, although a few designs have capacity to provide smaller TVs (<50 mL). Rodent and small mammal specific models have been created to adapt needs of exceedingly small patients (**Table 6**).[53]

Table 5 Common anesthetic circuits used in veterinary medicine		
Common Anesthetic Circuits	**Attributes**	**Type**
T-piece/Mapleson E	Low resistance, limited dead space, allows positive pressure ventilation	Non-rebreathing
Bain coaxial/Mapleson D	Low resistance, allows positive pressure ventilation, preservation of heat with coaxial system	Non-rebreathing
Circle system	High resistance, allows positive pressure ventilation, preservation of heat due to low fresh gas flow rates	Rebreathing
Universal F	High resistance, allows positive pressure ventilation, preservation of heat due to coaxial system	Rebreathing

RESTRAINT AND ROUTES OF ADMINISTRATION

The restraint required for safety of both patient and handler depends on patient demeanor. Restraint should allow for ease of drug administration and limit physiologic stresses. Even a quick transfer out of a cage may change heart rate (HR), blood pressure, and circulating cortisol/corticosterone levels for hours after the event. It is important to be aware of handling techniques that limit this stress, because they may have an impact on overall anesthetic outcome. Specifically designed rodent restraint tubes permit low stress handling during injections and venipuncture (**Fig. 2**).[54] See **Table 7** for common injection sites.[3]

CANNULATION

Venous access may be gained after sedation to provide more control of vital parameters during anesthesia and recovery. Due to small vessels and length of catheters, alternative routes may be sought. Typical venous sites include jugular, cephalic, saphenous (lateral or medial), and tail veins, if species permits. Preclipping and applying a topical anesthetic cream (lidocaine or prilocaine) for 60 minutes prior to cannulation diminishes pain and movement. In the authors' experience, applying a warm water bottle or heat lamp near the cannulation site allows for better visualization and blood flow. Caution should be used when clipping fur and securing catheters because these patients are prone to torn skin.

Alternatively, the placement of an intraosseous (IO) catheter is rapid and allows consistent vascular access in patients of all sizes. It is contraindicated in patients with sepsis, fractures of the target bone, and osteomyelitis. A human study showed that IO catheters had equal response in return of spontaneous circulation as when an intravenous (IV) catheter was used during cardiopulmonary resuscitaiton.[55] IO catharization also showed a higher success of first attempt placement compared with IV.[55] In patients where peripheral catharization is challenging, this is a safe and efficient route for fluid and drug administration. Common sites include the tibial crest, intertrochanteric fossa of the femur, ileal crest, and proximal humerus. Anatomically, the tibial crest is the easiest site due to easily palpable landmarks and limited soft tissues. After clipping and aseptic preparation of the location, local anesthetic (lidocaine, 2 mg/kg) is injected at the level of the periosteum. Using an 18-gauge to 25-gauge sterile hypodermic needle for initial penetration, the needle then can be replaced

Table 6
Commercially available small animal ventilators

Name	Weight Limit/Tidal Volume Ability
Anesto Merlin (Vetronic; Devon, England)	1–40 mL
Conduct Science VentStar (Conduct Science; Skokie, IL)	0.05–5 mL
CWE Small Animal Ventilators (CWE Inc.; Ardmore, PA)	1–2 kg
Hallowell Anesthesia WorkStation (Hallowell EMC; Pittsfield, MA)	0–100 mL
Kent Scientific: RoVent and RoVent Jr (Kent Scientific Corporation; Torrington, CT)	3–1250 g
MiniVent Ventilator for Mice (Model 845) (Harvard Apparatus; Holliston, MA)	1–50 g
TOPO Small Animal Ventilator (STEMart; Shirley, NY)	1–10 kg

Note this list should not be considered exhaustive.

with either a slightly smaller needle or the same needle after flushing. An injection cap, extension set, or fluid line can be attached directly to the needle.

This article does not permit an extensive review of fluid therapy in rodents. Perianesthetic fluid therapy should be used, however, for replacement of ongoing losses, support of cardiovascular function, counteracting negative physiologic effects associated with anesthetic agent administration (eg, vasodilation and hypotension), and prevention of clot formation in the catheter. Standard isotonic fluids administered at rates between 3 mL/kg/h to 15 mL/kg/h often are used in each of these species.[3] Some

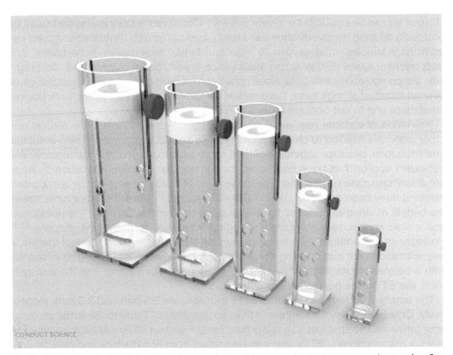

Fig. 2. Rodent restraint tubes. (With permission from ConductScience.com, by Louise Corscadden, PhD.).[54]

Table 7
Routes of medication administration for selected rodent species

Route of Administration	Species Type	Needle Size	Site	Additional Considerations
IM	Rodents (all)	25–27 gauge	Quadriceps, epaxials, and triceps muscles	Small muscle mass, avoid sciatic nerve
IV	Mice, rats	23–26 gauge	Lateral tail, saphenous, and cephalic vein	Use EMLA cream
	Gerbils	23–26 gauge	Lateral tail, saphenous, and cephalic vein	
	Guinea pigs	23–26 gauge	Aural, cephalic, saphenous, and penile vein	
Intraperitoneal	Mice, hamsters	25–27 gauge		Avoid liver and kidneys

literature advocates for a low concentration (2.5%–5%) of dextrose be added to isotonic solutions during longer procedures.[2] Warming IV fluids can help preserve body temperature. Due to the low volumes of fluids required, best accuracy is obtained using an infusion pump. Subcutaneous (SC) fluids can be administered if cannulation is unsuccessful.

INTUBATION

Oxygen should be available for rodent patients. Occult respiratory issues and sedation protocols causing hypoventilation can rapidly lead to hypoxia. Anesthetic circuits can administer supplemental oxygen to induction tanks, face masks, nose cones, and endotracheal tubes (ETTs). Small masks (size 0 and rodent masks) and diaphragm sets are commercially available. Nose cones can be modified by securing a latex glove over an adapted syringe case. Care should be taken to limit dead space from tailored equipment and to not occlude patient nares.

Intubation of rodents has variation depending on size and anatomy. Swabs and other materials needed to clean out oral cavities should be on hand during induction and intubation, because aspiration of food can lead to rapid demise. Transluminal and cut-down approaches have been described in rats for effective intubation.[56] Traditional laryngoscope blades often are too large to fit inside the oral cavity, and custom versions have been made for use in rats with success.[57] Recent studies have shown the benefit of video-endoscopy for proper placement of the ETT.[58–61] It is possible to use a rigid endoscope, otoscope, or vaginal speculum for the same purpose.[62,63] Positioning for endotracheal intubation can be facilitated by using rodent stands to help with alignment and opening of the oral cavity. Intubation is challenging in species with a palatal ostium (**Fig. 3**).[60] Stylets or wires can be advanced into the airway to allow the ETT to be positioned correctly.[64]

The smallest cuffed and uncuffed ETTs available are 2.5 mm and 2.0 mm, respectively. Cole ETTs allow for a tighter fit than an uncuffed ETT due to the larger proximal end; however, the smallest size is 2.0 mm. Mouse and rat ETTs can be purchased by various manufacturers. ETTs also can be crafted from IV catheters and directly connected to the circuit with low dead space ETT connectors (**Fig. 4**).[65] These adaptors have a side port for end-tidal carbon dioxide ($ETCO_2$) sampling. Delicate tissues and

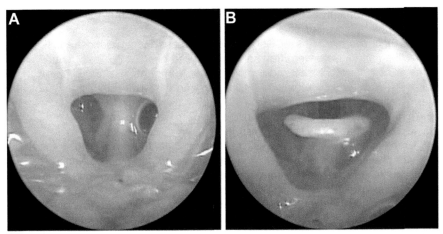

Fig. 3. (*A*) Palatal ostium in the guinea pig visualized using rigid endoscopy. (*B*) Palatal ostium in the guinea pig with the epiglottis disengaged from the soft palate. (*From* Johnson DH. Endoscopic intubation of exotic companion mammals. Vet Clin North Am Exot Anim Pract 2010;13(2):273-289.[60])

small airways put rodents at risk of blood obscuring the view, aspiration of blood, trauma to airway tissues, and tracheal tears. Swelling of airway tissues can lead to respiratory distress in recovery once the ETT is removed.

MONITORING

Monitoring vital signs under general anesthesia is paramount to success and risk reduction. Trends in anesthetic depth, cardiopulmonary values, and body temperature should be graphed and evaluated from the time of sedation through recovery. Corneal and palpebral reflexes may not be reliable, because drugs can cause a central pupil and changes to the pupil size. Pedal withdrawal and auricular reflexes are good indicators of depth and analgesia.

Minor changes in HR and RR are indicators of changes in depth and early signs of complications. Prevention of hypercapnia, hypoxemia, bradycardia, and hypotension is crucial. Simple equipment, such as a stethoscope and Doppler ultrasound probe,

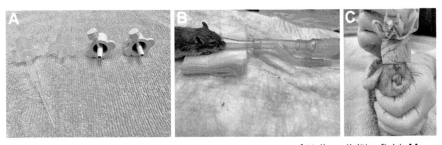

Fig. 4. (*A*) Low dead space ETT connectors. Image courtesy of Hallowell (Pittsfield, Massachusetts).[65] (*B*) Modified nose cone used in a rat to provide gas inhalant anesthesia. (*C*) Low dead space rodent non-rebreathing circuit being used in a Mongolian gerbil.

can provide a breadth of information without the necessity of sophisticated equipment. Doppler placement on the thorax can allow audible monitoring of both HR and RR. Electrocardiograms (ECGs) are used to assess rhythm changes and HRs. Alligator clips can cause severe trauma when applied directly. To limit trauma, small-diameter needles can be placed through the skin and the clips attached. High HR makes assessment of the rhythm challenging and the machine itself may not read rates greater than 350 beats/min. Both RR and character must be assessed to determine hypoventilation. Respiratory monitors increase work of breathing and add to mechanical dead space. They can assess TVs in patients as small as 300 g[66]

Pulse oximetry assesses global systemic oxygenation. Normally, readings above 95% are present if red blood cells are fully saturated and blood oxygen pressures are adequate. The percentage correlates to a partial pressure of oxygen in the arterial blood. The pulsatile flow of red blood cells past the probe is required to develop a measurement. HR greater than 400 beats/min may cause difficulties in acquiring readings. Both transmittance and reflectance probes are available for monitoring (**Fig. 5**).[67] The spring mechanism of the transmittance probes may occlude peripheral capillaries, which can prevent readings. The reflectance probe can be placed on fur-bearing skin and distal extremities to get a signal. Both types of probes have limitations, depending on patient temperature, ambient lighting, drugs administered to the patient, and patient size. Pulse oximetry is still a useful, audible tool for monitoring cardiopulmonary function in rodents. **Fig. 6** provides examples of rodent species' monitoring equipment placement in clinical cases.

Carbon dioxide (CO_2) is the by-product of aerobic metabolism. It is an indicator of ventilation, oxygenation, perfusion, and cardiac output. $ETCO_2$ is the CO_2 registered at the end of expiration. Normal $ETCO_2$ values are 35 mm Hg to 45 mm Hg but under

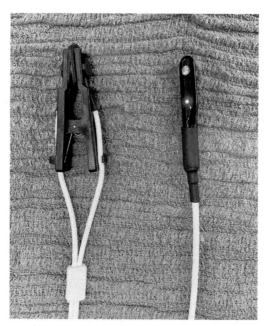

Fig. 5. Transmittance (left) versus reflectance (right) pulse oximetry probes.[67]

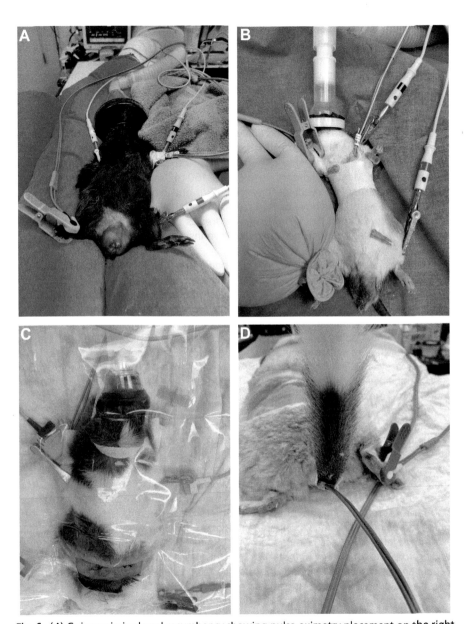

Fig. 6. (*A*) Guinea pig in dorsal recumbency showing pulse oximetry placement on the right pelvic limb, Doppler placement on the left thoracic limb, and ECG. (*B*) Rat in dorsal recumbency showing pulse oximetry placement on the right thoracic limb, Doppler placement over the heart, and ECG attached to transcutaneous hypodermic needles. (*C*) Guinea pig in sternal recumbency with clear drape allowing anesthesia personnel to visualize the patient. (*D*) Long-tailed chinchilla in sternal recumbency showing the Doppler placement on the ventral tail and pulse oximetry placement on the right pelvic limb.

anesthesia/deep sedation values up to 55 mm Hg are acceptable. $ETCO_2$ can be monitored with sidestream or mainstream capnography units. Mainstream units must be used in intubated patients and readings are from gases moving past the in-line sensor. Mainstream units add dead space and resistance to anesthetic equipment. Because rodents generally are not intubated with cuffed ETTs, this piece of equipment does not have accurate readings. High RRs and low TVs contribute further to inadequate data.[68] The sidestream unit offers more flexibility because it draws a portion of exhaled gases away to be analyzed and it does not require an intubated patient for readings. The unit can be attached to needles inserted directly into ETTs, onto catheters placed inside masks, or directly into the oral/nasal cavity of a heavily sedated patient. Most sidestream units recruit 150 mL/min to 200 mL/min of gases; this leads to falsely low readings given low TVs and high RRs. New low-flow (50-mL/min) sidestream units have been developed for human neonates but share similar inaccuracies in rodents. It is better to follow trends of $ETCO_2$ readings during monitoring. The resultant capnograph also can give insight into character and frequency of breath.

Blood pressure, in general, for conscious patients is 120/85 (95) mm Hg for systolic, diastolic, and mean arterial pressures, respectively. Under anesthesia, 95/60 (75) mm Hg is acceptable. Organs receiving substantial portions of cardiac output are perfused at pressures of 80/50 (60) mm Hg; drugs and concurrent disease may alter actual blood flow in these areas. Blood pressure can be assessed through a variety of methods. Manual palpation of pulses does not give a precise measurement but is a tactile assurance of systemic blood flow. In general, the presence of a femoral pulse suggests a systolic arterial pressure (SAP) greater than 60 mm Hg and more distal pulses (tail, tibial, pedal, and lingual) suggest an SAP greater than 80 mm Hg. Oscillometric blood pressure monitors and Doppler ultrasound probes coupled with a sphygmomanometer are 2 methods used for noninvasive blood pressure monitoring. Given the size of most rodents, there are constraints with adequate blood pressure cuff sizes and placement locales. High HR can decrease accuracy in oscillometric blood pressure readings, because the machine may struggle to read high-frequency oscillations. Doppler ultrasound probes and sphygmomanometers have similar constraints with cuff size and placement, although the limitation of discerning readings at high HR is set on the user. Invasive blood pressure monitoring is the gold standard to obtain blood pressure. Finding an artery for catheterization is challenging in rodents. Increased risk of blood loss, contamination, and occluding blood flow to cannulated extremities are reasons to use caution with this technique. It also is technically challenging to place an arterial catheter for the same reasons as venous catheterization. Benefit and risk must be weighed when adding the time spent attempting arterial catheters to the overall sedation/anesthesia period.

Other parameters that contribute to the overall outcome are body position, blood glucose, eye protection, and pain scoring. Body position can have an impact on respiratory efforts, especially in dorsal recumbency. The weight of abdominal organs can put pressure on the diaphragm, limiting appropriate depth of breath. Elevating the thorax can help direct organs caudally in the abdomen. Straightening the head and neck can allow better airflow in nonintubated patients. Eyes should be lubricated often, and care should be taken that eyes are not rubbing on masks or other nearby equipment. The eyelids often remain open under anesthesia and are at risk of corneal ulceration. Blood glucose should be monitored in the perioperative period for at-risk patients, and supplementation of dextrose can be considered. Postoperative pain scoring is vitally important to the overall success of the patient. Grimace scores in rats and mice are reliable in assessing pain.[69,70]

THERMOREGULATION

There are 4 forms of heat loss: conduction, convection, radiation, and evaporation. Each must be considered when maintaining body temperature in small patients. The hypothalamus regulates body temperature by feedback mechanisms, such as vaso-dilation, vasoconstriction, changes in ventilation (eg, panting), and shivering. Body temperature is finely controlled within $\pm0.4^\circ$C of normal. Anesthetic drugs widen that to $\pm4^\circ$C.[3] It should be taken into consideration that drug effects, durations, and metabolism may be altered at low body temperatures. Using warmed scrub, IV fluids, and saline irrigation during surgery are ways of preventing conductive losses.[71] Warming equipment, such as forced air blankets or circulating warm water blankets, should be near the patient from sedation through recovery, because these diminish radiative and convective losses. Body and extremity wraps prevent radiative losses. The authors have used cut portions of incontinence pads to cover exposed portions of the patient during the perianesthetic period. Fresh gas flow rates affect evaporative losses from the respiratory tract so lowest flow rates should be used. The Darvall system is an ultra–low-flow, heated anesthetic delivery system that can help maintain body temperature.[56] Prewarming rats has been shown to delay hypothermia under anesthesia.[72,73] Patients heated to 40°C in a warming chamber for 10 minutes achieved the expected rise in temperature.[72]

INDUCTION

Whether using a volatile agent or IV drugs, there are 4 stages of anesthesia. Stage 1 and stage 2 exhibit excitement phases associated with catecholamine release. Stage 3 is a surgical plane of anesthesia, which is required for intubation. The surgical anesthetic plane ranges from I to IV (light to deep surgical anesthesia). The final phase (stage 4) of anesthesia is brainstem paralysis and subsequent cardiopulmonary arrest. Given the initial excitement periods, it is wise to move rapidly through these phases to limit surges in catecholamines.

Gas inhalants frequently are used for inductions to limit stress of handling. There are several volatile anesthetic agents available, but isoflurane and sevoflurane are the most commonly used. Both agents cause cardiopulmonary depression, which progressively worsen at higher concentrations. They provide minimal analgesia with rapid onset and recovery. Isoflurane causes irritation to mucous membranes, so sevoflurane may be preferred. Rapidly filling chambers using high fresh gas flows decrease the duration of the involuntary excitement phase. Rodents commonly are placed in a large facemask or small chamber for anesthetic induction. The patient also can be restrained and a nose cone or small face mask placed during induction; it it important to be mindful of force of restraint during excitement phases. Species-specific minimum alveolar concentration (MAC) can be found in **Table 8**. Premedication is recommended, as previously reviewed.

IV administration of drugs also can be used for induction of general anesthesia. Alfaxalone is a neuroactive steroid exerting effect on the γ-aminobutyric acid type A (GABA$_A$)receptor. It has an onset of action of 30 seconds and peak duration of action of 15 minutes. It causes respiratory depression and vasodilation, dependent on both rate of administration and dose. It does not suppress the baroreceptor response to hypotension and, therefore, is thought to be cardioprotective. It is metabolized by the liver and excreted by the kidney. Induction doses are 2 mg/kg to 4 mg/kg IV.[3]

Propofol is a sedative-hypnotic agent also acting on the GABA$_A$ receptor. It has a similar onset, duration, and action to alfaxalone but does not allow reflex tachycardia to occur in the face of hypotension. It is metabolized mainly by the liver, but a portion is

Table 8
Minimum alveolar concentration of inhalant anesthetics in selected rodent species

Species	Isoflurane Minimum Alveolar Concentration (%)	Sevoflurane Minimum Alveolar Concentration (%)
Mice[3]	1.3–1.77	2.7
Rats[3]	1.17	2.99
Guinea pigs[76,77]	1.15	2[a]
Gerbils[74]	1.55	2.9
Hamsters[75]	1.62	2.31

[a] Extrapolated data.

metabolized by the lungs. The egg and soy emulsion give the distinct white color, which can support bacterial growth and hence has a short shelf-life. Induction doses are 3 mg/kg to 8 mg/kg IV.[3]

Ketamine is a dissociative with action on the N-methyl-ᴅ-aspartate receptor. The onset of action is 60 seconds. With an induction dose, 15 minutes of surgical anesthesia can be achieved. Duration of analgesia can persist up to 2 hours. Ketamine increases catecholamine release, causing increased cardiac output, normal to increased blood pressures, and variable changes to RR and pattern. Ketamine also produces muscle rigidity and often is paired with a benzodiazepine. It can decrease seizure thresholds and increase heart sensitivity to catecholamine induced arrhythmias. Induction doses are 2 mg/kg to 15 mg/kg IV.[3] Co-inductions can be used with various combinations. Propofol and alfaxalone can be paired with either ketamine or a benzodiazepine to decrease doses required of either drug, which diminishes deleterious side effects. Ketamine causes a central eye position and maintains palpebral response, which may make the patient appear at a lighter plane of anesthesia. Caution should be used when selecting inhalant concentrations for maintenance anesthesia.

MAINTENANCE

Anesthesia may be required for noninvasive procedures as well as surgical procedures. Depending on the duration of the procedure, expected pain levels, and physical limitations, a maintenance protocol can be selected. There are 3 fundamental options: volatile gas anesthesia, partial IV anesthesia (PIVA), and total IV anesthesia (TIVA). Infusions are excellent, but lengthy procedure times can lead to drug accumulation and prolonged recoveries.

Volatile gas agents can be used to maintain general anesthesia. Sevoflurane and isoflurane both have an impact on cardiac output by decreasing contractility, vasodilation, and to some degree HR. They are eliminated rapidly from the body and have minimal metabolism. These agents have a wide spectrum of utility. Volatile agents combined with continuous rate infusions (CRIs) to reduce inhalant requirements and MAC are known as PIVAs. Multiple studies have shown improved cardiopulmonary parameters when inhalant concentrations can be reduced with use of CRIs. Drugs with short elimination half-lives are best suited for infusions. Available options are detailed in **Table 9**.[78–81]

The goals of general anesthesia are immobilization, amnesia, and analgesia. Through a combination of drugs, these can be achieved with injectable agents alone. TIVA often is used in small animal anesthesia with nearly endless combinations of both drugs and rates of infusions. The primary downside of TIVA is accumulation of drugs in

Table 9
Percent reduction of minimum alveolar concentration of isoflurane and/or sevoflurane with use of adjunct drugs in dogs and rodents

Drug	Minimum Alveolar Concentration Reduction (%)	Application
α_2-Agonists	18–59	Infusion[78,79]
Benzodiazepines	30	Injection[80]
Opioids	17–70	Opioid specific, rate-dependent[79]
Propofol	48	Infusion[80]
Maropitant	30	Injection[81]
Lidocaine	30	Infusion[81]
Ketamine	>90	Infusion, rate-dependent[81]

the body and longer recoveries because of their metabolism. Combinations that include analgesia, sedation, and unconsciousness are most routine. Intermittent boluses of anesthetic drugs increase morbidity and mortality rates in rodents, so CRIs are the preferred method of anesthesia maintenance. A drug steady state must be achieved by overcoming the elimination or metabolism rate with an infusion rate and then titrating to affect. It takes approximately 5 times the half-life of a drug to provide a 97% steady state.[52] A loading dose can be used to offset the delay in achieving steady state.

Infusion rates can be surmised with a general calculation based on a drug's standard dose and duration of action. For example, if propofol's loading dose is 10 mg/kg and propofol has an average duration of 15 minutes, then it requires 4 boluses of propofol in an hour or 40 mg/kg/h for an infusion rate. Understanding basic doses and properties of anesthetics allows infusion rates to be calculated for most rodent species. See **Table 10** for a review of CRI dosing recommendations.

LOCAL ANESTHESIA

A full discussion of the topic of local anesthetic blocks is not within the scope of this article. Local anesthetics are the only drugs that prevent pain and nociception and should be used during any painful procedure. Knowledge of anatomy helps translate blocks used in small animals to rodents. The safe dose of lidocaine for rodents is 7 mg/kg and for bupivacaine, 8 mg/kg.[91] Local anesthetics can be diluted by 50% with sterile saline to allow for more volume.

RECOVERY

Recovery from sedation/anesthesia is highly variable, depending on the protocol used, the length of the procedure, and the condition of the patient. Prolonged recovery typically is a result of hypothermia, hypoperfusion due to hypotension, hypoglycemia, or impaired drug elimination. Postoperative losses make up a significant volume of morbidity in small mammals, so it is vital to monitor closely during this time. It is important to continue ventilating the patient after the anesthetic gas has been discontinued and until it is breathing independently. As discussed previously, the high metabolic rate of rodents does not allow for a buffer of hypoxic damage, and cardiac arrest rapidly follows respiratory arrest. Patients should be assessed continually by an anesthetist or technician until they have been extubated, are swallowing and breathing independently, and are able to lift their head. The authors

Table 10
Constant rate infusions in rodents.

Drug	Loading Dose	Infusion Rate	Comments
Alfaxalone[82]	N/A	10 mg/kg/h	Rats: premedicated with ketamine 80 mg/kg + xylazine 8 mg/kg; alfaxalone bolus 2–5 mg/kg IV produced apnea
Buprenorphine[83]	5 mg/kg	0.0125 mg/h/mouse	Mice: no change in immune function with chronic infusion
Butorphanol[84]	0.2–0.4 mg/kg 0.2–0.4 mg/kg	0.2–0.4 mg/kg/h 0.2–0.4 mg/kg/h	Guinea pigs Rats
Dexmedetomidine[85]	N/A	0.004–0.02 mg/kg/h	Rats: premedicated with fentanyl 0.3 mg/kg + medetomidine 0.3 mg/kg IP; higher rates required for analgesia
Fentanyl[83,84]	0.005–0.01 mg/kg 0.25 mg/kg 0.005–0.01 mg/kg	0.01–0.03 mg/kg/h (intraoperative) 0.00125–0.005 mg/kg/h (postoperative) 0.0075 mg/h/mouse 0.015–0.06 mg/kg/h (intra-perative) 0.00125–0.005 mg/kg/h (postoperative)	Guinea pigs Mice: acute immune suppression with bolus Rats: MAC reduction 10%–60%; respiratory depression
Hydromorphone[84]	0.05 mg/kg 0.05 mg/kg	0.025–0.05 mg/kg/h 0.025–0.05 mg/kg/h	Guinea pigs Rats
Ketamine[84,86]	0.5–2.5 mg/kg 80 mg/kg IM 30 mg/kg 0.5–2.5 mg/kg	0.3–1.2 mg/kg/h (intraoperative); 0.1–0.4 mg/kg/h (postoperative) 40–80 mg/kg/h IP 60–90 mg/kg/h 0.3–1.2 mg/kg/h (intraoperative); 0.1–0.4 mg/kg/h (postoperative)	Guinea pigs Mice: premedicated with ketamine + xylazine ± acepromazine Rats: vasoconstriction throughout administration Rats: clinical experience/reviews
Lidocaine[84]	1–2 mg/kg 1–2 mg/kg	0.05–0.1 mg/kg/min 0.05–0.1 mg/kg/min	Guinea pigs: Lethal Dose (LD50) 24 mg/kg Rats
Medetomidine[87]	0.12 mg/kg SC	0.08 mg/kg/h SC	Rats: allowed reduction of isoflurane to 0.5%

Drug	Dose	Dose	Notes
Morphine[88]	12 mg/kg IP	5 mg/kg/h	Rats and mice: awake animals/pain tolerance
Nalbuphine[89]	2 mg/kg SC	1–5 mg/kg/h	Rats: sepsis model, grimace scoring
Propofol[84,87]	20–30 mg/kg 10–20 mg/kg	20–60 mg/kg/h 0.6–1 mg/kg/min	Rats: vasodilation increases throughout maintenance Rats
Remifentanil[84]	N/A	0.06–0.12 mg/kg/h	Rats: MAC reduction 10%–60%; respiratory depression
Xylazine[90]	8 mg/kg IM	4 mg/kg/h IP	Mice: premedicated with ketamine + xylazine ± acepromazine

All routes of administration are intravenous, unless otherwise noted.

maintain monitoring equipment, including Doppler and pulse oximeter, on patients until they can ambulate. Fluid therapy should continue during this time, and, if vascular access was not obtained, warmed SC fluids can assist with temperature regulation and hydration.

Postoperative blood glucose measurement is not performed routinely, but in cases of a patient inappetent prior to the procedure or when a sustained anesthetic period is required, it is indicated. Care must be taken when rewarming patients that are questionably hypovolemic or hypoglycemic, because warming causes increased metabolic demand for glucose and allows for dilation of vasoconstricted peripheral vessels. It has been postulated that this may explain some of the sudden death appreciated postoperatively in rodents.[22]

Reversal agents can be administered to antagonize the action of some sedative drugs and allow faster recovery. In most rodent patients, a swift recovery is desirable to normalize body temperature and appetite as soon as possible to reduce chances of ileus or hypoglycemia. As the patient is recovering, evidence of pain, such as hunched posture, bruxism, grimace, or tachycardia, should be assessed for. Analgesia should be provided to ensure continual pain coverage.

A recovery cage should be provided that contains a source of supplemental heat capable of maintaining an ambient temperature of 80°F to 85°F. Warming devices that are demonstrably safest include circulating water blankets, forced air warmers, hotdog warming blankets, internal floor cage warmers, and heat lamps positioned outside the cage. Any warming device carries a risk of thermal injury to the patient, and following manufacturer instructions while ensuring close monitoring and protection from direct contact ia imperative. Warming devices, such as heated fluid bags, gloves, or microwavable discs, carry an increased risk for thermal burns due to uneven heating and a lack of knowledge of the internal temperature of the device. Recovering patients may be prone in 1 position long enough for a burn to occur even from a device that has been warmed to an appropriate temperature. The risk of thermal burns is increased with wet fur, fur removal, or pressure points. It is recommended to check the temperature every 15 minutes to 20 minutes until within 1° of normal and then reduce warming measures. In the authors' experience, small rodents fluctuate body temperature rapidly in response to external warming measures, and heat stress from overwarming is a consequence. A notable exception to the recommended recovery cage temperatureiss are chinchillas, which require lower ambient temperatures if their coat is intact. Hyperthermia in chinchillas can occur easily at temperatures greater than 75°F.

The recovery cage should be in a quiet, visible area. The floor and lower portion of the walls should be padded with towels or blankets because patients often are unsteady when they begin to ambulate. Particulate substrate, such as paper pulp bedding, is not recommended until a patient is fully recovered because it can obscure the view of the patient or obstruct respirations. If the recovery area is not directly visible and a staff member cannot be delegated for monitoring, a camera can be placed in the cage with the patient (ideally with audio capability to hear the Doppler) and observed remotely using a monitor screen.

SUMMARY

In conclusion, rodent sedation and anesthesia are a continually developing discipline with unique challenges. With some specialty equipment, dedication, and practice, the zoologic companion animal practitioner can mitigate many of the inherent dangers of rodent anesthesia and attain a successful outcome.

REFERENCES

1. AVMA. U.S. pet ownership statistics. 2017-2018 U.S. Pet Ownership & Demographics Sourcebook.
2. Longley L. Anaesthesia of exotic pets. 1st edition. New York: Elsevier Health Sciences; 2008.
3. Grimm, Lamont L, Tranquilli W, et al. Veterinary anesthesia and analgesia: the Fifth Edition of Lumb and Jones. Wiley-Blackwell; 2015. p. 1072.
4. Quesenberry K, Carpenter JW. Surgery. Anesthesia, Analgesia, and Sedation of Small Mammals. Found in: Rabbits, Rodents, and Ferrets Clinical Medicine and Surgery Third Edition. St. Louis, Missouri: Elseiver; 2012:429-451.
5. Boehmer E. Anesthesia and Analgesia. Found in: Dentistry in Rabbits and Rodents 2015:89-96
6. Brodbelt D. Perioperative mortality in small animal anaesthesia. Vet J 2009; 182(2):152-61.
7. West G, Heard D, Caulkett N. Rodents. Found in: Zoo Animal and Wildlife Immobilization and Anesthesia. 2007:665-664.
8. Yarto-Jaramillo E. Respiratory system anatomy, physiology, and disease: Guinea pigs and chinchillas. Vet Clin North Am Exot Anim Pract 2011;14(2):339-vi.
9. Cantwell SL. Ferret, Rabbit, and Rodent Anesthesia. Vet Clin North Am Exot Anim Pract 2001;4(1):169-91.
10. Jekl V, Hauptman K, Knotek Z. Diseases in pet degus: a retrospective study in 300 animals. J Small Anim Pract 2011;52(2):107-12.
11. Heatley JJ. Cardiovascular Anatomy, Physiology, and Disease of Rodents and Small Exotic Mammals. Vet Clin North Am Exot Anim Pract 2009;12(1):99-113.
12. Pignon C, Sanchez-Migallon Guzman D, Sinclair K, et al. Evaluation of heart murmurs in chinchillas (Chinchilla lanigera): 59 cases (1996-2009). J Am Vet Med Assoc 2012;241(10):1344-7.
13. Martel A, Donnelly T, Mans C. Update on Diseases in Chinchillas: 2013-2019. Vet Clin North Am Exot Anim Pract 2020;23(2):321-35.
14. Horn CC, Kimball BA, Wang H, et al. Why Can't Rodents Vomit? A Comparative Behavioral, Anatomical, and Physiological Study. PLoS One 2013;8(4):e60537.
15. Kling MA. A Review of Respiratory System Anatomy, Physiology, and Disease in the Mouse, Rat, Hamster, and Gerbil. Vet Clin North Am Exot Anim Pract 2011; 14(2):287 337.
16. Mancinelli E, Capello V. Anatomy and Disorders of the Oral Cavity of Rat-like and Squirrel-like Rodents. Vet Clin North Am Exot Anim Pract 2016;19(3):871-900.
17. Johnson D. Prairie Dog Medicine & Surgery. In: Atlantic Coast Veterinary Conference; Raleigh, NC, 2004.
18. Bonis A, Anderson L, Talhouarne G, et al. Cardiovascular resistance to thrombosis in 13-lined ground squirrels. J Comp Physiol B 2019;189(1):167-77.
19. Mayer J, Schnellbacher R, Rich E, et al. Use of a Commercial Continuous Interstitial Glucose Monitor in Rabbits (Oryctolagus cuniculus). J Exot Pet Med 2016;25(3):220-5.
20. Allweiler SI. How to Improve Anesthesia and Analgesia in Small Mammals. Vet Clin North Am Exot Anim Pract 2016;19(2):361-77.
21. Lu KH, Cao J, Oleson ST, et al. Contrast-Enhanced Magnetic Resonance Imaging of Gastric Emptying and Motility in Rats. IEEE Trans Biomed Eng 2017;64(11): 2546-54.
22. Johnson DH. Anesthesia, Surgery, & Postoperative Care of Exotic Companion Mammals. In: Western Veterinary Conference; Los Vegas, February 18, 2020.

23. Rondeau A, Langlois I, Pang DS, et al. Development of a sedation assessment scale for comparing the sedative effects of alfaxalone-hydromorphone and ketamine-midazolam-hydromorphone for intravenous catheterization in the domestic rat (Rattus norvegicus). J Exot Pet Med 2020;35:117–22.
24. Plumb DC. Plumb's 9th Edition veterinary drug Handbook. Wiley Blackwell; 2018.
25. Beiglböck C, Zenker W. Evaluation of Three Combinations of Anesthetics For Use in Free-Ranging Alpine Marmots (Marmota Marmota). J Wildl Dis 2003;39(3): 665–74.
26. Jones KL. Therapeutic Review: Alfaxalone. J Exot Pet Med 2012;21(4):347–53.
27. Hanusch C, Hoeger S, Beck GC. Anaesthesia of small rodents during magnetic resonance imaging. Methods 2007;43(1):68–78.
28. Keeble E, Meredith A. BSAVA manual of rodents and Ferrets. Hoboken: Wiley Blackwell; 2009.
29. Doerning CM, Bradley MP, Lester PA, et al. Effects of subcutaneous alfaxalone alone and in combination with dexmedetomidine and buprenorphine in guinea pigs (Cavia porcellus). Vet Anaesth Analg 2018;45(5):658–66.
30. Morgan RJ, Eddy LB, Solie TN, et al. Ketamine-acepromazine as an anaesthetic agent for chinchillas (Chinchilla laniger). Lab Anim 1981;15(3):281–3.
31. Carpenter J, Marion C. Exotic Animal Formulary. 5th Edition. St. Louis, Missouri: Elseiver; 2017.
32. Tsukamoto A, Uchida K, Maesato S, et al. Combining isoflurane anesthesia with midazolam and butorphanol in rats. Exp Anim 2016;65(3):223–30.
33. Boehm CA, Carney EL, Tallarida RJ, et al. Midazolam enhances the analgesic properties of dexmedetomidine in the rat. Vet Anaesth Analg 2010;37:550–6.
34. Higuchi S, Yamada R, Hashimoto A, et al. Evaluation of a combination of alfaxalone with medetomidine and butorphanol for inducing surgical anesthesia in laboratory mice. Jpn J Vet Res 2016;64:131–9.
35. Kawai S, Takagi Y, Kaneko S, et al. Effect of three types of mixed anesthetic agents alternate to ketamine in mice. Exp Anim 2011;60(5):481–7.
36. Tsukamoto A, Niino N, Sakamoto M, et al. The validity of anesthetic protocols for the surgical procedure of castration in rats. Exp Anim 2018;67(3):329–36.
37. Bellini L, Banzato T, Contiero B, et al. Evaluation of three medetomidine-based protocols for chemical restraint and sedation for non-painful procedures in companion rats (Rattus norvegicus). Vet J 2014;200(3):456–8.
38. Albrecht M, Henke J, Tacke S, et al. Effects of isoflurane, ketamine-xylazine and a combination of medetomidine, midazolam and fentanyl on physiological variables continuously measured by telemetry in Wistar rats. BMC Vet Res 2014; 10:198.
39. Wixson SK, White WJ, Hughes HC Jr, et al. The effects of pentobarbital, fentanyl-droperidol, ketamine-xylazine and ketamine-diazepam on core and surface body temperature regulation in adult male rats. Lab Anim Sci 1987;37(6):743–9.
40. Parkinson L, Mans C. Anesthetic and Postanesthetic Effects of Alfaxalone-Butorphanol Compared with Dexmedetomidine-Ketamine in Chinchillas (Chinchilla lanigera). J Am Assoc Lab Anim Sci 2017;56(3):6.
41. Doss GA, Mans C, Stepien RL. Echocardiographic effects of dexmedetomidine-ketamine in chinchillas (Chinchilla lanigera). Lab Anim 2017;51(1):89–92.
42. Fox L, Snyder LB, Mans C. Comparison of Dexmedetomidine-Ketamine with Isoflurane for Anesthesia of Chinchillas (Chinchilla lanigera). J Am Assoc Lab Anim Sci 2016;55(3):312–6.
43. Siriarchavatana P, Ayers JD, Kendall LV. Anesthetic Activity of Alfaxalone Compared with Ketamine in Mice. J Am Assoc Lab Anim Sci 2016;55(4):426–30.

44. Lau C, Ranasinghe MG, Shiels I, et al. Plasma pharmacokinetics of alfaxalone after a single intraperitoneal or intravenous injection of Alfaxan(®) in rats. J Vet Pharmacol Ther 2013;36(5):516–20.
45. Eshar D, Beaufrère H. Anesthetic Effects of Alfaxalone-Ketamine, Alfaxalone-Ketamine-Dexmedetomidine, and Alfaxalone-Butorphanol-Midazolam Administered Intramuscularly in Five-striped Palm Squirrels (Funambulus pennantii). J Am Assoc Lab Anim Sci 2020;59(4):384–92.
46. Pachon RE, Scharf BA, Vatner DE, et al. Best anesthetics for assessing left ventricular systolic function by echocardiography in mice. Am J Physiol Heart Circ Physiol 2015;308(12):H1525–9.
47. Tanaka DM, Romano MM, Carvalho EE, et al. Effect of different anesthetic agents on left ventricular systolic function assessed by echocardiography in hamsters. Braz J Med Biol Res 2016;49(10):e5294.
48. Olson ME, McCabe K. Anesthesia in the Richardson's ground squirrel: comparison of ketamine, ketamine and xylazine, droperidol and fentanyl, and sodium pentobarbital. J Am Vet Med Assoc 1986;189(9):1035–7.
49. Aguiar J, Mogridge G, Hall J. Femoral fracture repair and sciatic and femoral nerve blocks in a guinea pig. J Small Anim Pract 2014;55(12):635–9.
50. Adelsperger AR, Bigiarelli-Nogas KJ, Toore I, et al. Use of a low-flow digital anesthesia system for mice and rats. J Vis Exp 2016;115:54436.
51. Grune J, Tabuchi A, Kuebler WM. Alveolar dynamics during mechanical ventilation in the healthy and injured lung. Intensive Care Med Exp 2019;7:34.
52. Vreugdenhil HA, Heijnen CJ, Plötz FB, et al. Mechanical ventilation of healthy rats suppresses peripheral immune function. Eur Respir J 2004;23:122–8.
53. Kleinman LI, Radford EP Jr. Ventilation standards for small mammals. J Appl Physiol 1964;19(2):360–2.
54. Photo credit: Broome Rodent Restrainers. Conduct Science 2021. Available at: https://conductscience.com/lab/broome-rodent-restrainers/. Accessed February 28, 2021.
55. Clemency B, Tanaka K, May P, et al. Intravenous vs. intraosseous access and return of spontaneous circulation during out of hospital cardiac arrest. Am J Emerg Med 2017;35:222–6.
56. Zheng J, Xiao Z, Zhang K, et al. Improved blind tracheal intubation in rats: a simple and secure approach. J Vet Med Sci 2020;82(9):1329–33.
57. Vongerichten A, Aristovich K, dos Santos GS, et al. Design for a three-dimensional printed laryngoscope blade for the intubation of rats. Lab Anim (Ny) 2014;43(4):140–2.
58. Konno K, Shiotani Y, Itano N, et al. Visible, safe and certain endotracheal intubation using endoscope system and inhalation anesthesia for rats. J Vet Med Sci 2014;76(10):1375–81.
59. Konno K, Itano N, Ogawa T, et al. New Visible Endotracheal intubation method using the endoscope system for mice inhalational anesthesia. J Vet Med Sci 2014;76(6):863–8.
60. Johnson DH. Endoscopic intubation of exotic companion mammals. Vet Clin North Am Exot Anim Pract 2010;13(2):273–89.
61. Miranda A, Pêgo JM, Correia-Pinto J. Animal facility videoendoscopic intubation station: tips and tricks from mice to rabbits. Lab Anim 2017;51(2):204–7.
62. Thomas JL, Dumouchel J, Li J, et al. Endotracheal intubation in mice via direct laryngoscopy using an otoscope. J Vis Exp 2014;86:50269.
63. Alzaben KR, Abu-Halaweh SA, Aloweidi AK, et al. Use of the Nasal Speculum for Rat Endotracheal Intubation. Am J Appl Sci 2009;6(3):507–11.

64. Kujime K, Natelson BH. A method of endotracheal intubation of guinea pigs (Cavia porcellus). Lab Anim Sci 1981;31(6):715–6.
65. Photo credit: Low dead space endotracheal tube connectors. Hallowell (Pittsfield, MA) Product Catalog 2021. Available at: https://www.hallowell.com/index.php?pr=z152A1261. Accessed May 24, 2021.
66. Flecknell PA. Anaesthesia of common laboratory species. In: Flecknell P, editor. Laboratory animal Anaesthesia. Boston: Academic Press; 1996.
67. Lafferty K, Pollock C. Pulse oximetry in exotic animal species. Cornell, IL: Lafeber Vet Online; 2018.
68. Schmalisch G. Current methodological and technical limitations of time and volumetric capnography in newborns. Biomed Eng Online 2016;15(1):104.
69. Leung V, Zhang E, Pang DS. Real-time application of the Rat Grimace Scale as a welfare refinement in laboratory rats. Sci Rep 2016;6:31667.
70. Rojas-Mota D, Olmos-Hernandez A, Verduzco-Mendoza A, et al. The Utility of Grimace Scales for Practical Pain Assessment in Laboratory Animals. Animals (Basel) 2020;10(10):1838.
71. Skorupski AM, Zhang J, Ferguson D, et al. Quantification of Induced Hypothermia from Aseptic Scrub Applications during Rodent Surgery Preparation. J Am Assoc Lab Anim Sci 2017;56(5):562–9.
72. Rufiange M, Leung VSY, Simpson K, et al. Pre-warming before general anesthesia with isoflurane delays the onset of hypothermia in rats. PLoS One 2020; 15(3):e0219722.
73. Schuster CJ, Pang DSJ. Forced-air pre-warming prevents peri-anaesthetic hypothermia and shortens recovery in adult rats. Lab Anim 2018;52(2):142–51.
74. Gomez de Segura IA, Benito de la Vibora J, Criado A. Determination of minimum alveolar concentration for halothane, isoflurane, and sevoflurane in the gerbil. Lab Anim 2009;43(3):239–42.
75. Vivien B, Langeron O, Coriat P, et al. Minimum alveolar anesthetic concentration of volatile anesthetics in normal and cardiomyopathic hamsters. Anesth Analg 1999;88(3):489–93.
76. Seifen AB, Kennedy RH, Bray JP, et al. Estimation of minimum alveolar concentration (MAC) for halothane, enflurane and isoflurane in spontaneously breathing guinea pigs. Lab Anim Sci 1989;39(6):579–81.
77. Heindl B, et al. Sevoflurane and isoflurane protect the reperfused guinea pig heart by reducing postischemic adhesion of polymorphonuclear neutrophils. Anesthesiology 1999;91(2):521–30.
78. Sinclair MD. A review of the physiological effects of alpha2-agonists related to the clinical use of medetomidine in small animal practice. Can Vet J 2003;44(11): 885–97.
79. Teixerira Neto FJ. Dexmedetomidine: A New Alpha 2 Agonist for Small Animal Practice. WSAVA. World Congress Proceedings, Sao Paulo, Brazil, July, 2009.
80. Reed R, Doherty T. Minimum alveolar concentration: Key concepts and a review of its pharmacological reduction in dogs. Part 1. Res Vet Sci 2018;117:266–70.
81. Reed R, Doherty T. Minimum alveolar concentration: Key concepts and a review of its pharmacological reduction in dogs. Part 2. Res Vet Sci 2018;118:27–33.
82. Heng K, Marx JO, Jampachairsi K, et al. Continuous Rate Infusion of Alfaxalone during Ketamine-Xylazine Anesthesia in Rats. J Am Assoc Lab Anim Sci 2020; 59(2):170–5.
83. Martucci C, Panerai AE, Sacerdote P. Chronic fentanyl or buprenorphine infusion in the mouse: similar analgesic profile but different effects on immune responses. Pain 2004;110(1–2):385–92.

84. Schnellbacher R, Comolli J. Constant Rate Infusions in Exotic Animals. J Exot Pet Med 2020;35:50–7.
85. Frankem ND, van Oostrom H, Stienen PJ, et al. Evaluation of analgesic and sedative effects of continuous infusion of dexmedetomidine by measuring somatosensory- and auditory-evoked potentials in the rat. Vet Anaesth Analg 2008;35(5):424–31.
86. Brookes ZL, Brown NJ, Reilly CS. Intravenous anaesthesia and the rat microcirculation: the dorsal microcirculatory chamber. Br J Anaesth 2000;85(6):901–3.
87. Kint LT, Seewoo BJ, Hyndman TH, et al. The Pharmacokinetics of Medetomidine Administered Subcutaneously during Isoflurane Anaesthesia in Sprague-Dawley Rats. Animals (Basel) 2020;10(6):1050.
88. Cox BM, Ginsburg M, Willis J, et al. The Offset of Morphine Tolerance in Rats and Mice. Br J Pharmacol 1975;53(3):383–91.
89. Jeger V, et al. Improving animal welfare using continuous nalbuphine infusion in a long-term rat model of sepsis. Intensive Care Med Exp 2017;5(1):23.
90. Erickson RL, Terzi MC, Jaber SM, et al. Intraperitoneal Continuous-Rate Infusion for the Maintenance of Anesthesia in Laboratory Mice (Mus musculus). J Am Assoc Lab Anim Sci 2016;55(5):548–57.
91. Office of the IACUC. In: Vertebrate Animal Research. Analgesia (Guideline). 2020. Available at: https://animal.research.uiowa.edu/iacuc-guidelines-analgesia. Accessed March 10, 2021.

African Pygmy Hedgehog (*Atelerix albiventris*) and Sugar Glider (*Petaurus breviceps*) Sedation and Anesthesia

Grayson Doss, DVM, DACZM[a],*,
Cristina de Miguel Garcia, DVM, MSc, MRCVS, DECVAA[b]

KEYWORDS

- Anesthesia • Petauridae • Erinaceidae • Supraglottic airway device • Hypothermia
- Insectivore • Intraosseous catheter • Marsupial

KEY POINTS

- Aggressive thermal support is important to prevent rapid development of hypothermia when immobilizing hedgehogs and sugar gliders.
- Sedation provides an alternative to general anesthesia and can be partially to fully reversible, depending on the agents used.
- Intravascular access in these species can be challenging; intraosseous catheters are commonly used and placed in the proximal femur or tibia.
- Induction and maintenance of anesthesia is most commonly performed using inhalant anesthetics, such as isoflurane and sevoflurane.
- Due to their small size and unique anatomy, endotracheal intubation can be challenging in hedgehogs and sugar gliders, and requires small internal diameter endotracheal tubes; a supraglottic airway device designed for small rabbits can be used in hedgehogs.

 Video content accompanies this article at http://www.vetexotic.theclinics.com.

INTRODUCTION

African pygmy hedgehogs and sugar gliders are common zoologic companion animals that commonly require chemical immobilization for examination and diagnostic procedures. Because of their small size, veterinarians must take into account several

The authors do not have any commercial or financial conflicts of interest or any funding sources to disclose.
[a] Department of Surgical Sciences, School of Veterinary Medicine, University of Wisconsin-Madison, 2015 Linden Drive, Madison, WI 53706, USA; [b] Department of Clinical Sciences, Cornell University College of Veterinary Medicine, 602 Tower Road, Ithaca, NY 14853, USA
* Corresponding author.
E-mail address: gdoss@wisc.edu

Vet Clin Exot Anim 25 (2022) 257–272
https://doi.org/10.1016/j.cvex.2021.08.005
1094-9194/22/© 2021 Elsevier Inc. All rights reserved.
vetexotic.theclinics.com

key factors when planning for immobilization of these popular pet species. Major challenges include obtaining intravascular access, intubation, and monitoring, as well as rapid onset of hypothermia.

SPECIES AND ANATOMIC PARTICULARITIES RELEVANT TO SEDATION AND ANESTHESIA

African pygmy hedgehogs (*Atelerix albiventris*), or 4-toed hedgehogs, are solitary, nocturnal insectivores that are widespread throughout West, Central, and East Africa.[1] This species is part of the family Erinaceidae, part of the order Eulipotyphla, which contains other small insectivores including shrews, moles, and solenodons. Hedgehogs possess a unique dorsal covering of keratinaceous spines, known as the mantle, which contains a thick layer of adipose tissue. When startled, hedgehogs readily adopt a characteristic defensive posture, rolling into tight ball in which the entire body is wrapped protectively by the spiny mantle. This combination of peculiar anatomy and behavior can result in an inability to perform even a physical examination without chemical immobilization. A cursory examination can be performed in some individuals through scruffing, although this is likely stressful.

Hedgehogs have a narrow oropharyngeal cavity with a caudally located pharynx, as well as a prominent tongue base and large tonsils. The epiglottis is broad with a prominent apex (**Fig. 1**) and is normally dorsal to the soft palate (Video 1); it must be gently displaced to visualize the glottis (Video 2).

Sugar gliders (*Petaurus breviceps*) are small, arboreal, nocturnal marsupials native to New Guinea and Australia with patagia used for gliding short distances.[2,3] A limited physical examination can be performed with manual restraint; however, for a complete physical and an oral examination, chemical immobilization is generally required. The normal oropharyngeal anatomy of sugar gliders is poorly described. Unlike in African pygmy hedgehogs, the epiglottis does not normally sit dorsal to the soft palate (see **Fig. 1**, Video 3).

Hypothermia is a common concern when anesthetizing small mammals because of their relatively large surface area in relation to body mass. Rapid onset of hypothermia has been documented with both injectable sedation and inhalant anesthesia in hedgehogs, with rectal temperatures as low as 91.1°F (32.8°C) reported within 5 minutes of

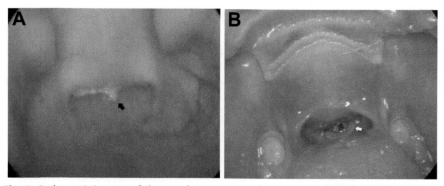

Fig. 1. Endoscopic images of the oropharynx in an African pygmy hedgehog (*A*) and sugar glider (*B*). Note the large tonsils (dorsolateral) and the prominent apex of the epiglottis (*arrow*) after it is displaced from its normal position behind the soft palate in African pygmy hedgehogs (*A*). Note how the epiglottis (*arrow*) of sugar gliders is visible and not normally positioned behind the soft palate (*B*).

injection or induction, despite thermal support.[4-7] Therefore, aggressive thermal support consisting of a combination of methods (eg, forced air warmers, circulating water blankets, microwaveable heat pads) should be used when anesthetizing hedgehogs and sugar gliders along with regular monitoring of rectal temperature. Hedgehog spines can easily penetrate circulating water blankets and the surface should be adequately protected (eg, layers of cloth) to prevent damage and water leakage. Expect normal body temperatures to be lower than most small mammal species, and the cloacal temperature of normal sugar gliders is significantly lower than the rectal temperature (**Table 1**). Considering the relatively high metabolic rates of these species, fasting times should be short to prevent complications.[8,9] Normal gastrointestinal transit times have not been established for either species.

Given their small size, placing intravenous (IV) catheters for cardiovascular support under anesthesia can be challenging in hedgehogs and sugar gliders. Commonly used IV catheter placement sites in hedgehogs are the cephalic and saphenous veins (**Fig. 2**) using a 24-gauge to 26-gauge or similarly sized over-the-needle catheter. Placing IV catheters in even the largest sugar gliders can be difficult to impossible. Intraosseous (IO) catheters are commonly used in both species, and short, small-gauge (22–25g) spinal needles (**Fig. 3**) can be placed in the proximal femur or proximal tibia (**Fig. 4**). Hypodermic needles also can be used in small individuals, but blockage with cortical bone can occur during placement (**Fig. 5**). Aspiration of bone marrow is helpful for determining if the needle is seated in the intramedullary cavity (see **Fig. 4**). Proper placement should be verified with orthogonal radiographs, and IO catheters can be used for both fluid and drug administration. Depending on the length of needle used, it may not be able to be fully seated to the hub but should still be effective for use. The IO catheter can be secured in place with tape along with a piece of wooden tongue depressor incorporated for rigidity (see **Fig. 5**). One benefit of tibial IO catheters in hedgehogs is they often remain accessible even when the hedgehog rolls up into a defensive posture.[10]

SEDATION

Injectable sedation can facilitate minor procedures including physical examination, venipuncture, imaging, and diagnostic sample collection without the need for general anesthesia (**Fig. 6**). The sedation protocol may be partially to fully reversible, depending on the agents used. The subcutaneous (SC) route is often used for injections, as

Table 1
Select physiologic parameters for normal African pygmy hedgehogs and sugar gliders[3,4,25,30,31]

Parameter	African Pygmy Hedgehogs	Sugar Gliders
Heart rate[a]	170–250 beats/min	100–200 beats/min
Respiratory rate[a]	18–90 breaths/min	16–40 breaths/min
Rectal temperature	95.7°F–98.6°F (35.4°C–37.0°C)	97.3°F (36.3°C)[b]
Cloacal temperature	—	89.6°F (32°C)[b]
Body weight		
Female	300–400 g	80–130 g
Male	400–600 g	100–160 g

[a] Values recorded in normal animals anesthetized with isoflurane anesthesia.
[b] Mean value.

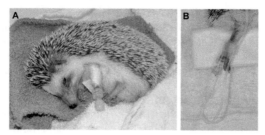

Fig. 2. IV catheter placement in hedgehogs. The most commonly used sites are the cephalic (*A*) and saphenous (*B*) veins. A 26ga catheter was used in both animals.

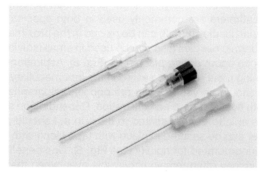

Fig. 3. Spinal needles are preferred for IO catheters in hedgehogs and sugar gliders, as the included stylet helps prevent bone coring and blockage. Short, small (22–25-gauge), spinal needles are most useful; 20-gauge (*yellow*), 22-gauge (*black*), and 25-gauge (*blue*) spinal needles are shown (BD, Franklin Lakes, NJ). Note the removable stylet partially retracted in the 20-gauge needle.

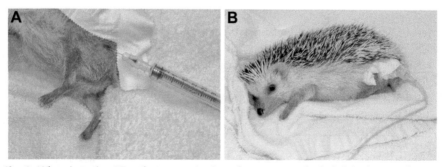

Fig. 4. When inserting IO catheters, aspiration of marrow can be helpful when confirming proper placement. Aspiration of bone marrow during placement of an IO catheter in the proximal femur using a 25-gauge spinal needle in a hedgehog (*A*). The same hedgehog once the intraosseous catheter has been secured in place (*B*).

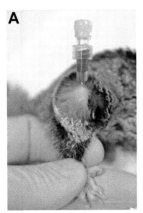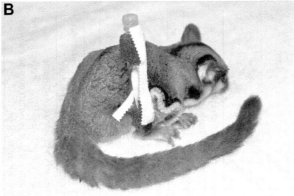

Fig. 5. Hypodermic needles can be used as IO catheters in small species, such as sugar gliders, but can obstruct with bone during insertion. Use of a 25-gauge hypodermic needle as an IO catheter placed in the proximal tibia of a sedated sugar glider (*A*). The IO catheter is secured in place with tape along with a piece of wooden tongue depressor incorporated for rigidity (*B*).

available muscle bellies are small in sugar gliders, and hedgehogs routinely ball-up when stimulated, making this route more easily accessible.

African Pygmy Hedgehogs

Drugs commonly used for sedation in hedgehogs are reported in **Table 2**. Various injectable sedative and anesthetic drugs have been anecdotally recommended for use in African pygmy hedgehogs, including dissociatives, benzodiazepines, opioids, alfaxalone, and alpha$_2$-agonists.[11,12] Midazolam and butorphanol can be combined for mild sedation; ketamine can be added to the protocol to deepen the level of sedation. In the authors' experience, small volumes of midazolam can be administered intranasally in hedgehogs for mild sedation; this is facilitated by use of concentrated forms (ZooPharm, Inc, Fort Collins, CO).

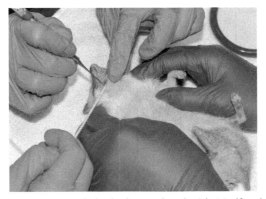

Fig. 6. Dental examination in a male hedgehog sedated with SC alfaxalone-midazolam. In this case, sedation was preferred over general anesthesia to fully examine the mouth with a decreased risk of exposure to waste gases.

Table 2
Selected drugs used for sedation and anesthesia in African pygmy hedgehogs[4,5,7,32–34]

Drug	Dose	Loss of Righting Reflex	Loss of Jaw Tone	Recovery Time Following SC Flumazenil (0.05 mg/kg)	Comments
Midazolam	1–2 mg/kg intranasal	No	No	Rapid	Mild sedation; administration volumes significantly smaller with concentrated midazolam forms
Midazolam + butorphanol	0.5 mg/kg (M) + 0.5 mg/kg (B) SC	No	No	Rapid	Mild sedation; can be used as preanesthetic
Midazolam + buprenorphine	0.5–1 mg/kg (M) + 0.03–0.05 mg/kg (Bup) SC	No	No	Rapid	Mild sedation; can be used as preanesthetic for mild-moderately painful procedures; long-lasting analgesia
Midazolam + butorphanol + ketamine	0.5 mg/kg (M) + 0.5 mg/kg (B) + 3–5 mg/kg SC	No	No	Rapid	Moderate sedation
Alfaxalone + midazolam	30 mg/kg (A) + 1 mg/kg (M) SC	Yes	~ 50% animals	Rapid	Heavy sedation to light anesthesia
Alfaxalone + midazolam	5 mg/kg (A) + 1 mg/kg (M) SC	Yes	>50% animals	Rapid	Deeper, longer duration of immobilization than with lower alfaxalone dose
Ketamine + midazolam	3 mg/kg (A) + 1 mg/kg (M) SC	>75% animals	~ 50% animals	Rapid	Light sedation to light anesthesia; premature and hyperactive recoveries and drop in food intake when compared with alfaxalone-midazolam
Tiletamine + zolazepam	10 mg/kg SC	>75% animals	Reduced but not lost	Prolonged	Heavy sedation to light anesthesia; recovery times slightly faster following flumazenil
	30 mg/kg SC	Yes	Reduced but not lost	Very prolonged	Light anesthesia; significantly longer recovery times vs lower tiletamine-zolazepam dose; no effect of flumazenil on recovery times
Isoflurane	Induction: 3%–5% Maintenance: 2%–3%	Yes	Yes	NA	General anesthesia
Sevoflurane	To effect	Yes	Yes	NA	General anesthesia

None of the listed injectable sedative protocols resulted in consistent loss of the pelvic limb withdrawal reflex and should not be used for painful procedures without provision of analgesia.

There are only a handful of studies investigating sedative agents in hedgehogs. A combination of alfaxalone (3 mg/kg) and midazolam (1 mg/kg) administered SC into the mantle produced heavy sedation in hedgehogs.[5] One author (GD) routinely uses a combination of alfaxalone (5 mg/kg) and midazolam (1 mg/kg) injected SC into the mantle of hedgehogs when a deeper level of immobilization is required. Recovery following administration of flumazenil (0.05 mg/kg) SC is usually quick (<20 minutes) for alfaxalone-midazolam combinations.

A combination of ketamine (30 mg/kg) and midazolam (1 mg/kg) SC provided a similar depth of immobilization to alfaxalone-midazolam, but hedgehogs experienced premature and rougher recoveries. In addition, hedgehogs sedated with ketamine-midazolam had a significant decrease (>50%) in food intake for 2 days post-sedation.[5]

Subcutaneous tiletamine-zolazepam (Telazol; Zoetis, Inc, Kalamazoo, MI) produces dose-dependent heavy sedation to light anesthesia in African pygmy hedgehogs. However, when compared with alfaxalone-midazolam and ketamine-midazolam immobilization, recovery length was significantly longer and dose-dependent.[7] Flumazenil (0.05 mg/kg) administration did not have a significant effect on reversal of the zolazepam; however, recovery times were slightly faster for the lower dose (10 mg/kg) studied.[7]

Sugar Gliders

There is limited information regarding sedation in sugar gliders, as inhalant anesthesia is the most common form of chemical immobilization used in this species. Different injectable sedative and anesthetic drugs have been anecdotally recommended, including combinations of benzodiazepines, opioids, alpha$_2$-agonists, and ketamine (**Table 3**). Midazolam can be administered intranasally for mild sedation.[13]

Various injectable combinations aimed at providing postoperative sedation and analgesia in an attempt to reduce the incidence of self-mutilation following surgical procedures have been reported (see **Table 3**).[13–15] Tiletamine-zolazepam use is controversial in sugar gliders. In one report, administration of tiletamine-zolazepam at 10 mg/kg resulted in neurologic signs and death in squirrel gliders (*Petaurus norfolcensis*).[16] However, another report used tiletamine-zolazepam at 8.4 to 12.8 mg/kg in sugar gliders without mention of adverse effects.[17] Additional information is needed before tiletamine-zolazepam can be recommended for chemical immobilization in sugar gliders.

PREMEDICATION

Premedication is an integral part of any balanced anesthetic procedure. The authors routinely use a combination of a benzodiazepine and opioid administered intramuscularly (IM) or SC for premedication of hedgehogs and sugar gliders, to provide enhanced muscle relaxation, anxiolysis, and preemptive analgesia, which helps reduce the amount of inhalant anesthesia required, subsequently reducing the risk of associated complications like hypotension and hypothermia. Although butorphanol has sedative effects in both hedgehogs and sugar gliders, it is not an ideal analgesic option for procedures that are moderately or severely painful. For these cases, μ-agonist opioid agents should be prioritized.

Atropine and glycopyrrolate have been recommended in hedgehogs and sugar gliders as a preanesthetic to reduce the level of hypersalivation noted with isoflurane anesthesia.[18–20] However, as anticholinergics increase the viscosity of salivary and airway secretions, and negatively affect gastrointestinal motility and lower esophageal sphincter function, its adverse effects may outweigh perceived benefits.[21]

Table 3
Selected drugs used for sedation and anesthesia in sugar gliders[3,13,15,35]

Drug	Dose	Comments
Midazolam	0.1–0.5 mg/kg SC, IM, intranasal	Mild sedation
Midazolam + butorphanol	0.5 mg/kg (M) + 0.5 mg/kg (B) SC	Mild sedation
Buprenorphine + midazolam + meloxicam	0.01 mg/kg (Bup) + 0.1 mg/kg (Midaz) + 0.2 mg/kg (Melox) IM	May be useful for reducing postoperative self-mutilation
Flumazenil	0.05 mg/kg SC, IM	For reversal of midazolam
Acepromazine + butorphanol	1.7 mg/kg (A) + 1.7 mg/kg (B) SC	Hypotension common adverse effect of acepromazine documented in multiple species
Acepromazine + ketamine	1 mg/kg (A) + 10 mg/kg (K) SC	Potential hypotension with acepromazine; may be useful for reducing postoperative self-mutilation
	2 mg/kg (A) + 30 mg/kg (K) SC, IM	Heavy sedation to light anesthesia
Ketamine + midazolam	10–20 mg/kg (K) + 0.35–0.5 mg/kg (M) SC, IM	Heavy sedation to light anesthesia
Isoflurane	Induction: 5% Maintenance: 1%–3%	General anesthesia
Sevoflurane	1%–5% to effect	General anesthesia

Abbreviations: IM, intramuscular; SC, subcutaneous.

INDUCTION

Hedgehogs and sugar gliders are most commonly induced in a chamber using an inhalant anesthetic although injectable agents may be used alternatively by various routes (SC, IM, IV, IO). Anesthetic chambers can be commercial models or improvised (eg, a canine facemask) (**Fig. 7**). Monitoring animal posture can identify induction of anesthesia in animals inside a chamber. Sugar gliders will become recumbent; hedgehogs will no longer adopt a defensive posture (eg, roll up) when stimulated. For lidded chambers, slowly tipping the enclosure to check for loss of the righting reflex can be helpful to prevent premature opening and additional exposure to waste gases. Sugar gliders and sedated hedgehogs also may be induced with inhalants via facemask. Muscle relaxation and loss of limb withdrawal and righting reflexes are helpful parameters to monitor for successful induction.

Isoflurane is the most commonly reported inhalant anesthetic used in these species, although sevoflurane also has been described.[3,11] In the authors' experience, sugar gliders may vomit when chamber-induced with isoflurane (see **Fig. 7**). Conversely, hedgehogs rarely vomit during anesthetic events.

Emergency drug (eg, epinephrine, atropine) as well as reversal drug (eg, flumazenil, naloxone, atipamezole) doses, if applicable, should be calculated and drawn up before induction; recommended doses for small mammal emergencies have been summarized elsewhere.[22]

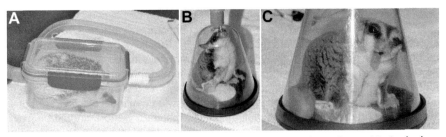

Fig. 7. Chamber induction with inhalant anesthetics is routinely performed in hedgehogs and sugar gliders. Altered plastic containers (*A*), canine facemasks (*B, C*), or commercially available chambers can be used in hedgehogs and sugar gliders. Vomiting is not uncommon in sugar gliders during chamber induction (*C*); note the obvious ptyalism.

MAINTENANCE

Inhalant anesthetics are most commonly used for anesthetic maintenance in hedgehogs and sugar gliders and should be administered via non-rebreathing systems. The use of circle systems in small species with low tidal volumes is not recommended, as they increase the effort required to move gases during respiration (eg, increase resistance to flow from unidirectional valves, large-bore hoses).[23] Suggested non-rebreathing systems include the Mapleson D systems (Co-axial bain and Ayre's T-piece) and the Mapleson F system (Ayre's T-piece with Jackson Rees modification).

Intubation of hedgehogs and sugar gliders is challenging and requires small-sized endotracheal tubes (**Fig. 8**) or modified IV catheters. Endoscopy using rigid (eg, 2.7 mm, 30°) or smaller, semi-rigid, fiberoptic endoscopes and use of stylets can expedite intubation. Stylets can be commercial or improvised (eg, unfolded metal paper clip) (see **Fig. 8**). Small (size 00, 0) Miller laryngoscope blades are also helpful for visualization if endoscopy is not available. Both over-the-endoscope and side-by-side intubation are possible, depending on the size of the endoscope and endotracheal

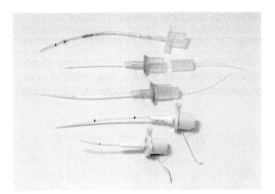

Fig. 8. Commercially available, 1.0-mm to 2.0-mm internal diameter, noncuffed endotracheal tubes. Note the small diameter, which increases airway resistance and the risk of blockage with airway secretions. The endotracheal tubes can be trimmed (see bottom tube) to decrease their length. Note the low dead space adapters for attaching sidestream capnography present on the 2 bottom tubes, as well as the top tube. Commercial and improvised (unfolded metal paper clip) stylets are inserted in the bottom 4 tubes. Internal diameter size in order from top to bottom: 2.0 mm, 1.0 mm, 1.5 mm, 1.5 mm, 1.0 mm.

tube needed.[24] If visualization is limited, a soft stylet can be passed into the trachea and the endotracheal tube guided over it. For hedgehogs, 1.0-mm to 2.0-mm internal diameter endotracheal tubes are recommended.[9,25] Smaller tubes (1.0–1.5 mm internal diameter) are used for sugar gliders.[3,24] Commercial tubes are often long (see **Fig. 8**) and may require trimming before use. Determine the insertion depth before trimming by measuring the distance from the incisors to the thoracic inlet. Bilateral lung sounds should be audible on auscultation following a manual breath.[26] Endotracheal tubes and capnography, as well as patient respiratory effort, should be monitored closely as small diameter tubes are prone to blockage with respiratory secretions. Also, as commercially available 1.0-mm to 2.0-mm internal diameter endotracheal tubes are uncuffed, they may leak at lower peak inspiratory pressures and will not protect the airway against regurgitation.[26]

Because of the challenges associated with intubation in these species, a facemask is often used for anesthetic maintenance. Options include facemasks with snug-fitting plastic diaphragms (**Fig. 9**) or nose cones designed for rodents (see **Figs. 9** and **10**); however, facemasks do not provide any airway protection during regurgitation or vomiting events and may not permit positive pressure ventilation. In addition, as hedgehogs and sugar gliders are not described as obligate nasal breathers, some personnel exposure to waste gases could occur if the animal's nose and mouth are not covered by the facemask. Additional research into the normal oronasal anatomy and function of these species is needed.

A supraglottic airway device designed for small rabbits (v-gel R1; Docsinnovent, Hempstead, UK) (**Fig. 11**) is an alternative option for airway maintenance in hedgehogs.[6,27] Recent research demonstrated that this supraglottic airway device was quickly and easily placed and atraumatic in African pygmy hedgehogs weighing 360 to 700 g.[6] In addition, unlike facemasks, the supraglottic airway device permitted administration of positive pressure ventilation up to 10 cmH$_2$0.[6] Using a supraglottic airway device avoids the tracheal mucosal damage that can occur when using modified IV catheters as endotracheal tubes, and may be less likely to obstruct with respiratory secretions compared with small internal diameter endotracheal tubes. A newer, single-use model (v-gel ADVANCED R1; Docsinnovent) recently has been introduced (see **Fig. 11**) and has been used successfully by one author (GD) for anesthetic maintenance in adult hedgehogs weighing between 370 and 600 g.

Anesthetic Monitoring

Physiologic variables including heart rate, respiratory rate, and rectal temperature, as well as reflexes (palpebral, limb withdrawal), eye position, and jaw tone should be regularly monitored in anesthetized animals to gauge patient stability and anesthetic

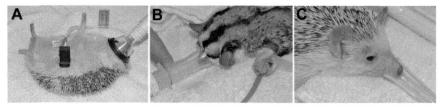

Fig. 9. Facemasks with tight-fitting diaphragms (*A*) and rodent nose cones (*B, C*) can be used for anesthetic maintenance or oxygen supplementation in hedgehogs and sugar gliders. Note the placement of pulse oximetry (*A*) and Doppler (*B*) probes on a forelimb paw for monitoring.

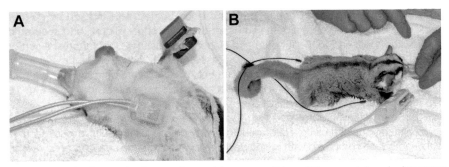

Fig. 10. Anesthetic monitoring equipment in sugar gliders. When peripheral placement fails, a Doppler probe can be placed on the thorax adjacent to the heart; be careful not to restrict normal thoracic excursions (*A*). Commercial electrocardiography needle probes are useful to prevent tissue damage that can occur with strong clamps (*B*). Note the pulse oximetry probe placed on a forelimb paw and rodent cone used for anesthetic maintenance.

depth. Normal physiologic parameters for hedgehogs and sugar gliders are reported in **Table 1**.

Recommended routine anesthetic monitoring equipment for hedgehog and sugar glider anesthesia includes pulse oximetry, Doppler, electrocardiography, and capnography. Serial noninvasive blood pressure measurements using a sphygmomanometer and size 1 cuff may be performed to monitor trends; however, this methodology has not been validated in either species. Advances in veterinary anesthetic equipment have made items suitable for use in small species, including sugar gliders, readily available. Some commercially available portable devices (eg, Vetcorder, Sentier, Waukesha, WI) permit measurement of electrocardiography and pulse oximetry readings simultaneously, even at the high resting heart rates of hedgehogs and sugar gliders.

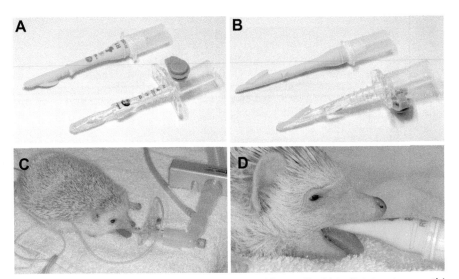

Fig. 11. A supraglottic airway device (SGAD) designed for small rabbits (R1, Docsinnovent) is an alternative option for airway maintenance in hedgehogs. Dorsal (*A*) and ventral (*B*) aspects of multi-use (bottom; v-gel R1) and single-use (top; v-gel ADVANCED R1) SGADs are shown. Use of SGADs for anesthetic maintenance in hedgehogs (*C*, *D*); note the use of sidestream capnography (*C*).

Following hair clipping, Doppler probes can be coated with transducer gel and applied to peripheral vessels of the limbs, or the tail in sugar gliders, and secured in place with tape (see **Fig. 9**). If peripheral placement fails, the Doppler crystal can be placed on the thorax, adjacent to the heart (see **Fig. 10**); however, be careful not to restrict normal thoracic excursions. Placement of electrocardiography clamps onto needles inserted through the skin or use of specialized needle probes (see **Fig. 10**) can help protect the skin from damage.

Sidestream capnography (see **Fig. 11**) is preferred in intubated hedgehogs and sugar gliders, or when using a supraglottic airway device, as it results in less mechanical dead space compared with in-line devices; low dead space adapters are available for endotracheal tubes (see **Fig. 8**). Rebreathing of dead space gases can be prevented by increasing the fresh gas flow rate; however, this can result in erroneously low end-tidal carbon dioxide readings secondary to the dilution of expired gases by fresh gas flow.[28,29] Furthermore, as the fresh gas flow increases, the patient is exposed to cooler and drier gases, potentially compromising their pulmonary function, and more agent and inhaled gases are wasted.

Intravascular fluid support (IV, IO) should be provided during the anesthetic event, with administration rates and fluid type depending on the patient's health status (ie, systemically ill, healthy animal undergoing elective surgical procedure). Fluids should be warmed before administration. If intravascular access cannot be obtained, then SC fluid therapy should be provided.

RECOVERY

Recovery from inhalant anesthesia in healthy hedgehogs and sugar gliders (eg, immobilization for preventive health examination) is often rapid, and patient arousal commonly occurs during brief removal of the facemask to complete an oral examination. Recovery times can be longer following prolonged anesthetic events (eg,

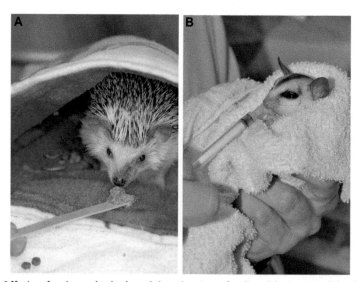

Fig. 12. Offering food to a hedgehog (A) and syringe-feeding (B) a sugar glider following anesthetic recovery. Hedgehogs and sugar gliders should be provided food shortly after recovery to provide nutrients and promote a quick return of normal gastrointestinal tract function.

Box 1
Equipment list for hedgehog and sugar glider anesthesia

Restraint
  Plastic-coated woven work gloves (hedgehogs)
  Small towel (sugar gliders)

Anesthetic equipment
  Machine, vaporizer, oxygen, waste gas scavenger system
  Breathing system (eg, Mapleson)

Anesthetic and emergency drugs
  Premedication agents (eg, benzodiazepines, opioids, anticholinergics)
  Reversals (eg, flumazenil, naloxone, atipamezole)
  Inhalant anesthetic (eg, isoflurane, sevoflurane)
  Precalculated emergency doses of epinephrine, atropine, glycopyrrolate

Induction
  Induction chamber (eg, canine face mask)

Intubation
  Cotton-tipped applicators for cleaning oral cavity
  Gauze squares to grasp and extend tongue
  Laryngoscope with small Miller blade (size 00, 0) or rigid endoscope
  1-mm to 2-mm internal diameter endotracheal tubes
  Ties for securing endotracheal tube around head

Maintenance (if not intubated)
  Small facemask or rodent nose cone
  Supraglottic airway device (hedgehogs)

Thermal support
  Circulating water blanket
  Forced air warmer
  Small towels, plastic bubble wrap

Monitoring equipment
  Infant or pediatric stethoscope
  Doppler (with tape to secure probe)
  Pulse oximeter
  Electrocardiography (with hypodermic needles to attach clamps to)
  Thermometer
  Sphygmomanometer and size 1 cuff
  Sidestream capnography

Intravascular access
  Injection caps
  Clippers
  Topical antiseptics for skin prep
  White medical tape for securing catheter
  For IV catheters: 24 to 26 gauge or similarly sized over-the-needle catheter
  For IO catheters: 25 to 22ga spinal or hypodermic needles; lidocaine (2–4 mg/kg) for local
  anesthesia

Fluid therapy
  Warmed crystalloid ($\pm$ colloid) fluids at 10 to 15 mL/kg per hour (IV/IO) or 20 mL/kg SC, if
  stable
  Mini extension set used as fluid line
  Various sized syringes and hypodermic needles
  Fluid pump

Abbreviations: ID, internal diameter; IO, intraosseous; IV, intravenous; SC, subcutaneous.

laparotomy) or in debilitated animals. Hedgehogs recovering from anesthesia with a supraglottic airway device inserted will often bite down, or simultaneously retract their head and contract the mantle in an attempt to remove the device from their oropharynx (Video 4); a brief period of tachypnea often occurs immediately before arousal and attempted self-removal of the device.[6]

Sugar gliders should be monitored very closely during recovery from anesthesia, as self-mutilation following surgical procedures is common.[3]

Hedgehogs and sugar gliders should be provided aggressive thermal support, and physiologic parameters monitored until they are fully recovered or it is no longer possible (eg, hedgehog adopts defensive posture). If not required for continued fluid therapy and the patient is cardiovascularly stable, consider removal of peripheral IV or IO catheters before full arousal in hedgehogs, as later removal can require an additional anesthetic event to access the site.

Unless contraindicated, food should be offered immediately after hedgehogs and sugar gliders have recovered from anesthesia to provide nutrients and promote a quick return of normal gastrointestinal tract function (**Fig. 12**).

SUMMARY

Given their small size, and unique anatomy and behavior, hedgehogs and sugar gliders can be challenging anesthetic candidates. Hypothermia is a common adverse effect of immobilization in both species, making aggressive thermal support paramount during all phases of sedation and anesthesia. Studied injectable sedation protocols for these species are scarce, particularly for sugar gliders, but can provide an alternative to inhalant anesthesia for minor procedures. Intubation is challenging but can be aided by use of rigid endoscopy and small laryngoscope blades. Preparation of all necessary equipment before the sedative or anesthetic event will help improve patient care. **Box 1** contains a suggested equipment list for anesthetizing these species.

SUPPLEMENTARY DATA

Supplementary data to this article can be found online at https://doi.org/10.1016/j.cvex.2021.08.005.

REFERENCES

1. IUCN red list. 2021. Available at: https://www.iucnredlist.org/. Accessed January 15, 2021.
2. Johnson R, Hemsley S. Gliders and possums. In: Vogelnest L, Woods R, editors. Medicine of Australian mammals. Clayton South Vic: CSIRO Publishing; 2008. p. 395–438.
3. Johnson-Delaney CA. Sugar gliders. In: Quesenberry KE, Orcutt CJ, Mans C, et al, editors. Ferrets, rabbits, and rodents: clinical medicine and surgery. 4th edition. St. Louis: Elsevier; 2021. p. 385–400.
4. Hawkins SJ, Doss GA, Mans C. Postanesthetic effects of two durations of isoflurane anesthesia in African pygmy hedgehogs (*Atelerix albiventris*). J Exot Pet Med 2020;32:27–30.
5. Hawkins S, Doss G, Mans C. Evaluation of subcutaneous alfaxalone-midazolam and ketamine-midazolam sedation protocols in African pygmy hedgehogs (*Atelerix albiventris*). J Am Vet Med Assoc 2020;257:820–5.

6. Huckins G, Doss G, Ferreira T. Feasibility of supraglottic airway device use during maintenance of inhalant anesthesia in healthy African pygmy hedgehogs (*Atelerix albiventris*). Vet Anaesth Analg 2021;48:517–23.

7. Hausmann K, Doss G, Mans C. Subcutaneous tiletamine-zolazepam immobilization and effect of flumazenil reversal in African pygmy hedgehogs (*Atelerix albiventris*). J Exot Pet Med 2020;36:42–6.

8. Vogelnest L. Capture, physical and chemical restraint. In: Vogelnest L, Portas T, editors. Current therapy in medicine of Australian mammals. Clayton South Vic: CSIRO Publishing; 2019. p. 121–50.

9. Heard D. Insectivores (hedgehogs, moles, and tenrecs). In: West G, Heard D, Caulkett N, editors. Zoo animal and wildlife immobilization and anesthesia. 2nd edition. Ames: John Wiley & Sons; 2014. p. 529–31.

10. Lennox AM. Emergency and critical care procedures in sugar gliders (*Petaurus breviceps*), African hedgehogs (*Atelerix albiventris*), and prairie dogs (*Cynomys* spp). Vet Clin North Am Exot Anim Pract 2007;10:533–55.

11. Helmer PJ, Carpenter JW. Hedgehogs. In: Carpenter JW, editor. Exotic animal formulary. 5th edition. St. Louis: Elsevier; 2018. p. 443–58.

12. Lennox AM, Miwa Y. Anatomy and disorders of the oral cavity of miscellaneous exotic companion mammals. Vet Clin North Am Exot Anim Pract 2016;19:929–45.

13. Brust DM, Mans C. Sugar gliders. In: Carpenter JW, editor. Exotic animal formulary. 5th edition. St. Louis: Elsevier; 2018. p. 432–42.

14. Johnson S. Orchiectomy of the mature sugar glider (*Petaurus breviceps*). Exot Pet Pract 1997;2:71.

15. Ness RD, Johnson-Delaney CA. Sugar gliders. In: Quesenberry KE, Carpenter JW, editors. Ferrets, rabbits, and rodents: clinical medicine and surgery. 3rd edition. St. Louis: Elsevier; 2012. p. 393–410.

16. Holz P. Immobilization of marsupials with tiletamine and zolazepam. J Zoo Wildl Med 1992;23:426–8.

17. Bush M, Graves J, O'Brien SJ, et al. Dissociative anaesthesia in free-ranging male koalas and selected marsupials in captivity. Aust Vet J 1990;67:449–51.

18. Lightfoot T. Therapeutics of African pygmy hedgehogs and prairie dogs. Vet Clin North Am Exot Anim Pract 2000;3:155–72.

19. Johnson-Delaney C. Therapeutics of common marsupials. Vet Clin North Am Exot Anim Pract 2000;3:173–81.

20. Johnson-Delaney C. What veterinarians need to know about hedgehogs. Exot DVM 2007;9:38–44.

21. Lerche P. Anticholinergics. In: Grimm K, Lamont L, Tranquilli W, et al, editors. Lumb and Jones' veterinary anesthesia and analgesia. 5th edition. Ames: John Wiley & Sons; 2015. p. 178–82.

22. Gladden J, Lennox A. Emergency and critical care of small mammals. In: Quesenberry KE, Orcutt CJ, Mans C, et al, editors. Ferrets, rabbits, and rodents: clinical medicine and surgery. 4th edition. St. Louis: Elsevier; 2021. p. 595–608.

23. Flecknell P. Basic principles of anaesthesia. In: Laboratory animal anaesthesia. 4th edition. Waltham: Academic Press; 2015. p. 1–75.

24. Johnson DH. Endoscopic intubation of exotic companion mammals. Vet Clin North Am Exot Anim Pract 2010;13:273–89.

25. Doss G, Carpenter J. African pygmy hedgehogs. In: Quesenberry K, Orcutt C, Mans C, et al, editors. Ferrets, rabbits, and rodents: clinical medicine and surgery. 4th edition. St. Louis: Elsevier; 2021. p. 401–15.

26. Hillier S, McNiece W, Dierdorf S. Pediatric anesthesia systems and equipment. In: Ehrenwerth J, Eisenkraft J, Berry J, editors. Anesthesia equipment: principles and applications. 2nd edition. Philadelphia: Elsevier-Saunders; 2013. p. 353–76.
27. Baldo CF, Boelke R. Rabbit supraglottic airway device (V-GEL) for successful airway control in a hedgehog (*Atelerix albiventris*). Vet Anaesth Analg 2019;47: 141–3.
28. Schieber RA, Namnoum A, Sugden A, et al. Accuracy of expiratory carbon dioxide measurements using the coaxial and circle breathing circuits in small subjects. J Clin Monit 1985;1:149–55.
29. Gravenstein N, Lampotang S, Beneken JE. Factors influencing capnography in the Bain circuit. J Clin Monit 1985;1:6–10.
30. Black PA, Marshall C, Seyfried AW, et al. Cardiac assessment of African hedgehogs (*Atelerix albiventris*). J Zoo Wildl Med 2011;42:49–53.
31. Booth RJ. General husbandry and medical care of sugar gliders. In: Bonagura JD, editor. Kirk's current veterinary therapy XIII: small animal practice. Philadelphia: WB Saunders Co; 2000. p. 1157–63.
32. Smith A. General husbandry and medical care of hedgehogs. In: Bonagura JD, editor. Kirk's current veterinary therapy XIII: small animal practice. Philadelphia: WB Saunders Co; 2000. p. 1128–33.
33. Heatley J. Hedgehogs. In: Mitchell MA, Tully T, editors. Manual of exotic pet practice. St. Louis: Elsevier; 2009. p. 433–55.
34. Doss G, Mans C. Antinociceptive efficacy and safety of subcutaneous buprenorphine hydrochloride in African pygmy hedgehogs (*Atelerix albiventris*). J Am Vet Med Assoc 2020;257:618–23.
35. Plumb's veterinary drug handbook. 2021. Available at: https://www.plumbsveterinarydrugs.com/home2/. Accessed January 15, 2021.

Ferret Sedation and Anesthesia

Nathaniel Kapaldo, DVM, MPH, DACVAA*, David Eshar, DVM, DABVP (ECM), DECZM (SM & ZHM)

KEYWORDS

- Anesthesia • Small mammal anesthesia • Ferret anesthesia • Exotic anesthesia
- *Mustela putorius furo*

KEY POINTS

- Safe anesthetic management of ferrets relies on understanding of basic anesthetic principles applicable to all small mammals.
- Because of the ease of intubation, control of the airway should occur whenever possible following induction of anesthesia, regardless of anesthetic event duration.
- Ferrets are prone to significant thermoregulatory derangements perioperatively and thusso certain measures should be put in place to mitigate severe changes in core body temperature.
- Ferrets may experience severe respiratory depression when anesthetized with inhalant anesthetics and thus there should be constant evaluation of ventilatory status when anesthetized, especially postanesthetically while recovering.
- Blood pressure is difficult to accurately measure in ferrets; therefore, they may experience significant cardiovascular derangement secondary to anesthetics, and thus hypotension should be mitigated against.

INTRODUCTION

Domestic ferrets (*Mustela putorius furo*) are a common pet species that are also extensively used in research.[1,2] They often require either short or more prolonged periods of general anesthesia (GA) for noninvasive or invasive procedures. Relatively few new publications specific to the anesthetic management of ferrets have been introduced in the last 10 years. Regardless, rational anesthetic management relies on a working knowledge of species-specific anatomy, physiology, and pharmacologic idiosyncrasies. Among small mammals a veterinarian may need to anesthetize routinely, ferrets have the lowest relative anesthetic-related risk of death: 0.33%.[3] Anesthetic-

The authors do not have any commercial or financial conflicts of interest or any funding sources to disclose.
Department of Clinical Sciences, Veterinary Health Center, Kansas State University College of Veterinary Medicine, 1800 Denison Avenue, Manhattan, KS 66502, USA
* Corresponding author.
E-mail address: kapaldo@vet.k-state.edu

related risk of death is only lower in dogs and cats: 0.17% and 0.25%, respectively.[3] However, confidence in and knowledge regarding anesthetizing a specific species is associated with the frequency of interacting with it.[4]

General working knowledge of basic anesthetic principles is fundamental to administering safe anesthetic care to any species. The following review addresses phases of anesthetic care, such as the preanesthetic, intra-anesthetic, and postanesthetic phases, and focuses on fundamental anesthetic considerations. Several aspects of anesthetic management in ferrets and perioperative pain assessment and analgesia have been discussed elsewhere; these will be indicated and not expounded upon in this review.

PREANESTHETIC PHASE
Patient Assessment

A complete history and physical examination should be performed before any GA event. Stabilization of any overt free water deficits (eg, dehydration, hypovolemia) should be attempted before induction of anesthesia. Many induction and inhalant anesthetics will uncover, through vasodilation, even mild hypovolemia, resulting in significant hypotension. A complete blood cell count and biochemistry profile should be attained and assessed before GA in sick ferrets; however, depending on the patient's demeanor, this may not be achievable without sedation. Ferrets have a short gastric transit time of approximately 4 hours and are prone to hypoglycemia during this time.[5] Fasting before GA should occur for only 2 to 4 hours.[6]

Vascular Access

Vascular access is relatively easy to achieve in awake or lightly sedate individuals. It is the authors' opinion that vascular access should be attained in any ferret undergoing GA for a surgical or prolonged diagnostic procedure and should be considered for shorter procedures.

Sites for catheterization include the cephalic, saphenous (medial and lateral), femoral, and jugular (sedation required) veins.[2] A 24- or 26-gauge catheter is appropriate for most peripheral veins, and a 20- or 22-gauge catheter may be used for jugular catheterization. Ferrets have a thick epidermis; therefore, a small pilot hole made with a 20- to 22-gauge needle is helpful to mitigate catheter burring on penetration of the skin. Intraosseous catheterization can be a useful technique in select populations when peripheral veins are difficult to visualize. This technique has been described in detail.[2,6]

Arterial catheterization for monitoring of direct arterial blood pressure (BP) or sampling of arterial blood to assess acid-base status can be achieved but is challenging. Sites that can be catheterized include the dorsal pedal, saphenous, femoral, and coccygeal artery. A 26-gauge catheter is ideal for ferret arterial catheterization. Interpretation of arterial BP and arterial blood gas data has been described elsewhere.[7–9]

Premedication/Sedation

Premedication before an anesthetic event offers many advantages, including calming to facilitate handling and catheterization, reducing induction and maintenance anesthetic requirements, and facilitating a smoother induction of, and recovery from, anesthesia.[10] Premedicants may be described as a sedative, which reduces response to external stimuli, or a tranquilizer, which may reduce anxiety experienced by the ferret. The selection of premedicants and their route of administration should always take into consideration the patient's presenting problems, volume status, age, temperament, and cardiovascular (CV) effects (eg, effect on cardiac output [CO], stroke volume, systemic vascular resistance, BP, and myocardial contractility) in relation to the former factors. The CV effects may not be known in ferrets for a particular drug; however, these drugs often behave similarly in varying mammalian species, and thus the CV effects often will be known in another species. Benzodiazepines (eg, midazolam) and alpha-2 agonists (eg, dexmedetomidine) often in combination with an opioid (eg, butorphanol, buprenorphine, hydromorphone, methadone, fentanyl) are the most used premedications.[11] The authors commonly will administer 0.2 to 0.3 mg/kg each of midazolam and butorphanol with rapid onset (approximately 5 minutes), providing moderate sedation for 30 to 40 minutes. A full mu-agonist may be substituted if premedicating for an invasive surgical procedure.

The authors administer premedications 10 to 15 minutes before proposed attempts to gain vascular access and induce GA or perform short diagnostics. Intravenous (IV), subcutaneous (SC), or intramuscular (IM) are all possible routes of administration of premedications. Selection of route should be based on the patient's temperament, although in the authors' experience is primarily performed via IM or SC routes. If administering premedicants IV, peak plasma concentration of the administered drug, and subsequently the peak level of sedation, may be greater than if given IM or SC, and will be reached in a shorter time.

Benzodiazepines are gamma-aminobutyric acid (GABA) receptor (subtype A) agonists, increasing affinity for the inhibitory neurotransmitter, GABA, resulting in greater chloride conductance (ie, hyperpolarization) into postsynaptic neurons.[10] Midazolam is more commonly available in the United States; however, diazepam may be used in a similar manner. Diazepam should not be administered via IM or SC routes because of the propylene glycol used as a solvent, producing pain and potential local inflammation when given via these routes.[10] Benzodiazepines produce good-quality, dose-dependent, sedation (**Table 1**). Physiologic effects of benzodiazepines are not reported in ferrets but are considered similar to other mammals and may include minimal to no respiratory depression, a mild reduction in heart rate (HR) with preservation of CO and BP, and no adverse effects to acid-base status.[10,12] Reversal of benzodiazepines can be achieved with flumazenil administered IM or SC.[10,13]

Alpha-2 adrenergic receptors are present throughout the body in both neural and nonneural (eg, vascular smooth muscle) tissue.[10] These drugs provide centrally mediated sedation in a dose-dependent manner (see **Table 1**).[10] Dexmedetomidine is the most used alpha-2 agonist. Physiologic effects of alpha-2 agonists include peripheral vasoconstriction and subsequent increase in BP, often a dose-dependent reflex bradycardia, and in other species, such as cats, a significant reduction in CO, mediated by the bradycardia.[10] Peripheral effects of dexmedetomidine last approximately 30 to 45 minutes; however, they are dose-dependent.[10] The bradycardia and reduced vascular tone may continue beyond the peripheral effects because of centrally mediated reduction in sympathetic nervous system tone. Alpha-2 agonists may be reversed effectively using atipamezole (see **Table 1**).[10,11,13]

Opioids are commonly administered as part of a premedication protocol. Ferrets do not commonly experience emesis; however, opioid-induced nausea and emesis have been reported. The emetogenic effect of morphine has been documented when 0.1 and 0.3 mg/kg were administered SC resulting in emesis in 17% and 100% of ferrets after 9 and 3 minutes, respectively.[14] The authors suggest maropitant or ondansetron (see **Table 1**) be considered before premedication to inhibit the emetogenic effect of certain opioids (eg, hydromorphone, morphine).[14]

Opioids are also valuable in reducing the overall anesthetic requirement.[15,16] Opioids have been shown to significantly reduce minimum alveolar concentration

Table 1
Suggested injectable sedatives, tranquilizers, and induction anesthetics (mg/kg) for ferrets

Drug	Dose, Route	Comments
Dexmedetomidine	0.005–0.01 IV 0.008–0.02 IM, SC	Consider reduced doses when administered IV
Medetomidine	0.01–0.015 IV 0.015–0.04 IM, SC	See above[6]
Acepromazine	0.04–0.2 IV, IM, SC	May exacerbate hypotension when used at high doses and the ferret concurrently exposed to additional vasodilating agent
Midazolam	0.2–0.5 IV, IM, SC	Dose-dependent sedation Consider use as coinduction agent with ketamine
Atipamezole	—	Reversal of alpha-2 agonists; 10× or 5× dose in miligrams of dexmedetomidine or medetomidine, respectively[6]
Flumazenil	0.05–0.1 SC, IM	Reversal of benzodiazepines[6]
Propofol	3–8 IV	Never give SC or IM
Alfaxalone	3–5 IV,[14] IM	Consider similar doses IM for mild sedation
Ketamine	7–10 IV, IM, SC	Significant burning on IM or SC administration. If not sedate at time of induction, coinduction with 0.2–0.3 mg/kg midazolam
Propofol + ketamine	3 P/3 K	Titrate similar as if propofol alone[23]
Etomidate	2–3 IV	If not sedate at time of induction, coinduction with 0.2–0.3 mg/kg midazolam. Mild muscle tremors possible when administered to poorly sedated patients
Maropitant	1 IV, IM, SC	Not evaluated in ferrets
Ondansetron	3 IV[14]	

The above dosing recommendations are based on the authors' experience and other published data in ferrets and other species.

(MAC) of inhalants in dogs in a consistent and dose-dependent manner, for example, 20% to 50%.[15–17] This same MAC-sparing effect in ferrets has not been investigated in a similar manner; however, it is suspected of being similar. Ketamine and lidocaine may be used in conjunction with intermittent dosing, or constant rate infusions (CRIs) of opioids during surgical procedures (see **Table 6**).

Last, effective analgesia is vital to ensure appropriate postoperative recovery and wound healing and to facilitate quick return to normal function and behavior.[17] Full discussion of analgesia, the assessment and recognition of pain in ferrets, as well as common indications for surgical intervention have been discussed elsewhere.[17,18]

INDUCTION OF ANESTHESIA PHASE
Approach to Induction and Intubation

Induction of anesthesia should always occur in a controlled manner, and the number of personnel and noise in the room should be limited. Keeping the ferret quiet and calm is important to minimize the induction anesthetic dose required, which may minimize the magnitude of induction anesthetic associated adverse effects, such as respiratory depression and vasodilation. Before administration of induction anesthetics, ensure all equipment needed for intubation is present.

At minimum, thoracic auscultation should be performed to assess the HR and rhythm; however, electrocardiogram (ECG) lead placement and assessment ideally should be performed before induction of anesthesia. Assessment of the ECG before induction of anesthesia may identify cardiac rhythm disturbances before and after administration of induction anesthetics. A review of normal echocardiographic parameters in both awake and anesthetized ferrets and proper ECG placement, complex morphology, and interpretation cardiology principles has been described.[19-21] **Fig. 1** demonstrates a normal ECG tracing.

Preoxygenation

Preoxygenation with a high fraction of inspired oxygen (Fio_2) increases intrapulmonary oxygen reserves.[22] This process effectively delays the time to hypoventilation or apnea-induced desaturation of hemoglobin that may occur upon induction of anesthesia. Although desaturation of hemoglobin may occur in even healthy ferrets on induction of anesthesia, this is less common with a timely intubation following induction of anesthesia.[23] Indications for preoxygenation include ferret populations with any of the following:

1. Pulmonary parenchymal disease (eg, pneumonia of any cause)
2. Intrathoracic disease reducing functional residual capacity (eg, thymoma, mediastinal disease, pneumothorax, pleural effusion)
3. Challenging airways requiring longer time for intubation

Preoxygenation is most effective when a tight-fitting face mask with diaphragm is used.[22] However, depending on the patient's demeanor, placement of a facemask may induce excitement, anxiety, and poor handling circumstances. Therefore, preoxygenation by flow-by technique (ie, holding a circuit 2–3 cm away from the nose with 3–4 L/min of oxygen flow) can be used but is less effective at increasing the Fio_2 and intrapulmonary oxygen reservoir.[22]

Induction Anesthetics

Induction anesthetic selection should take into consideration the hemodynamic status, whether there is a suspected interstitial or intravascular volume deficit, and whether there is any cardiac or intracranial disease. IV induction anesthetics that may be considered include propofol, alfaxalone, ketamine, and the less commonly used etomidate.[6,10,24] Induction of anesthesia is ideally performed in a premedicated ferret. Premedication facilitates lower induction anesthetic doses being required and an overall smoother induction of anesthesia.[10] **Table 1** lists recommended doses for induction agents.

Propofol and alfaxalone both produce GA by acting as agonists of centrally located GABA gated chloride channels.[10] Propofol must be administered IV or intraossously,

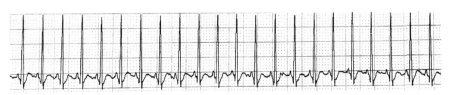

Fig. 1. Normal ECG tracing in lead II from a ferret premedicated with midazolam and maintained on isoflurane. Squared divisions = 0.5 mV; speed = 25 mm/s; HR = 222.

and its use may be limited if vascular access is not attained.[10] The respiratory and CV effects of propofol have not been evaluated in ferrets; however, they are suspected to be similar to those documented in other species. These include transient vasodilation, an increase in HR, and a dose-dependent respiratory depression that may result in apnea.[10,25] Propofol-induced negative inotropy reported in other species has not been reported in ferrets but may be present. Alfaxalone's CV effects have not been reported in ferrets; however, they are suspected to be similar to those seen from propofol. Reports in dogs and cats suggest alfaxalone produces less respiratory depression but, in the authors' experience, this agent produces a similar incidence of postinduction apnea compared with propofol.[25] A recent study evaluated alfaxalone in both premedicated (medetomidine) and unpremedicated ferrets.[24] They required a higher dose (eg, 5+ mg/kg) IV to allow intubation. This study reported 2 mortality events after high-dose IV alfaxalone, both 10 and 20 mg/kg IV; however, the study did not speculate as to the cause of these events.[24]

Ketamine is an NMDA antagonist and may induce GA when administered IV, IM, or SC.[10] Although not reported in ferrets, in other species, CV effects include a transient increase in HR, myocardial contractility, and systemic vascular resistance, secondary to increasing sympathetic tone transiently.[10] Because ketamine may transiently cause central excitation, this drug should always be used in an effectively premedicated individual or coadministered with midazolam. This practice will ensure a smoother induction. Ketamine may induce apnea at higher doses and may be associated with a breath-holding (apneustic) respiratory pattern transiently after administration.[10] Because of ketamine's aforementioned CV effects, this agent is considered to produce a more stable hemodynamic profile when inducing anesthesia in either an overtly dehydrated, hypotensive patient or a patient suspected of having dehydration or a volume deficit.[26] Alternatively, if hemodynamic instability is suspected, ketamine may be mixed in an equal mg/kg ratio with propofol and titrated to effect.[23,26] The addition of ketamine to propofol is suspected to counteract the negative inotropy and vasodilation imposed from propofol. This combination has not been evaluated in ferrets.

The effects of mask induction using an inhalant anesthetic in oxygen via facemask (mask induction) have been evaluated in other species.[27] Mask inductions are associated with central excitation during the induction process, increased cardiopulmonary depression, and longer times until endotracheal intubation and have been associated with a greater odds ratio of anesthetic-related death in sick dogs and cats (6 and 1.5, respectively) compared with IV techniques.[26,27] Many of the aforementioned studies have not been repeated in ferrets. However, it is safe to assume that mask inductions of unpremedicated individuals should be approached judiciously with the understanding that this method produces a substantial degree of stress, potentially greater cardiopulmonary alterations during the induction of anesthesia, and that in other species mask inductions have been associated with a greater complication rate.[27] Whenever possible, ferrets should have appropriate premedication before mask induction to reduce both the stress of and the time required to produce GA from mask induction.

Rarely mentioned are the effects of mask inductions and maintenance via face mask on room contamination and exposure of personnel to trace gas levels, which may have significant health effects.[28] There are double facemask scavenge systems, which reduce room exposure to trace anesthetic levels, available in veterinary medicine; however, their use has not become widespread in veterinary medicine yet.[28] Last, induction of anesthesia via a chamber induction method has been discussed elsewhere; this practice may intermittently be required. However, it leads to substantial room contamination and patient risks that must be considered.[29]

Intubation

Intubation is straightforward; therefore, intubation should be performed whenever GA is required, regardless of duration.[13,30,31] Control of the airway is vital to

1. Mitigate against aspiration of foreign material
2. Allow administration of intermittent positive pressure ventilation (IPPV)
3. Minimize room contamination from inhalant anesthetics
4. Administer a higher Fio_2
5. Allow airway control in the case of cardiopulmonary arrest

While the patient is in sternal recumbency, the head and neck should be extended, mandible gently detracted ventrally, and tongue pulled rostrally. Extension of the neck is important to facilitate laryngeal visualization (**Fig. 2**). Ferrets are not prone to laryngospasm; however, it may still occur. Therefore, before intubation, the laryngeal structures can be sprayed with a local anesthetic (LA) via atomizer, and at least 30 to 60 seconds allowed before intubation attempt.[32] When using an atomizer, the dose of LA should be considered (eg, 0.1 mL per spray of 2% lidocaine = 2 mg/kg if patient weighs 1 kg). **Table 2** lists recommended airway control devices sizes. Cuffed endotracheal tubes (ETT) should be used whenever possible and are available in sizes down to 2.5 mm (internal diameter; www.medis-medical.com, www.tri-anim.com). A guide tube may be used to facilitate intubation, especially when upper airway anatomy is abnormal; however, it is not necessary with normal anatomy.

Intubation is successful as demonstrated by an $Etco_2$ waveform or value, fogging of the ETT, or obvious sensation of expired tidal volume (V_T) by hand. The ETT should be advanced to the level of the thoracic inlet to ensure endobronchial intubation does not occur. The end of the ETT should extend approximately to the incisors or just past, to limit circuit dead space. The ETT should be secured behind the head and the forelimbs because of the ferret's craniocervical anatomy (**Fig. 3**). Laryngeal mask airways (LMA) can be used successfully (see **Table 2**).[30] Careful attention must be paid when moving patients with LMAs, as they are more difficult to secure and easily become dislodged, resulting in an upper airway obstruction.

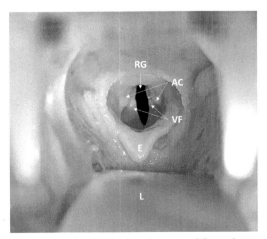

Fig. 2. Oral laryngoscopy image demonstrating the normal ferret laryngeal apparatus with labeled rima glottidis (RG), vocal folds (VF), arytenoid cartilages (AC), epiglottis (E), and laryngoscope (L) observed before tracheal intubation.

Table 2 Suggested endotracheal tube and laryngeal mask airway sizes for ferrets under anesthesia		
Weight	**ETT (Internal Diameter)**	**LMA**
<1 kg	Uncuffed 2.0–3.5 mm Cuffed 2.5–3.0 mm	Size 1
>1 kg	Uncuffed 2.5–3.5 mm Cuffed 2.5–3.5 mm	Size 1

MAINTENANCE PHASE
Inhalants

Use of inhalants, most commonly isoflurane or sevoflurane, is popular because of their ease in titratability, relatively quick onset and recovery, and negligible hepatic metabolism and renal excretion make them ideal for a wide range of patient populations. Relative anesthetic dose of inhalants required to effectively anesthetize an animal is defined in terms of MAC.[15] The MAC value is the anesthetic dose required for 50% of anesthetized ferrets to have no gross, purposeful motor response to a noxious stimulus.[15] The MAC of isoflurane and sevoflurane is 1.5% to 1.7% and 2.6%, respectively.[33–35] Many factors affect MAC and subsequently the anesthetic requirement, and the reader is encouraged to investigate this topic discussed at length elsewhere.[15,16,36] It may be desirable to reduce the anesthetic requirement for a given procedure (MAC reduction), and an appropriate plane of anesthesia must still be achieved. The anesthesia provider is encouraged not to fixate on achieving a certain perceived ideal vaporizer dial setting at the cost of titrating anesthetics to an appropriate anesthetic plane.

Cardiovascular Effects

Both isoflurane and sevoflurane are potent negative inotropes. In vitro assessment of isoflurane and sevoflurane on ferret ventricular myocardium demonstrates that indicators of contractility may be reduced by 50% at 1.5 to 2 and 1.7 to 2.5 MAC, respectively.[37–39] It is important to consider that (1) this is an in vitro and not an in vivo assessment of ventricular myocardium, (2) it is uncommon that a veterinarian would

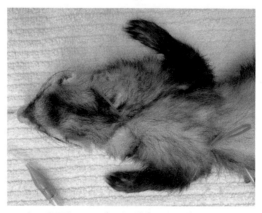

Fig. 3. Method of securing ETT in anesthetized ferrets. The tie is secured around the ETT, passed around the back of the neck, crossed over and wrapped around, caudally, in the axillary regions, and secured at the dorsum.

need to maintain these high anesthetic doses, and (3) based on this negative inotropy effect, in ferrets maintained on inhalant anesthetics and concurrently hypotensive, a positive inotrope such as dobutamine may be beneficial (see section entitled, Hypotension).

Both inhalants are also potent vasodilators, a mechanism thought to underlie much of the hypotension induced by these drugs. Unpremedicated ferrets anesthetized with isoflurane at 0.8 MAC at a mean arterial pressure (MAP) of 75 mm Hg became hypotensive (MAP = 57 mm Hg) at 1 MAC, and progressively more hypotensive at 1.5 (MAP = 38 mm Hg) and 2 MAC (MAP = 36 mm Hg), respectively.[33] The importance of this latter study is apparent when considering the often-unknown inspired percent concentration of isoflurane in the setting of brief periods of anesthesia maintained by mask, when short diagnostics or procedures are performed. It would be unsurprising that many of these ferrets often experience brief or prolonged periods of hypotension. Last, both isoflurane and sevoflurane will cause splenic capsule relaxation and a subsequent sequestration in red blood cells. At 1 MAC, packed cell volume (PCV) decreased by 38% and 43% for isoflurane and sevoflurane, respectively, 15 minutes following induction and returned to normal 2 hours following recovery.[34]

Respiratory Effects

Inhalant anesthetics are potent respiratory depressants.[33] Respiratory depression is defined as a reduced sensitivity to arteriolar carbon dioxide partial pressure (Pa_{CO_2}).[36] Whereas at the same level of Pa_{CO_2}, minute ventilation (Respiratory rate $\times$ V_T) is reduced in a ferret anesthetized with an inhalant anesthetic, subsequently leading increased Pa_{CO_2}.[36] Unpremedicated ferrets, intubated with a 3-mm cuffed ETT, breathing spontaneously, and anesthetized with isoflurane at 0.8, 1.0, 1.5, and 2.0 MAC, Pa_{CO_2} was 71 mm Hg, 78 mm Hg, 83 mm Hg, and 158 mm Hg, respectively.[33] Despite an increased RR of 25 to 40 breaths/min across these anesthetic doses, overt hypoventilation occurred.[33] This emphasizes that a significant degree of respiratory depression occurs in ferrets maintained on isoflurane across doses routinely administered in clinical practice. Data are not available for sevoflurane; however, data are suspected of being similar to isoflurane.

Nonrebreathing Circuits

Mapleson D and Bain modification are examples of commonly used nonrebreathing circuits.[40] These circuits lack unidirectional valves and carbon dioxide (CO_2) absorber canisters and rely instead on high fresh gas flow to ensure there is no rebreathing of CO_2. High fresh gas flow pushes previously expired gases down the circuit so as not inhaled on the next subsequent inspired V_T. Fresh gas flows should be approximately 200 mL/kg/min to achieve nonrebreathing; however, at higher RR (less time in between each expired breath), this flow may need to be elevated.[40] Failure to achieve nonrebreathing can be detected on a capnograph with the waveform not returning to baseline or inspired CO_2 increasing (eg, >3–4 mm Hg). Unique to a nonrebreathing circuit, when used appropriately, every single breath is 100% fresh gas. This means that when the vaporizer dial is changed, the respective change is reflected at the level of the patient immediately, and therefore, changes in depth can occur rapidly when adjusting vaporizer dial settings.

Intravenous Maintenance Protocols

IV maintenance of GA can either be performed in addition to inhalant anesthesia for the goal of MAC reduction or independent of inhalant anesthetics. Total intravenous anesthesia (TIVA) has increased in popularity; however, it is important to realize this may be a different experience than managing patients on inhalant anesthetics. Interpreting subjective parameters of the plane of anesthesia and making changes to the depth of anesthesia may be different and occur less quickly. Experience in managing ferrets anesthetized with TIVA techniques will improve satisfaction and comfort in assessing depth.

Anesthetics considered for TIVA include either propofol or alfaxalone; however, other combinations of sedatives, opioids, and general anesthetics may be used as well (**Table 3**; see **Table 6**). Continuous rate infusions of either of these agents and their respective CV and pulmonary effects in ferrets have not been reported. However, in dogs, each of these agents may provide appropriate anesthetic depth without substantial CV depression.[41] Dogs maintained on propofol CRIs do have moderate hypoventilation.[41] Like ferrets managed with inhalant anesthetics, first ensure an appropriate plane of anesthesia is achieved, then any adverse effects (eg, hypoventilation, hypotension) should be subsequently managed appropriately.

Logistical Considerations

The importance of patient access is vital and cannot be overstated. When considering positioning a ferret on a surgical table, access and visualization should be maximized. Clear drapes can be used for the purpose of visualization and can be helpful in monitoring respiratory rate and character. Depending on the surgical procedure, many clear drapes are not sized appropriately to offer sufficient sterile field. With traditional surgical drapes, an anesthesia screen should be used. Anesthesia screens allow for limited physical and visual access to the patient depending on positioning and procedure.

Because of a ferret's size, care should be taken to monitor for the presence of instruments, such as retractors, or surgeons resting their hands on the patient. Weight on the abdomen or thorax can easily result in compression to the degree of causing hypoventilation if breathing spontaneously or make mechanical ventilation more difficult resulting in the need for greater peak inspiratory pressures (PIP) to provide an adequate V_T.

Ferrets may need to be moved between recumbencies or locations numerous times during their anesthetic event. Movement provides opportunities for accidental deinstrumentation, ETT kinking, movement, or overt extubation.[42,43] In dogs, cats, and humans, simple manipulation of the cervical region can result in ETT migration within the trachea.[43,44] In dogs, extension of the neck results in cranial migration of the ETT tip by approximately 1 vertebral space; however, during flexion of the neck, ETTs are noted to migrate caudally by 3 to 4 vertebral spaces with migration to the extent of endobronchial intubation intermittently occurring.[43]

Vital Parameter Monitoring

The degree of anesthetic monitoring may vary depending on equipment availability and the environment where the anesthetic event occurs (eg, radiographs, MRI). It is the authors' opinion that anesthetized ferrets have the following monitored: ECG, core body temperature, pulse oximetry, $EtCO_2$, BP, and intermittent subjective depth evaluation. **Table 4** provides acceptable physiologic parameters. The following is a brief discussion on these parameters.

Anesthetic Depth Monitoring

Monitoring of depth is an important aspect of administering GA in that it allows the clinician to ensure that an appropriate depth is achieved before surgical stimulation; depth of anesthesia should be tracked over time to mitigate adverse effects from

Table 3
Suggested constant rate infusion doses for IV maintenance and adjunct anesthetics for ferrets

Drug	Dose (mg/kg/h)	Comments
Propofol	10–20	
Alfaxalone	5–15	
Ketamine[a]	0.6–1.8 0.5–1 mg/kg loading dose	Consider combining with fentanyl when administered as CRI
Dexmedetomidine[a]	0.001–005 1–2 μg/kg loading dose	
Lidocaine[a]	1–3 1–2 mg/kg loading dose	Bolus loading dose for ventricular arrythmias

The above doses are recommendations only and based on the authors' experience in ferrets and other species.
[a] CRIs should be prepared with a carrier rate of at least 3 mL/h in the authors' opinion. Lower carrier flows result in delayed onset of effect when starting a CRI or changing the CRI dose rate.

anesthetics administered in excess.[7] Eye position is relatively constant at an appropriate plane of anesthesia and will appear central; ventral eye position may indicate a lighter plane of anesthesia. The palpebral reflex is only present at a very light plane of anesthesia and is quick to disappear at deeper planes of anesthesia. Lacrimation and nystagmus are not appreciated in this species at even light planes of anesthesia. Pupil diameter is difficult to assess; however, it increases in diameter at deeper planes of anesthesia. Perhaps one of the most telling indicators of depth is jaw or masseter muscle tone, which may be significant at lighter planes of anesthesia but more relaxed at deeper planes of anesthesia. BP may become lower at progressively greater MAC multiples. However, the anesthesia provider is encouraged not to treat hypotension by continuously reducing the vaporizer dial setting. The patient should be assessed for anesthetic plane, and if deemed excessively anesthetized, the vaporizer dial setting may be reduced. However, if depth is deemed appropriate and hypotension is present, this should be addressed differently (see section entitled, Hypotension). Last, autonomic responses (eg, increased HR and BP) to surgical stimuli may be present at adequate planes of anesthesia; when observed, assess the other parameters of depth to determine if the ferret is adequately or inadequately anesthetized.

Blood Pressure
Given the CV effects of inhalant anesthetics, any ferret anesthetized should ideally have BP routinely monitored. Doppler flow probe placement on the tail with a number 1 neonatal size cuff tightly wrapped at the base of the tail, with sphygmomanometer, is the most consistent method to measure BP indirectly. This method aims to estimate systolic blood pressure (SBP); however, it has been documented to underestimate true SBP, when compared with direct SBP via arterial catheterization.[7,45,46] This is likely due to a number 1 cuff being relatively too large for the tail. This method is still valuable in detecting trends in BP over the anesthetic event. The authors recommend treating a Doppler BP less than 90 mm Hg as hypotension. Oscillometric methods of detecting BP are not accurate, often do not detect a flow signal, and are not recommended by the authors. There has been a report of high-definition oscillometric methods of detecting BP in ferrets with good correlation compared with direct BP measurements.[47] However, these high-definition oscillometric units are costly and not routinely available.

Table 4
Recommended acceptable physiologic and monitoring parameter values for ferrets under general anesthesia

Parameter	Range	Comments
Heart rate	180–260 beats/min	HR may vary directly following induction of anesthesia
Respiratory rate	20–40 breaths/min	
Temperature	99–101°F	
Blood pressure (Doppler)	>90 mm Hg	
Blood pressure (mean arterial pressure)	>60 mm Hg	
End-tidal co_2	35–55 mm Hg	See section discussing ventilation
Hemoglobin saturation of oxygen (Spo_2)	>93%	

Pulse Oximetry

Pulse oximetry can concurrently give information about saturation of hemoglobin with oxygen (Spo_2) and pulse rate.[46] There is significant value in use of this monitor perioperatively in ferrets. Principles of pulse oximetry have been described thoroughly elsewhere and should be understood. Results of arterial blood gas analysis have demonstrated good correlation between Spo_2 and calculated hemoglobin saturation of oxygen (SaO_2) as expressed by the oxygen-hemoglobin dissociation curve, in isoflurane anesthetized ferrets.[46]

Ventilation

The elimination of CO_2 is directly proportional to minute ventilation (RR $\times$ V_T); therefore, a change in either V_T or RR will indirectly influence $Paco_2$ (ie, reduced minute ventilation = increased $Paco_2$ or hypercapnia).[48] Many anesthetic drugs used cause respiratory depression. Respiratory depression is defined by a reduced central sensitivity to $Paco_2$ resulting in a lessened drive for ventilation.[36] As mentioned above, isoflurane and opioids are potent respiratory depressants resulting in progressively elevated $Paco_2$; because of this, anesthetized ferrets are very likely to severely hypoventilate because of respiratory depression.

Ventilation may be subjectively monitored through assessment of the RR. However, RR alone, without knowing the V_T of each breath, tells the anesthesia provider nothing regarding what minute ventilation is at any given time. This is supported by the aforementioned study in ferrets documenting significant hypoventilation while only at 1 MAC isoflurane.[33] The latter fact emphasizes the benefit of monitoring $Etco_2$ as an indicator of the degree of hypoventilation occurring. For prolonged diagnostic or surgical procedures, $Etco_2$ monitored via side-stream or mainstream capnograph should occur; however, these both require endotracheal intubation.[40]

An important consideration in monitoring $Etco_2$ in any anesthetized animal with small V_T is understanding a monitor's limitations. The authors routinely use side-stream capnographs with small patients, and these monitors sample at constant rates (eg, 50 mL/min). A ferret's V_T may be 5 to 15 mL, and any additional circuit dead space will inhibit a capnograph's ability to display an accurate Eto_2. **Fig. 4** represents capnogram tracings from an anesthetized ferret breathing spontaneously, demonstrating the absence of a complete expiratory plateau and a peak, representing a true end-tidal sample.[40] The latter means that an accurate $Etco_2$ is not being displayed, and the

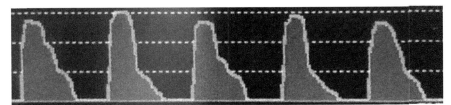

Fig. 4. Capnogram tracings from a side-stream capnograph of a ferret anesthetized with iso-flurane in 200 mL/kg/min oxygen via nonrebreathing circuit (Bain). Note that there is not a complete expiratory plateau or peak displayed due to (1) high fresh gas flow and (2) circuit dead space resulting in dead-space sampling and washout of the end-expiratory phase of the capnogram. This results in a displayed end-tidal co_2 (Etco$_2$), which underreports the true Etco$_2$, which is some unknown higher value. Side-stream capnograph sampling at 50 mL/min.

true ECO_2 is some unknown value higher than the one displayed. Depending on the capnograph sampling rate (ideal sampling rate for small mammals is 50 mL/min), cir-cuit dead space, and fresh gas flow, the displayed Etco$_2$ values may be underreporting true $EtCO_2$.[40,49,50]

The use of adapters and elbows may contribute to circuit dead space unnecessarily and exacerbate hypoventilation. Increases in circuit dead space volume will reduce the effective V_T that reaches the alveoli. The effect of circuit dead space on small mammals has been discussed at length.[50]

IPPV should bo instituted if a spontaneously breathing ferret cannot maintain Etco$_2$ < 55 mm Hg. Controlled ventilation can be performed manually or with the use of a mechanical ventilator. Important considerations in ventilating ferrets is under-standing their species-specific pulmonary mechanics and lung volumes.[51] V_T, RR, and acceptable PIP during IPPV are expressed in **Table 5**. An important consideration when delivering IPPV is their compliant respiratory system. Ferrets may require a PIP of less than 5 cmH$_2$O to deliver an adequately sized V_T; however, a PIP of up to 10 to 15 cmH$_2$O can be reached without significant adverse effect. A complete discus-sion of mechanical ventilation can be read elsewhere, and general principles apply to ferrets.[48,52]

The importance of monitoring and controlling ventilatory status may be explained briefly by examining the physiologic effects of hypercapnia. Elevated Paco$_2$ will result in an indirect reduction in plasma pH and respiratory acidosis and has certain direct effects on body systems.[48,53] Physiologic effects secondary to respiratory acidosis are dependent on the magnitude of derangement.[53] However, acidosis may be asso-ciated with reduced responsiveness to circulating catecholamines, subsequent re-ductions in cardiac contractility, and an increase in plasma potassium.[48,53] The increase in plasma potassium may be relevant in cases whereby ferrets are sus-pected, or known, to have an elevated plasma potassium before GA. Other body sys-tem effects of elevated CO$_2$ include stimulation of the sympathetic nervous system, increased circulating plasma catecholamines, and cerebral vasodilation, potentially increasing intracranial pressure.[48] Those suspected of having intracranial disease should be intubated under GA and hyperventilated (Etco$_2$ = 30–35 mm Hg) to mitigate this latter effect.

Regional Anesthesia

Lumbosacral (LS) epidurals should be considered for any invasive procedure involving the tail, perineal region (eg, rectal prolapse), pelvic limbs, or abdomen.[54] The

Table 5
Lung volumes, pulmonary mechanics, acceptable mechanical ventilation parameters, and acceptable acid-base ranges for an anesthetized ferret

Variable	Range	Comments
Tidal volume (V_T)	10–12 mL/kg	A 0.5 kg ferret has an approximately 6 mL V_T[51]
		Important consideration if wanting to safely administer manual or mechanical IPPV
Respiratory rate	20–40 bpm	
Minute volume	150–400 mL/kg/min[51]	
Peak inspiratory pressure (PIP)	2–8 cmH$_2$O	These are not upper limits but PIPs that may produce adequate V_T delivery
		Do not exceed 20 cmH$_2$O PIP
Inspiratory time	1–1.5 s	Time over which a V_T is administered either manually or mechanically

The above are suggested parameter ranges based on the authors' opinions and published data in ferrets or similar mammalian species.

technique has been described in ferrets.[55,56] For perineal or pelvic limb procedures (eg, fracture fixation), cranial spread of the administered drugs should reach at least L3-L4. When considering this technique, the volume of infusate must be increased to ensure cranial spread within the epidural compartment up to T9-10 (**Table 6**).

Drugs commonly used for this purpose are LAs or opioids, such as preservative-free lidocaine, ropivacaine, and morphine. Duration of LAs is dependent on the drug, 1 to 2 and 4 to 6 hours, respectively, for lidocaine or ropivacaine/bupivicaine. Epidural morphine may produce effective segmental analgesia for 12 to 18 hours.[54]

Considerations when performing an LS epidural should include self-limiting LA-induced motor paralysis (eg, 1–2 hours for lidocaine, 3–4 hours for bupivacaine or ropivacaine), or epidural opioid-induced urine retention reported in people, dogs, and cats can result in urine retention for up to 12 to 18 hours.[54] Although considered low in incidence, ferrets should be observed for urination following LS epidural administration. Last, epidural LAs may produce regional sympathetic blockade (eg, blocking regionally the sympathetic trunk).[54–56] Although the latter is relatively uncommon, it may be more likely if an LS epidural is performed for an abdominal procedure (ie, more cranial spread of the LA). Should a sympathetic block occur, regional vasodilation and subsequent hypotension could occur; this can be addressed with the use of vasopressors or IV crystalloids boluses.

Fluid Therapy

The goal of administering maintenance rate IV fluids (IVF) should achieve 3 objectives: (1) to maintain a patent catheter; (2) to provide a means to administer necessary medications or IVF boluses, if indicated; and (3) to supplement insensible free fluid loss (eg, evaporation from body cavities, urine production).[57,58] Maintenance rates will not contribute significantly to a calculated volume deficit over a short period of time; therefore, if a volume deficit is suspected, then a bolus (10–20 mL/kg) should be considered. Otherwise, higher IVF rates (10+ mL/kg/h) may be considered to correct a volume deficit throughout the anesthetic event. Failure to appropriately volume resuscitate or manage intravascular volume may result in significant hypotension and renal damage.[59,60] The choice of fluids should be a balanced electrolyte solution (eg,

Table 6
Systemic injectable and locoregional analgesic drug doses (mg/kg or mg/kg/h for CRI doses) for ferrets

Drug	Dose, Route	Frequency	Comments
Butorphanol	0.2–0.5 IV, IM, SC (0.1–0.3 mg/kg/h CRI with 0.1–0.2 mg/kg loading dose)	Every 1–2 h[a]	Mild sedation alone, consider combining with alpha-2 agonist or midazolam when used as premedicants
Buprenorphine	0.02–0.03 IV, IM, SC	Every 2–4 h	Mild sedation alone, consider combining with alpha-2 agonist or midazolam when used as premedicants
Fentanyl	0.005–0.01 IV, IM, SC (0.005–0.015 CRI with 0.003–0.005 loading dose)	Every 20–45 min (bolus)	Mild sedation alone, consider combining with alpha-2 agonist or midazolam when used as premedicants Consider combining with ketamine when administered as CRI
Hydromorphone	0.1–0.2 IV, IM, SC	Every 2–3 h	
Methadone	0.2–0.5 IV, IM, SC	Every 2–3 h	
Morphine	0.2–0.5 IV, IM, SC	Every 2–3 h	
Preservative-free morphine (1 mg/mL)	1.1 mg/kg epidurally		When combined with 2 mg/kg lidocaine or 0.5 mg/kg ropivacaine or bupivacaine for pelvic limb or perineal procedures[b]
	0.2 mg/kg epidurally		When combined with 4 mg/kg lidocaine or 1 mg/kg ropivacaine or bupivacaine abdominal procedures[b] Administered alone for pelvic limb or perineal procedures when local anesthetic is not administered concurrently

The above dosing recommendations are based on the authors' experience and other published data.
[a] The authors recommend redosing at least every 60 min during a stimulating procedure.
[b] See text for epidural opioid or local anesthetic duration of effects.

lactated Ringer, Plasmalyte, Normosol-R). Any additives (eg, dextrose, potassium chloride) to the IVF should be added as needed based on the veterinarian's discretion.

Management of anesthetic problems

Light Plane of Anesthesia

If a ferret becomes light under GA, it may manifest as an autonomic response (increase in HR, BP) with or without changes in subjective parameters of depth (eg, increased jaw tone). If HR and BP increase suddenly, depth of anesthesia should be first assessed. If the anesthetic plane is deemed appropriate, based on subjective parameters, then the maintenance anesthetic should be increased (ie, increase vaporizer dial setting). If the ferret is subjectively adequately anesthetized, then inadequate analgesia should be considered, taking into account recent analgesics administered and whether this makes clinical sense given the external stimulus present.

Hypoventilation

Hypoventilation is almost a ubiquitous anesthetic problem in any anesthetized mammal on inhalant anesthetics. This common problem is discussed above in the section entitled, Ventilation.

Hypotension

Hypotension is the most common adverse events to occur under GA in ferrets. If hypotensive, as measured via Doppler flow probe or direct arterial catheterization, the first consideration is to assess the plane of anesthesia. If the depth of anesthesia is adequate, it should not be lightened further for risk of emergence. In a simplified description, BP is a result of complex interactions between intravascular volume, vascular tone, and CO (CO = HR × stroke volume). In addition, measurement factors often lead to a falsely decreased measured BP.

The anesthetic provider should consider which factors are contributing most to the measured BP. A bolus of crystalloid fluids should be considered if there is suspicion of a volume deficit. A bolus of 10 to 20 mL/kg over 5 to 10 minutes of a crystalloid fluid is acceptable and may improve BP transiently; however, crystalloids redistribute quickly out of the vascular space, and a bolus' effect may be short lived. If not suspected of having a volume deficit, then the major factor contributing to hypotension is likely either secondary to reduced CO or reduced vascular resistance. If there is mild bradycardia (eg, <160 bpm), an anticholinergic may be considered (**Table 7**). If HR is normal, consider either a vasopressor or a positive inotrope. Ferrets anesthetized with inhalant anesthetics may have reduced vascular resistance from vasodilation and reduced contractility, and subsequent reduced stroke volume. Therefore, drugs, such as ephedrine, norepinephrine, dopamine, or dobutamine, may be considered.

Hypothermia

Derangements in body temperature perioperatively are common in anesthetized small mammals.[61,62] Perioperative inadvertent hypothermia (PIH) has been defined in dogs and cats as being a core temperature less than 97.7°F (36.5°C) with an incidence of 32.1% and 70.9%, respectively.[63] No similar study assessing the incidence of hypothermia in ferrets has been conducted; however, considering their small body mass, the authors suspect PIH incidence would approach or exceed the reported incidence in cats. High risk for PIH is likely due to having a large surface-area-to-mass ratio, which facilitates substantial radiant heat loss. In addition, veterinarians may not have standardized protocols to address PIH once present or attempt to mitigate PIH from developing.[64,65] It has been suggested that a core temperature perioperatively less than 96.8°F (36°C) be considered an adverse anesthetic event.[64,65] The

Table 7
Intervention drugs for ferrets under anesthesia

Drug	Dose, Route	Comments
Atropine	0.02 mg/kg IV 0.02–0.04 mg/kg IM, SC	Onset of action 5–10 min following IV, 10–15 min following IM, SC; duration 15–20 min (IV) and 20–45 min (IM, SC)
Glycopyrrolate	0.005–0.01 mg/kg IV, IM, SC	Onset of action 5–10 min following IV, 10–15 following IM, SC; subjectively longer duration compared with atropine
Ephedrine	0.1–0.25 mg/kg IV bolus (10–20 ug/kg/min IV as CRI[a])	Repeat boluses as needed every 5–15 min to effect, if repeat dosing required, consider CRI for maintenance Controlled drug
Phenylephrine	0.001–0.005 mg/kg IV bolus (0.1–0.5 µg/kg/min IV as CRI[a])	Repeat bolus doses as needed every 5–15 min to effect, if repeat dosing required, consider CRI for maintenance ECG required when administering bolus doses due to potential reflex bradycardia
Norepinephrine	0.05–0.5 µg/kg/min IV as CRI[a]	Authors' first choice following minimal to no response to ephedrine
Dopamine	5–20 µg/kg/min IV as CRI[a]	Higher-dose rates may produce more alpha-1 (vasoconstriction) effects, poorly understood
Hypertonic saline (7.2%)	2–4 mL/kg	Administer over 5–10 min for low volume resuscitation. Ideally, have ability to monitor plasma [Na]
Metoclopramide	1 mg/kg IV, SC[77] 1 mg/kg/h as CRI with the above dose for load[77]	For mitigating regurgitation perioperatively. If regurgitation preoperatively, administer loading dose before induction of anesthesia

The above doses are from the authors' experience from the use of these drugs in ferrets and other species.
[a] CRIs should be prepared with a carrier rate of at least 3 mL/h in the authors' opinion. Lower carrier flows result in delayed onset of effect when starting a CRI or changing the CRI dose rate.

authors suggest that a core body temperature of less than 97.0°F (36.1°C) should be considered PIH.

Heat loss occurs fastest in the first hour of anesthesia because of a redistribution of heat from the core to the periphery, secondary to vasodilation.[65] Complications associated with PIH are dependent on the magnitude and duration of hypothermia and are well documented in people.[65] Fewer studies have assessed complications in veterinary species. However, complications include hypocoagulopathies resulting in increased transfusion rates, prolonged recovery from anesthesia, and discomfort during recovery.[66-68] Although perioperative hypothermia in people has been associated with increased surgical site infections secondary to immunomodulatory effects of PIH, this was not documented when assessed in dogs and cats that experienced PIH and has not been assessed in ferrets.[63,66]

Heat loss often cannot be prevented; however, there are several methods recommended to mitigate the occurrence of PIH. At a minimum, barriers such as blankets or towels should be placed over top and between the patient and cold surfaces to mitigate conductive loss.[65] Recommended external heat sources are warm water and forced air blankets.[65] Both types of heat sources are most effective when more body surface area is covered. These are designed to have little difference in temperature in different locations, mitigating against heat concentration points. Similar to studies in human infants, a single veterinary study showed that increasing the operating room temperature to at least 75°F (23.9°C) reduced the incidence of PIH by approximately 50%.[67] Methods that are not recommended include warmed IVF bags, warmed bags of cereal grains, or placement of a forced air blanket hose in proximity to the anesthetized ferret, as this can concentrate heat, which may lead to burns.[65]

Historically, cool anesthetic gases have been considered a significant contributing cause of PIH; however, evaporation and loss of heat from the airway are suspected to be negligible in comparison to other mechanisms of heat loss.[65] A study using nonrebreathing circuits in cats demonstrated they did not result in faster onset, or more significant, PIH.[67]

Recommendations for Mitigating Against Perioperative Inadvertent Hypothermia

- Core temperature should be collected at least every 10 to 15 minutes.
- Barriers should be provided between premedicated, anesthetized, or recovering ferrets and cold surfaces.
- supplemented, whenever possible, using warm water or forced air blankets.
- Operating room temperatures should be increased to at least 75°F (23.9°C).
- Supplemental heat should be discontinued or reduced if core temperature increases more than 99°F (37.2°C).

Hyperthermia

Perioperative hyperthermia (eg, >102°F [38.9°C]), in the authors' experience, appears to be equivocally or more common than PIH. However, hyperthermia is more likely to be a problem when sources of heat supplementation are instituted. This is likely a product of small body mass and prolonged surgical procedures where the ferrets are draped and exposed to either warm water or forced air blankets. The authors recommend discontinuing or decreasing supplementation when core temperature measures greater than 99.5°F (37.5°C). If hyperthermia occurs, discontinue all heat supplementation. Active cooling may be required; however, this topic is discussed elsewhere.

Hypoglycemia

Ferrets are prone to hypoglycemia during preanesthetic fasting or if they have endocrine diseases (eg, insulinoma). Blood glucose (BG) should be measured routinely. If there is a history of hypoglycemia or known insulinoma, the authors suggest evaluation every 30 to 60 minutes under GA and supplementing as needed. The authors supplement with 2.5% dextrose solution administered at 5 to 10 mL/kg/h to ensure BG is 70 to 150 mg/dL.

Box 1
Ferret anesthesia: clinical case example: hypoventilation-induced hypoxemia

What is the significance of the hypoventilation for the ferret entering into the recovery cage? To answer this, the alveolar gas equation will be introduced. The alveolar gas equation (Eq. 1) allows a veterinarian to calculate what the partial pressure of oxygen is expected to be at the level of the alveolus (P_{AO_2}), considering the 2 other major gases present in the alveolus: water vapor and CO_2. The P_{AO_2} is ultimately the partial pressure of oxygen, which can saturate hemoglobin passing by the alveolus. Equation 2 (Eq. 2) exemplifies what the P_{AO_2} is in a normal awake ferret breathing room air (Fio_2 = 0.21 or 21% oxygen) and normal $Paco_2$. Note that the P_{AO_2} is 106 mm Hg, assuming that there is no significant intrapulmonary shunting of blood, then Pao_2 is approximately 10 to 15 mm Hg less than P_{AO_2} (90–95 mm Hg). Now consider the case example:

Eq. 1: Alveolar gas equation[77] $\qquad$ $P_{AO_2} = Fio_2(Patm - P_{H2O}) - Paco_2/Q$

Eq. 2: Normal ventilation on room air $\qquad$ $P_{AO_2} = 0.21(760 - 47) - 35/0.8$
$\qquad\qquad\qquad\qquad\qquad\qquad\qquad = 150 - 44$
$\qquad\qquad\qquad\qquad\qquad\qquad\qquad = 106$ mm Hg

Case example: a postoperative ferret has just been weaned from IPPV, is now breathing spontaneously, and has been breathing an Fio_2 of 1.0 (ie, 100% oxygen). The ferret recently has had systemic opioid redosed to ensure a comfortable recovery. The isoflurane was just turned off; the $Etco_2$ on the capnograph is registering 67 mm Hg consistently with an RR of 30 breaths per minute, and the ferret is then moved into the recovery cage. Five minutes later, the ferret is still intubated, $Etco_2$ is still 63 to 65 mm Hg, and Spo_2 now reads 84% to 85% while it is breathing room air (Fio_2 = 0.21). Why is the ferret not no longer saturating?

Equation 3 shows the alveolar gas equation calculated in this new context, assuming $Paco_2$ to be about 65 mm Hg. Note that the P_{AO_2} is now approximately 69 mm Hg, which assuming no significant intrapulmonary shunting of blood results in a Pao_2 of 55 to 60 mm Hg. A Pao_2 less than 60 mm Hg is the definition of hypoxemia and explains the SpO_2 reading. Note that the additional partial pressure of CO_2 in the alveolus due to hypoventilation results in a reduction in the P_{AO_2}, producing a hypoxic mixture of gas.

This ferret was connected back to the circuit and provided oxygen, increasing the Fio_2, P_{AO_2}, Pao_2, and subsequently the SpO_2. The ferret was later extubated when ready, saturating normally on room air.

Eq. 3: Hypoventilating on room air $\qquad$ $P_{AO_2} = 0.21(760 - 47) - 65/0.8$
$\qquad\qquad\qquad\qquad\qquad\qquad\qquad = 150 - 81$
$\qquad\qquad\qquad\qquad\qquad\qquad\qquad = 69$ mm Hg

[a] Pao_2, alveolar partial pressure of oxygen; Patm, atmospheric pressure; P_{AO_2} arteriolar partial pressure of co_2 (estimating true alveolar or end-tidal partial pressure of co_2); P_{H2O}, alveolar partial pressure of water vapor; Q, respiratory quotient.

[b] Atmospheric pressure assumed to be 760 mm Hg; P_{H2O} = 47 mm Hg, Q = 0.8.

Hemorrhage

Blood loss may occur in a variety of surgical procedures. Ferrets have approximately 60 mL/kg, or 6% of their body weight, in blood volume.[69] Blood loss of 10% may be tolerated without a need for transfusion. However, this is dependent on the starting hematocrit, and the anesthesia provider should consider replacing the lost blood volume itself. Blood lost is volume that is no longer filling the intravascular compartment, and ferrets may benefit from either a crystalloid fluid bolus or 2 to 4 mL/kg of hypertonic (7.2%) saline. When blood loss approaches or exceeds 20% of blood volume, initiate or consider transfusion of whole blood. Consider iatrogenic reduction in PCV owing to inhalant anesthetics.[34]

There are no documented blood types in ferrets; therefore, any ferret may be a blood donor.[70,71] Approximately 10% to 15% of the donor's blood volume may be sampled without undue harm incurred. Collection of blood for transfusions has been discussed elsewhere.[71] Xenotransfusion using feline blood may be considered as last resort.[72]

POSTANESTHESIA PHASE
Recovery

Like induction, recovery from anesthesia should always occur in a controlled environment. Before discontinuing maintenance anesthetic drugs, collect a final rectal temperature. If the ferret does have a severely deranged temperature (eg, <94°F or >104°F), this derangement should start to be addressed before discontinuing anesthetic agents. Consider the last time the ferret received an analgesic and ensure appropriate redosing is conducted in recovery to ensure it does not emerge from GA in discomfort.

If mechanically ventilated, the patient must regain spontaneous ventilation before being extubated. Weaning from mechanical ventilation is recommended as follows: discontinue maintenance anesthetic agents, reduce minute ventilation through reduction of the RR to deliver 2 to 3 breaths/min. With a reduced minute ventilation, $Paco_2$ will be allowed to increase until the ferret resumes spontaneous ventilation.

General anesthetics and analgesics often result in profound reduction in the drive for ventilation, and adequate ventilation when recovering from GA is important. The alveolar gas equation is valuable in evaluating the effect of hypoventilation on the risk for developing hypoxemia in recovery.[73] **Box 1** demonstrates a case example of a hypoventilating ferret in recovery. In this scenario, pulse oximetry identified the patient no longer had normal hemoglobin saturation. Despite Spo_2 being a monitor for hemoglobin saturation with oxygen, it can be used in recovery to identify desaturation, often secondary to continued hypoventilation after being placed in a recovery cage.[23,74,75] Respiratory depression secondary to inhalant anesthetic will continue until the ferret ventilates out the anesthetic. In addition, redosed opioid also contributes to respiratory depression in this scenario and needs to be considered. The authors recommend pulse oximetry on every postanesthesia recovering ferret until it is demonstrated that their Spo_2 is consistently (eg, >5 minutes) higher than 93%. If the Spo_2 is less than 93%, provide oxygen supplementation via face mask at 2 to 3 L/min or attach the circuit back to the ETT, if still intubated.

SUMMARY

GA can be achieved safely if appropriate considerations are taken. Many fundamental principles to safe administration of GA are applicable to ferrets. How a person, dog, or cat is managed during an anesthetic event is known to have potential long-term impacts beyond the anesthetic event.[6,60,76] As ferrets are anesthetized more frequently, these same long-term impacts of adverse events under anesthesia may become more apparent. The anesthesia provider should strive for the highest possible care of the anesthetized ferret, regardless of anesthetic event duration.

REFERENCES

1. American Veterinary Medical Association. AVMA pet ownership and demographics sourcebook : 2017-2018 Edition.

2. Ko J, Marini RP. Anesthesia. In: Fox JG, Marini RP, editors. Biology and diseases of the ferret. 3rd edition. Ames (IA): John Wiley & Sons, Inc.; 2014. p. 259–83.
3. Brodbelt DC, Blissitt KJ, Hammond RA, et al. The risk of death: the confidential enquiry into perioperative small animal fatalities. Vet Anaesth Analg 2008;35: 365–73.
4. Wills A, Holt S. Confidence of veterinary surgeons in the United Kingdom in treating and diagnosing exotic pet species. Vet Rec 2020;186:e20.
5. Schwarz LA, Solano M, Manning A, et al. The normal upper gastrointestinal examination in the ferret. Vet Radiol 2003;44:165–72.
6. Hawkins MG, Pascoe PJ. Anesthesia, analgesia, and sedation of small mammals. In: Carpenter J, editor. Ferrets, Rabbits, and Rodents. 4th edition. Philadelphia: Elsevier; 2021. p. 536–58.
7. Haskins S. Monitoring anesthetized patients. In: Grimm K, Lamont L, Tranquilli W, et al, editors. Veterinary anesthesia and analagesia: the fifth edition of Lumb and Jones. 5th edition. Ames (IA): John Wiley & Sons, Inc; 2015. p. 86–113.
8. Bateman S. Making sense of blood gas results. Vet Clin Small Anim 2008;38: 543–57.
9. Yuschenkoff D, Graham J, Sharkey L, et al. Reference interval determination of venous blood gas, hematologic, and biochemical parameters in healthy sedated, neutered ferrets (Mustela putorius furo). J Exot Pet Med 2021;36:25–7.
10. Rankin D. Sedatives and tranquilizers. In: Grimm K, Lamont L, Tranquilli W, et al, editors. Veterinary anesthesia and analagesia: the fifth edition of Lumb and Jones. 5th edition. Ames (IA): John Wiley & Sons, Inc; 2015. p. 196–206.
11. Lichtenberger M, Ko J. Anesthesia and analgesia for small mammals and birds. Vet Clin North Am Exot Anim Pract 2007;10:293–315.
12. Smith AC, Zellner JL, Spinale FG, et al. Sedative and cardiovascular effects of midazolam in swine. Lab Anim Sci 1991;41:157–61.
13. Morrisey JK, Matthew SJ. Ferrets. In: Carpenter J, editor. Exotic animal formulary. 5th edition. Philadephia: Elsevier; 2017. p. 532–57.
14. Wynn RL, Essien E, Thut PD. The effects of different antiemetic agents on morphine-induced emesis in ferrets. Eur J Pharmacol 1993;241:47–54.
15. Reed R, Doherty T. Minimum alveolar concentration: key concepts and a review of its pharmacological reduction in dogs. Part 1. Res Vet Sci 2018;117:266–70.
16. Reed R, Doherty T. Minimum alveolar concentration: key concepts and a review of its pharmacological reduction in dogs. Part 2. Res Vet Sci 2018;118:27–33.
17. van Oostrom H, Schoemaker NJ, Uilenreef JJ. Pain management in ferrets. Vet Clin North Am Exot Anim Pract 2011;14:105–16.
18. d'Ovidio D, Adami C. Locoregional anesthesia in exotic pets. Vet Clin North Am Exot Anim Pract 2019;22:301–14.
19. Bublot I, Randolph WR, Chalvet-Monfray K, et al. The surface electrocardiogram in domestic ferrets. J Vet Cardiol 2006;8:87–93.
20. Dudás-Györki Z, Szabó Z, Manczur F, et al. Echocardiographic and electrocardiographic examination of clinically healthy, conscious ferrets. J Small Anim Pract 2011;52:18–25.
21. Wagner RA. Ferret cardiology. Vet Clin North Am Exot Anim Pract 2009;12: 115–34.
22. Ambros B, Carrozzo MV, Jones T. Desaturation times between dogs preoxygenated via face mask or flow-by technique before induction of anesthesia. Vet Anaesth Analg 2018;45:452–8.
23. Henao-Guerrero N, Riccó CH. Comparison of the cardiorespiratory effects of a combination of ketamine and propofol, propofol alone, or a combination of

ketamine and diazepam before and after induction of anesthesia in dogs sedated with acepromazine and oxymorphone. Am J Vet Res 2014;75:231–9.

24. Giral M, García-Olmo DC, Gómez-Juárez M, et al. Anaesthetic effects in the ferret of alfaxalone alone and in combination with medetomidine or tramadol: a pilot study. Lab Anim 2014;48:313–20.

25. Keates H, Whittem T. Effect of intravenous dose escalation with alfaxalone and propofol on occurrence of apnoea in the dog. Res Vet Sci 2012;93:904–6.

26. Fayyaz S, Kerr CL, Dyson DH, et al. The cardiopulmonary effects of anesthetic induction with isoflurane, ketamine–diazepam or propofol–diazepam in the hypovolemic dog. Vet Anaesth Analg 2009;36:110–23.

27. Brodbelt DC, Vetmb MA, Dipecva D. The confidential enquiry into perioperative small animal fatalities. 2006. (Dissertation)

28. Friembichler S, Coppens P, Säre H, et al. A scavenging double mask to reduce workplace contamination during mask induction of inhalation anesthesia in dogs. Acta Vet Scand 2011;53:1–5.

29. Schmid R, Hodgson D, McMurphy R. Comparison of anesthetic induction in cats by use of isoflurane in an anesthetic chamber with a conventional vapor or liquid injection technique. J Am Vet Med Assoc 2008;233:262–6.

30. Brietzke SE, Mair EA. Laryngeal mask versus endotracheal tube in a ferret model. Ann Otol Rhinol Laryngeal 2001;110:827–33.

31. Kircher SS, Murray LE, Juliano ML. Minimizing trauma to the upper airway: a ferret model of neonatal intubation. J Am Assoc Lab Anim Sci 2009;48:780–4.

32. Dyson DH. Efficacy of lidocaine hydrochloride for laryngeal desensitization: a clinical comparison of techniques in the cat. J Am Vet Med Assoc 1998;192:1286–8.

33. Lrnai A, Steffey EP, Farver TB, et al. Assessment of isoflurane-induced anesthesia in ferrets and rats. Am J Vet Res 1999;60:1577–83.

34. Lawson A, Lichtenberger M, Day T, et al. Comparison of sevoflurane and isoflurane in domestic ferrets (Mustela putorius furo). Vet Therap 2006;7:207–12.

35. Murat I, Housmans PR. Minimum alveolar concentration (MAC) of halothane, enflurane, and isoflurane in ferrets. Anesthesiology 1988;68:783–6.

36. Steffey EP, Mama K, Brosnan R. Inhalant anesthetics. In: Grimm K, Lamont L, Tranquilli W, et al, editors. Veterinary anesthesia and analagesia: the fifth edition of Lumb and Jones. 5th edition. Ames (IA): John Wiley & Sons, Inc; 2015. p. 277–96.

37. Housmans PR, Murat I. Comparative effects of halothane, enflurane, and isoflurane at equipotent anesthetic concentrations on isolated ventricular myocardium of the ferret. Contractility Anesthesiol 1988;69:451–63.

38. Bartunek AE, Housmans PR. Effects of sevoflurane on the contractility of ferret ventricular myocardium. J Appl Physiol 2000;89:1778–86.

39. Baele P, Housmans PR. The effects of halothane, enflurane, and isoflurane on the length-tension relation of the isolated ventricular papillary muscle of the ferret. Anesthesiology 1991;74:281–91.

40. Dorsch J, Dorsch S. Mapleson breathing system. In: Dernoski N, editor. Understanding anesthesia equipment. Philadelphia: Lippincott Williams & Wilkins; 2008. p. 209–22.

41. Ambros B, Duke-Novakovski T, Pasloske K. Comparison of the anesthetic efficacy and cardiopulmonary effects of continuous rate infusions of alfaxalone-2-hydroxypropyl-βcyclodextrin and propofol in dogs. Amer J Vet Res 2008;69:1391–8.

42. Campoy L, Hughes J, McAllister H, et al. Kinking of endotracheal tubes during maximal flexion of the atlanto-occipital joint in dogs. J Small Anim Prac 2003; 44:3–7.
43. Quandt J, Robinson E, Walter P, et al. Endotracheal tube displacement during cervical manipulation in the dog. Vet Surg 1993;22:235–9.
44. Kim JT, Kim HJ, Ahn W, et al. Head rotation, flexion, and extension alter endotracheal tube position in adults and children. Can J Anesth 2009;56:751–6.
45. Mark J. Arterial blood pressure: direct versus indirect measurement. In: Houston M, editor. Atlas of cardiovascular monitoring. New York: Churchill Livingstone Inc.; 1998. p. 81–98.
46. Olin JM, Tracy D, Smith J, et al. Evaluation of noninvasive monitoring techniques in domestic ferrets (Mustela putorius turo). Am J Vet Res 1997;58:1065–9.
47. van Zeeland YR, Wilde A, Bosman IH, et al. Non-invasive blood pressure measurement in ferrets (Mustela putorius furo) using high definition oscillometry. Vet J 2017;228:53–62.
48. Lumb A. Anesthesia. In: Nunn's applied respiratory physiology. 8th edition. Philadelphia: Elsevier; 2012. p. 291–313.
49. Duke-Novakovski T, Fujiyama M, Beazley SG. Comparison of mainstream (Capnostat 5) and two low-flow sidestream capnometers (VM-2500-S and Capnostream) in spontaneously breathing rabbits anesthetized with a Bain coaxial breathing system. Vet Anaesth Analg 2020;47:537–46.
50. Pearsall MF, Feldman JM. When does apparatus dead space matter for the pediatric patient? Anesth Analg 2014;118:1404–8
51. Vinegar A, Sinnett EE, Kosch PC, et al. Respiratory mechanics of a small carnivore: the ferret. J Appl Phys 1982;52:832–7.
52. Evassilev M. An overview of positive pressure ventilation. J Vet Emer Crit Care 2004;14:15–21.
53. Handy JM, Soni N. Physiological effects of hyperchloraemia and acidosis. Br J Anaesth 2008;101:141–50.
54. Campoy L, Read M, Peralta S. Canine and feline local anesthetic and analgesic techniques. In: Grimm K, Lamont L, Tranquilli W, et al, editors. Veterinary anesthesia and analagesia: the fifth edition of Lumb and Jones. 5th edition. Ames (IA): John Wiley & Sons, Inc; 2015. p. 827–56.
55. Sladky K, Horne W, Goodrowe K, et al. Evaluation of epidural morphine for postoperative analgesia in ferrets (Mustela putorius furo). J Am Assoc Lab Anim Sci 2000;30:33–8.
56. Eshar D, Wilson J. Epidural anesthesia and analgesia in ferrets. Lab Anim 2010; 39:339–40.
57. Gaynor SJ, Wertz ME, Kesel ML, et al. Effect of intravenous administration of fluids on packed cell volume, blood pressure, and total protein and blood glucose concentrations in healthy halothane-anesthetized dogs. J Am Vet Med Assoc 1996;208:2013–5.
58. Muir W, Kijtawornrat A, Ueyama Y, et al. Effects of intravenous administration of lactated Ringer's solution on hematologic, serum biochemical, rheological, hemodynamic, and renal measurements in healthy isoflurane-anesthetized dogs. J Am Vet Med Assoc 2011;239:630–7.
59. Lobetti R, Lambrechts N. Effects of general anesthesia and surgery on renal function in healthy dogs. Am J Vet Res 2000;61(2):121–4.
60. Ross L. Acute kidney injury in dogs and cats. Vet Clin North Am Sm Anim Pract 2011;41:1–14.

61. Redondo JI, Suesta P, Serra I, et al. Retrospective study of the prevalence of postanaesthetic hypothermia in dogs. Vet Rec 2012;171:1–5.
62. Redondo JI, Suesta P, Gil L, et al. Retrospective study of the prevalence of post-anaesthetic hypothermia in cats. Vet Rec 2012;170:1–5.
63. Mcmillan M, Darcy H. Adverse event surveillance in small animal anaesthesia: an intervention-based, voluntary reporting audit. Vet Anaesth Analg 2016;43: 128–35.
64. Díaz M, Becker DE. Thermoregulation: physiological and clinical considerations during sedation and general anesthesia. Anesth Prog 2010;57:25–33.
65. Grimm K. Perioperative thermoregulation. In: Grimm K, Lamont L, Tranquilli W, et al, editors. Veterinary anesthesia and analagesia: the fifth edition of Lumb and Jones. 5th edition. Ames (IA): John Wiley & Sons, Inc; 2015. p. 372–9.
66. Beal MW, Brown DC, Shofer FS. The effects of perioperative hypothermia and the duration of anesthesia on postoperative wound infection rate in clean wounds: a retrospective study. Vet Surg 2000;29:123–7.
67. Rodriguez-Diaz JM, Hayes GM, Boesch J, et al. Decreased incidence of perioperative inadvertent hypothermia and faster anesthesia recovery with increased environmental temperature: a nonrandomized controlled study. Vet Surg 2020; 49:256–64.
68. Kelly CK, Hodgson DS, McMurphy RM. Effect of anesthetic breathing circuit type on thermal loss in cats during inhalation anesthesia for ovariohysterectomy. J Am Vet Med Assoc 2012;240:1296–9.
69. Brown C. Blood collection from the cranial vena cava of the ferret. Lab Anim 2006;35:23–4.
70. Manning D, Bell J. Lack of detectable blood groups in domestic ferrets: implications for transfusion. J Am Vet Med Assoc 1990;197:84–6.
71. Pignon C, Donnelly TM, Todeschini C, et al. Assessment of a blood preservation protocol for use in ferrets before transfusion. Vet Rec 2014;174:277.
72. Bell AL, Gladden JN, Graham JE. Successful xenotransfusion in a domestic ferret with spontaneous hemoperitoneum using feline packed red blood cells. J Vet Emer Crit Care 2020;30:336–41.
73. Cruickshank S, Mb BA, Frca BS, et al. The alveolar gas equation. Br J Anaesth 2004;4:24–7.
74. Sarkar M, Niranjan N, Banyal PK. Mechanisms of hypoxemia. Lung India 2017;34: 47–60.
75. Williams AJ. ABC of oxygen: assessing and interpreting arterial blood gases and acid-base balance. Br Med J 1998;317:1213–6.
76. Eisenach JC. Long-term consequences of anesthetic management. Anaesthesiology 2009;111:1–4.
77. Wilson DV, Evans AT, Mauer WA. Influence of metoclopramide on gastroesophageal reflux in anesthetized dogs. Am J Vet Res 2006;67:6726–31.

Miniature Companion Pig Sedation and Anesthesia

Joe S. Smith, DVM, MPS, PhD, DACVIM(LAIM), DACVCP*, Reza Seddighi, DVM, MS, PhD, DACVAA

KEYWORDS

- Anesthesia • Miniature companion pig • Pot-bellied pig • Sedation • Surgery

KEY POINTS

- Miniature companion pigs (MCP) are increasing in popularity, and as such, there is an increased need for veterinarians trained in sedation and anesthesia for the species.
- MCPs have several species-specific qualities that can complicate injectable drug administration and create challenges for inhalational anesthesia (eg, with endotracheal intubation).
- General anesthetic complications, such as hypothermia and hypotension, are commonly described in miniature companion pigs, so monitoring of vital parameters during anesthetic procedures and recovery is crucial.

INTRODUCTION

Miniature companion pigs (MCPs, Sus scrofa domesticus) are rapidly increasing in popularity in North America. Originally, the Vietnamese pot-bellied pig was the most common MCP breed, but now multiple breeds are being kept as pets, including Kunekune, Juliana, Ossabaw Island, and others. With increasing numbers of animals and their longer (potentially 15–20 year) life spans,[1,2] there is a need for sedation and general anesthesia to perform a variety of procedures, such as routine hoof maintenance, tusk trimming, ovariohysterectomy, and castration, and more advanced techniques for diagnostic imaging and surgical interventions. This article discusses the considerations for sedation and anesthesia of MCPs, highlighting species specifics, and reviews the agents and their applications commonly used in these animals.

The authors declare that they have no relevant or material financial interests that relate to the research described in this article.

Large Animal Clinical Sciences, College of Veterinary Medicine, University of Tennessee, 2407 River Drive, Knoxville, TN 37996-4500, USA

* Corresponding author.

E-mail address: joesmith@utk.edu

ANATOMIC CONSIDERATIONS
Physical Examination

MCPs are often not the most tractable patients, and the ability to perform a thorough physical examination before sedation or anesthesia is challenging. A suspending sling is sometimes used to facilitate physical examination (**Fig. 1**). Alternative methods for calming pigs to facilitate physical examination may include such techniques as "forking" (**Fig. 2**).[3] In this technique, a pig is stroked with a back-scratching device or plastic fork and will move from standing position to lateral recumbency. Additional techniques to facilitate preanesthetic examination may include providing small treats, such as Cheerios, or encouraging the owner to train the pig to present in lateral recumbency for belly rubs. Other considerations for physical examination and restraint include the use of pig boards to guide them, and earplugs to protect the animal from hearing surrounding noises. In addition to the pig board, the authors have had success with holding a bucket around the head of a pig to facilitate them backing up and directing their movement. The use of a commercial hog snare for MCPs is discouraged[4] because when these snares are used, they may strain and undergo musculoskeletal damage leading to lameness.[5] Additionally, the facial conformation of some breeds of MCPs, such as the shortened face of the Vietnamese pot-bellied pig, makes restraint with snares further challenging, because they are designed for securing the elongated nose of commercial pigs.

Venous Access and Catheterization

Another consideration of MCP anatomy is the challenge of obtaining venous access. Typically, the auricular vein is the easiest location for venous access and

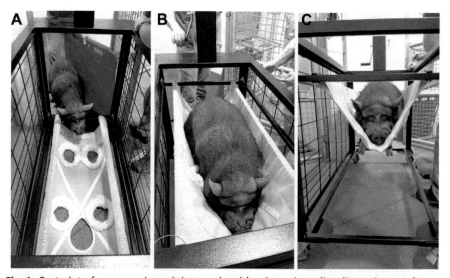

Fig. 1. Restraint of a companion miniature pig with a Panepinto sling (Panepinto and Associates). (*A*) The pig is directed into the sling with a pig board while the sling is lowered. (*B*) The sling is raised, capturing the limbs in the openings. (*C*) The sling is raised the entire way. At this point, required restraint for examination and injections is achieved. Care should be taken to ensure that all of the pig's limbs fall into the corresponding openings in the sling, and the appropriate-sized sling is used to minimize the chances of the pig moving out of the sling.

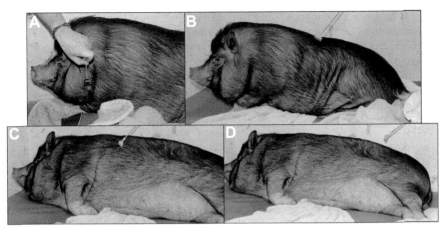

Fig. 2. Moving a pig into a lateral recumbency with tactile stimulation or "forking." (*A*) The skin around the neck is gently tapped or scratched with a fork. (*B*) The stimulation then moves to the dorsum. Alternatively a plastic "back-scratcher" is used for this purpose instead of an actual fork. (*C*) Stimulation is directed ventrally and/or caudally as the pig starts to lie down. (*D*) At the end the animal is presenting in lateral recumbency.

catheterization. This is done with the MCP in a sling or performed under sedation. A rubber band is placed around the base of the ear to aid in venous distention and identification. Topical lidocaine gel placed over the catheter site to desensitize the skin before antiseptic preparation is used for some animals if they are refractory to catheter placement. After catheter placement, it is recommended to tape a roll of gauze or an appropriately sized plastic syringe case inside the ear and incorporating the catheter into a wrapped bandage around the ear for security (**Fig. 3**). In addition to the auricular vein, catheterization of the cephalic and subcutaneous abdominal veins have been described in MCPs.[6,7] Catheterization of the jugular vein is possible, but this process

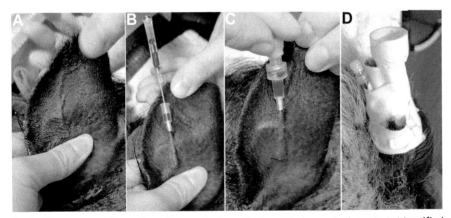

Fig. 3. Placement and securing of an auricular catheter. (*A*) The auricular vein is identified, clipped, prepared, and distended with digital pressure. (*B*) The catheter is placed in an auricular vein. (*C*) The catheter is capped before securing. (*D*) The catheter is secured with a white tape and a syringe case (alternatively, a rolled gauze is used) placed in the center of the ear to provide additional security.

typically requires a cutaneous "cutdown" approach in anesthetized patients. Multiple references exist for jugular catheter placement in commercial pigs without a cutdown approach, but these techniques are challenging in MCPs because the head conformation is typically shorter than commercial breeds. Some MCP breeds (eg, Vietnamese pot-bellied pigs) also have pronounced jowls that can complicate jugular catheterization without a cutdown. The use of ultrasound to guide jugular vein catheterization has been described for a Yucatan miniature pig.[8]

Injections

In MCPs, it is challenging to determine if injections are intramuscular (IM), subcutaneous, or potentially administered into fat deposits. To increase the likelihood of IM administration, a long needle (1.5–2 inch) is used for injection into the cervical musculature in an adult MCP.[9] A 1-inch needle may be adequate for smaller pigs.[1] The semimembranosus and semitendinosus muscles are also described for IM injection, with a 1.5-inch needle considered appropriate for most adult MCPs. When possible, the gluteal muscles should be avoided as injection sites because of the risk of injury to the sciatic nerve.[9] The intended drugs are administered via a needle connected to a 30-inch extension line with a syringe (**Fig. 4**). This prevents dislodgement of the needle and allows for the patient to relax before the injection is given to avoid trauma or incomplete injections. Alternately, a butterfly catheter can be used for IM injections in smaller pigs.

Laryngeal Anatomy

The anatomy of the porcine head and pharynx can present challenges for laryngeal visualization and endotracheal intubation. Additionally, pigs possess a separate bronchial branch (tracheal bronchus) that ventilates an accessory right lung lobe that presents a risk of being bypassed by the endotracheal tube (ETT), and thus bypassing ventilation of this lobe or intubation of the tracheal bronchus may occur.[10,11] Therefore, care should be taken to not advance the ETT too far past the level of the thoracic inlet. MCPs are also obligate nasal breathers and are prone to respiratory obstruction. Because of this, minimization of trauma during intubation should be a constant focus. Additional anatomic challenges for intubation include the elongated soft palate and the laryngeal diverticulum (discussed later in intubation section). A cadaveric image of the tracheal bronchus is presented in **Fig. 5**.

As a monogastric species, MCPs should have some degree of withholding of food, and possibly water, before anesthesia to reduce the risk of regurgitation and aspiration. Recommendations for withholding vary from ranges of food material for 6 to 12 hours before anesthesia,[6,9,12–14] and water for 2 to 6 hours prior.[1,6,9] The authors acknowledge previous water withholding recommendations, but recommend clinical judgment because water deprivation can lead to dehydration and increase stress in hospitalized patients. These time recommendations do not always lead to complete gastric emptying, especially in pigs with grazing habits or access to browse, so diet and environment should be taken into consideration when determining withholding time periods for MCPs. For pigs younger than 8 weeks of age undergoing anesthesia, it has been recommended to reduce access to food and water for a period of time of 1 to 4 hours before anesthesia,[9] with no withholding considered for suckling animals.

SEDATION

Multiple classes of agents may be considered for sedation in MCPs. A detailed chart of dosage, route, and particular considerations for sedation is listed in **Table 1**.

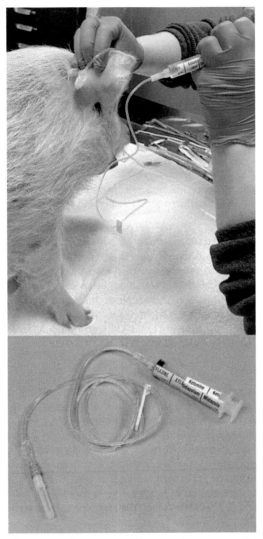

Fig. 4. Using a 30-inch extension line connected to an 18-gauge needle to administer anesthetic premedication/induction medications in a companion miniature pig by intramuscular injection in the neck (*top*). The *bottom* image displays the setup of 18-gauge syringe, extension line, and syringe.

Sedatives, such as acepromazine and benzodiazepines, may cause hypothermia in MCPs, so practitioners should monitor temperature during periods of extended sedation.

Benzodiazepines

Benzodiazepines, such as diazepam and midazolam, have been commonly used. Midazolam has higher affinity for receptors, quicker onset, and increased potency, but has a shorter duration of effect when compared with diazepam. Commonly administered at dosages of 0.2 to 0.5 mg/kg IM, midazolam can also be administered

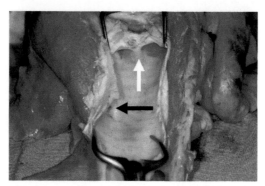

Fig. 5. Tracheal bronchus in a porcine cadaveric specimen. Opening of the tracheal bronchus (*black arrow*) is shown in proximity to the bronchial bifurcation (*white arrow*).

intranasally. This is achieved via a catheter with the stylet removed and injected during inspiration in small volumes. Although only rarely indicated (eg, overdosage), midazolam and diazepam can be reversed with flumazenil (0.01–0.02 mg/kg). Although repeated administrations of flumazenil may be necessary for complete reversal because of a short half-life. Benzodiazepines may cause unpredictable sedation when used as a single agent for sedation and require regulatory oversight for their use. For MCPs that require frequent sedation with benzodiazepines, tolerance may develop after long-term administration (28 days).[15]

α_2-Adrenergic Agonists

The α_2-adrenergic agonists, such as xylazine, dexmedetomidine, and medetomidine, have also been described for sedation in pigs.[16] These agents are commonly used in combination with an opioid and ketamine to induce heavy sedation or general anesthesia (dose-dependent). α_2-Agents result in sedation via central nervous system depression, analgesia, decrease in gastrointestinal function, bradycardia, hypotension, respiratory depression, and hypothermia. The authors have observed vomiting when α_2-agents are used, particularly at high doses. Currently, it is recommended to use α_2-agents in combination with other agents for multimodal sedation protocols. The α_2-agents in pigs are reversed with yohimbine or tolazoline.

Ketamine

Ketamine has been described as part of multiple agent protocols for sedation in MCPs. Ketamine is considered a dissociative sedative/anesthetic and induces analgesia via an N-methyl-D-aspartate antagonistic effect. Ketamine's sedative/anesthetic mechanism of action involves inhibiting γ-aminobutyric acid activity and potentially blocking serotonin, norepinephrine, and dopamine in the central nervous system. It does not generally cause profound cardiovascular depression, but it can result in apnea at higher doses. When the authors use ketamine for sedation, they typically incorporate it into a multiagent protocol with an opioid and α_2-agonist. Although rare, adverse reactions to ketamine have been reported in a case series of three MCPs. The signs observed ranged from erythema and tachycardia to respiratory and cardiac arrest.[17] All three pigs recovered well after implementation of epinephrine, fluid therapy, discontinuation of sedation, and supportive care. Because of the clinical appearance of these adverse effects it can be assumed that anaphylaxis to ketamine, an extremely rare phenomenon observed in people, could also be a possibility in

Table 1
Common sedative and anesthetic premedication agents in porcine

Drug	Mechanism of Action	Dose	Route	Comments	Reference
Acepromazine	Antagonism of post-synaptic dopamine receptors	0.05–1.0 mg/kg	IM, SC, IV	More sedative effect is achieved when used in combination with other drugs. Onset should be within 20-30 minutes with a duration of 30 min to several hours, depending on the dose used. Lower dosages should be considered for IV administrations.	Van Amstel[55]; Mitek[56]; Anderson & Mulon[16]
Alfaxalone	Neuroactive steroid; modulates chloride ion transport and binds to GABA receptors	1–2 mg/kg	IM, IV, intranasal	Concerns with apnea, volume required for sedation may be too large to achieve in all sizes of pigs, particularly for IM and intranasal administration.	Mitek[56]; Hampton et al[22]
Azaperone	Inhibition of dopamine and norepinephrine	1–2 mg/kg	IM	Doses >1 mg/kg may cause priapism in boars. Hypotension may be a concern for doses >1 mg/kg. IV administration is not recommended because of potential for excitation.	Van Amstel[55]; Anderson & Mulon[16]
Butorphanol	Opioid receptor agonist and antagonist	0.1–1.0 mg/kg	IM, IV	Usually used to provide sedation as part of a multiple agent protocol.	Mitek[56]; Østevik et al[12]
Dexmedetomidine	α_2-Agonist	10–20 µg/kg	IM	More effective as part of a multiple agent protocol. Cardiovascular effects are more significant at higher doses. May cause vomiting.	Mitek[56]; Carpenter[18]
Diazepam	Benzodiazepine; modulates chloride ion transport via binding to GABA$_A$ receptors	0.1–0.5 mg/kg	IV, PO	IM administration of diazepam is not recommended because of pain from injection and erratic absorption.	Bollen[10]; Carpenter[18]

(continued on next page)

Table 1
(continued)

Drug	Mechanism of Action	Dose	Route	Comments	Reference
Midazolam	Benzodiazepine; modulates chloride ion transport via binding to GABA$_A$ receptors	0.1–0.5 mg/kg	IM, SC, IV, intranasal	Can be administered intranasally via a catheter with the stylet removed and squirted during inspiration. The volume is challenging to administer intranasally in large pigs. Consider reversal with flumazenil when large doses are used.	Carpenter[18], Swindle & Sistino[57]
Morphine	Full opioid receptor agonist	0.1–1.0 mg/kg	IM, IV	May cause undesirable excitation in pigs. High doses may cause respiratory depression.	Booth[19], Mitek[56]
Tiletamine + zolazepam	Tiletamine: a dissociative and an NMDA receptor antagonist Zolazepam: benzodiazepine; modulates chloride ion transport via binding to GABA$_A$ receptors	1–2 mg/kg	IM	Considered for heavy sedation, may result in rough recovery afterward.	
Xylazine	α_2-Agonist	0.5–3.0 mg/kg	IM	Cardiovascular effects are more significant than dexmedetomidine. May cause vomiting.	Anderson & Mulon[16]
Combination of medications					
Midazolam + ketamine + dexmedetomidine	Ketamine: dissociative NMDA receptor antagonist	Midazolam: 0.2 mg/kg Ketamine: 5–20 mg/kg Dexmedetomidine: 0.01–0.02 mg/kg	IM		Mitek[56]

Agent	Mechanism of Action	Dose	Route	Comments	Reference
Dexmedetomidine + midazolam + butorphanol		Dexmedetomidine: 0.01–0.04 mg/kg; Midazolam: 0.1–0.3 mg/kg; Butorphanol: 0.2–0.4 mg/kg	IM	Can substitute xylazine (at 1 mg/kg) for dexmedetomidine.	Carpenter[18]
Azaperone + midazolam		Azaperone: 2–4 mg/kg; Midazolam: 0.5 mg/kg	IM	Sedation without analgesia.	Bollen et al[10]
Ketamine + butorphanol + midazolam		Ketamine: 5 mg/kg; Butorphanol: 0.2 mg/kg; Midazolam: 0.2 mg/kg	IM		Østevik et al[12]
Induction Combinations:					
Agent	**Mechanism of Action**	**Dose**	**Route**	**Comments**	**Reference**
Acepromazine + ketamine	As listed above	Acepromazine: 0.4 mg/kg; Ketamine: 15 mg/kg	IM	Approximate 5 min onset and 15–20 min duration.	Anderson & Mulon[16]
Alfaxalone	As listed above	0.9 mg/kg	IV	Induction was after premedication with: 4 mg/kg alfaxalone; 40 µg/kg medetomidine; and 0.4 mg/kg butorphanol IM.	Bigby et al[58]
Butorphanol	As listed above		IM	Induction for debilitated or compromised patients only.	Kerrie Lion Lewis, Personal Communication, 2021.
Ketamine		n/a	n/a	Not recommended as a sole induction agent. Recommended use involves combination therapy with other agents.	
Midazolam + ketamine	As listed above	Midazolam: 0.3–1 0 mg/kg; Ketamine: 10 mg/kg	IM	This combination can cause hypothermia.	Bollen et al[10]; Carpenter[18]; Østevik et al[12]
Diazepam + ketamine	As listed above	Diazepam: 0.2–0.5 mg/kg; Ketamine: 5–15 mg/kg	IV, titrated to effect	Anesthesia is prolonged with an additional 2–4 mg/kg of ketamine. High doses of ketamine car lead to increased risk of apnea.	Wheeler et al[29]; Carpenter[18]; Moon & Smith[32]; Østevik et al[12]

(continued on next page)

Table 1
(continued)

Induction Combinations:

Agent	Mechanism of Action	Dose	Route	Comments	Reference
Propofol	Hypnotic	0.4–5.0 mg/kg	IV, titrated to effect	Cardiorespiratory depression.	Dubois[59], Lagerkranser et al[60], Coutant et al[61], Moon & Smith[32], Østevik et al[12]

Inhalational Induction (not usually recommend as sole method for induction of anesthesia)

Isoflurane	CNS depression	3.0%–5.0%	Inhalation	Hypotension and respiratory depression are possible.	Anderson & Mulon[16], Trim & Braun[6], Needleman & Videla[62]
Sevoflurane	CNS depression	3.0%–5.0%	Inhalation	Rapid onset and recovery.	Carpenter[18]
Nitrous oxide			Inhalation	Not commonly used. Its use is described for relaxation before induction with isoflurane. Has to be administered with oxygen.	

Maintenance of Anesthesia:

Agent	Mechanism of Action	Dose	Route	Frequency	Comments	Reference
Inhalant						
Isoflurane	CNS depression	0.5%–2%	Inhalational	Entire procedure	Hypotension and respiratory depression are possible, particularly at higher doses.	Anderson & Mulon[16], Trim & Braun[6], Needleman & Videla[62]

Drug	Mechanism	Dose	Route	Frequency	Notes	Reference
Sevoflurane	CNS depression	1.0%–3.0%	Inhalational	Entire procedure	Rapid onset and recovery. Hypotension and respiratory depression are possible, particularly at higher doses.	Carpenter[18]
Halothane	CNS depression	n/a	n/a	n/a	No longer recommended because of unavailability and malignant hyperthermia concerns in commercial pigs.	
Injectable						
Fentanyl + propofol	Opioid receptor agonist and anesthetic	Fentanyl: 2.5–20 mic/kg/hr; Propofol: 11 mg/kg/h	IV (as continuous infusion)	CRI	Immediate onset.	Anderson & Mulon[16]
Propofol	Hypnotic (anesthetic)	0.4–2.5 mg/kg followed by CRI of 8–12 mg/kg/h	IV	CRI		Lagerkranser et al[60]
Xylazine, ketamine, midazolam		Xylazine: 2 mg/kg; Ketamine: up to 20 mg/kg; Midazolam: 0.25 mg/kg	IM	Once	10-min onset, approximate 60-min duration.	Anderson & Mulon[16]
Xylazine, ketamine, telazol		Xylazine: 4.4 mg/kg; Ketamine: 2.2 mg/kg; Telazol: 4.4 mg/kg	IM	Once	Short onset, approximately 60-min duration.	Anderson & Mulon[16]
Xylazine, butorphanol, ketamine		Xylazine: 2 mg/kg; Butorphanol: 0.2–0.22 mg/kg; Ketamine: 5–11 mg/kg	IM	Once	Short onset, approximately 60-min duration. For minor procedures.	Anderson & Mulon[16], Bollen et al[10], Calle & Morris[63]

Reversal Agents:

Agent	Mechanism of Action	Dose	Route	Comments	Reference
Atipamezole	α-Receptor antagonist	0.05–0.1 mg/kg; or same volume of dexmedetomidine (0.5 mg/mL)	IM	For reversal of α_2-adrenergic agonists. Typically dosed at the same volume of dexmedetomidine administered.	Mitek[56]; Carpenter[18]
Flumazenil	Benzodiazepine receptor antagonist	0.02–0.05 mg/kg	IV, IM	Useful for reversal of diazepam, midazolam.	Mitek[56]; Papich[64]
Naloxone	Opioid antagonist	0.5–2.0 mg/kg; 0.005–0.04 mg/kg	IV	Opioid reversal. May need to be administered multiple times as necessary. The authors recommend starting with a lower dosage (0.005–0.04 mg/kg) and repeating as necessary.	Mitek[56]; Swindle & Sistino[57]
Yohimbine	α-Receptor antagonist	0.1–0.5 mg/kg	IM, SC	Useful in the reversal of xylazine, dexmedetomidine. IV administration only in emergency situations or if diluted in saline solution.	Kim et al[65]

Abbreviations: CNS, central nervous system; CRI; GABA, γ-aminobutyric acid; IV, intravenously; NMDA, N-methyl-D-aspartate; SC, subcutaneously; CRI, constant rate infusion; n/a: not applicable.

MCPs.[17] An agent from the same drug class but with higher potency and duration of action is tiletamine, which is available in combination with zolazepam. Tiletamine-zolazepam is used at low doses (1–2 mg/kg) in MCPs for sedation or at higher doses and in combination with other agents (opioids, α_2-agonists) for induction of anesthesia. Both tiletamine and zolazepam are long-lasting drugs and may result in prolonged or rough recoveries.

Opioids

Opioids are used as sedatives for MCPs either as sole agents, or in combination with other agents. Butorphanol and morphine are the most common opioids used for this purpose. Butorphanol is primarily used as a sedative agent and is combined with: ketamine and xylazine, tiletamine-zolazepam, tiletamine-zolazepam and xylazine, and xylazine.[18] In contrast, morphine has an efficacious analgesic, and a sedative, effect. Nevertheless, a stimulatory effect has been described for some pigs after receiving morphine.[19] Excitatory effects of morphine are more likely if higher doses of morphine are used, particularly as a sole agent. Therefore, animals should be monitored after administration of morphine for increased activity. Opioids can typically be reversed by injections of naloxone.[20]

Alfaxalone

One of the newer agents available for MCPs is alfaxalone.[21] Alfaxalone is a neuroactive steroid that works by modulating chloride ion transport and binding to γ-aminobutyric acid receptors.[22,23] This agent is used for sedation and immobilization purposes, but unlike opioids and α_2-agonists, it is not thought to provide analgesia. Because of the risk of apnea, particularly after intravenous (IV) administration of alfaxalone or when used at higher doses, endotracheal intubation, oxygen support, and ventilation support may be necessary. Recent research has demonstrated sedative effects of alfaxalone after intranasal administration (1–2 mg/kg) in the miniature breed of Yucatan swine; however, considering the low concentration of alfaxalone, the use of this route is limited by the volume that is needed to achieve the sedative effects.[22] The authors recommend a combination of alfaxalone with a benzodiazepine administered IM to achieve preanesthetic sedation.

Azaperone

Azaperone is a neuroleptic agent with the ability to tranquilize or immobilize pigs in a dose-dependent manner.[16] Salivation, hypothermia, sensitivity to noise, and hypotension have been reported in pigs administered azaperone.[16] Priapism is another adverse effect of azaperone when administered in high doses to intact boars.[16] Azaperone has no intrinsic analgesic properties, and if analgesia is desired, it should be combined with analgesic agents.

PREMEDICATION

Most premedication protocols for MCPs are similar to the previously described agents used for sedation. These protocols usually include multiple agents to achieve the maximum effect with minimum adverse effects. In some references, addition of an anticholinergic, such as atropine, has been recommended to reduce salivation and bronchial secretions before surgery. However, anticholinergics should not be administered simultaneously with α_2-agonists, because the initial bradycardia induced by α_2-agonists is a physiologic reflex in response to increased peripheral blood pressure. Some example premedication protocols include: butorphanol, midazolam, and xylazine; butorphanol, midazolam, and medetomidine; or butorphanol, midazolam, and tiletamine-zolazepam.[6] An in-depth list of premedication protocols is provided in **Table 1**.

EPIDURAL ANESTHESIA

In MCPs, epidural anesthesia should be considered as an adjunct for procedures caudal to the thorax[20] involving the pelvic limbs and abdomen. In overconditioned animals, identifying the epidural space is challenging. Epidural anesthesia has improved the anesthetic plane in commercial pigs undergoing herniorrhaphy with injectable agents.[24] Lidocaine (2 mg/kg), bupivacaine (1 mg/kg), morphine (0.1–0.15 mg/kg), and xylazine (0.2 mg/kg) have been used for epidural anesthesia in pigs.[25–27] When considering formulations of morphine (or other medications) for epidural use, it is important to select a preservative-free formulation, because many preservatives have been associated with inflammation in other mammalian species when administered epidurally.[28]

INDUCTION

Although injectable agents are used for induction of anesthesia in MCPs, inhalational agents can also be used in premedicated animals to induce anesthesia. Induction of anesthesia in unsedated animals is not recommended because it may result in excitatory effects and cardiorespiratory compromise. Induction is achieved with a facemask and an oxygen flow rate of 3 to 4 L/min and 3% to 4% isoflurane. Standard veterinary anesthesia masks are used for MCPs, and for larger pigs, masks for induction are fashioned from gallon-sized jugs by cutting off the bottom and fixing the gas connection hose to the original opening. Drug dosages for induction and maintenance are located in **Table 1**.

ENDOTRACHEAL INTUBATION

Following induction, endotracheal intubation provides an efficient method of ventilatory support during anesthesia. A secured and sealed ETT also prevents the risk of aspiration pneumonia in the case of regurgitation. However, the anatomy of the pig can lead to some major challenges in intubation. Mainly, the jaws do not open widely, the soft palate is long, and the epiglottis frequently is trapped on top of the soft palate and needs to be repositioned. In addition, the trachea of the pig is narrow in diameter relative to body size. Pigs have a large ventral diverticulum located caudal to the glottis that can catch the ETT. Lateral laryngeal ventricles can also cause challenges for a successful intubation. A long-bladed laryngoscope is often necessary for intubation of pigs. Care should be taken to select an appropriately sized ETT, because too large of a tube can lead to trauma. ETT diameters of 6.5 to 14 mm have been recommended for MCPs.[6] **Table 2** shows a range of ETT sizes relative to body weight.

For intubation, with the pig in sternal recumbency, and after the administration of induction agents when the jaws are relaxed, the epiglottis should be released from the soft palate to visualize the glottis. The glottis should be sprayed with 0.5 to 1 mL of 2% lidocaine. An introducer or stylet is passed through the glottis and intubation attempted over the stylet. It is not uncommon for the ETT to enter the larynx and become trapped (usually at the laryngeal diverticulum). If this occurs, the tube should be rotated 90° and gently advanced again, with care to not force the tube to avoid trauma. With curved polyvinyl chloride ETT, intubation is facilitated by passing the tube down the glottis while the outward curvature of the tube is at either the 3- or

Table 2
Endotracheal tube sizes with associated weight ranges for miniature companion pigs presented to the Farm Animal Hospital at the University of Tennessee (2010–2021)

Endotracheal Tube Size (ID-mm)	4.5	5	5.5	6	6.5	7	7.5	8	8.5	9	9.5	10
Patient Weight (kg)	3.0–6.8	6.4–9.6	5.0–10.0	17.3–21.4	11.4–36.5	35–78	52.0–113	46.0–122.0	35.0–69.0	60.0–160.0	86.4–164.0	108.2–117.0

9-o'clock position to avoid entrapment of the tip of the tube in the laryngeal diverticulum. Laryngeal edema from trauma, regurgitation, aspiration, or perforation of the larynx are common complications during and after intubation.[29–32] Clinicians should be aware of these complications and favor restarting the intubation process rather than applying more pressure for challenging intubations. **Figs. 6** and **7** demonstrate intubation.

MAINTENANCE

The method used for maintenance of anesthesia for MCPs is determined by factors including the availability of the equipment and drugs, duration of the proposed procedure, and underlying condition of the animal. Generally, maintenance of anesthesia is achieved by inhalational anesthesia, total IV anesthesia (TIVA), or a combination of inhalational and injectable anesthetics in partial IV anesthesia (PIVA). The most commonly used method for maintenance of anesthesia is with inhalation agents, and this is used when a moderate to long duration of anesthesia is intended. Inhalation anesthetics are beneficial because they provide a more controlled plane of anesthesia[16]; however, almost all of the inhalational anesthetics cause a dose-dependent cardiorespiratory depression and lack analgesic effects. For swine patients of up to 140 kg, a small animal anesthetic machine system is adequate.[33] Isoflurane (1%–3%) and sevoflurane (2%–4%) are commonly used inhalant anesthetics in pet pigs.[18,34] Nitrous oxide administered by a mask has been described for calming an MCP before mask induction with isoflurane.[18]

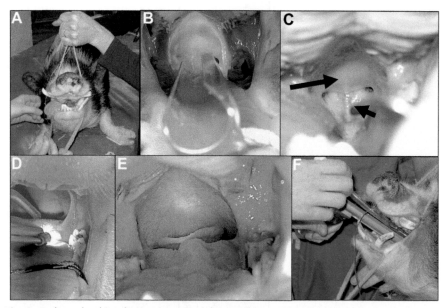

Fig. 6. Endotracheal intubation in a pig. (*A*) Animal is positioned in sternal recumbency and the jaws are gently pulled open using two appropriately sized fine ropes. (*B*) Initial placement of the laryngoscope. (*C*) Intraoral view of the epiglottis (*short arrow*) and the soft palate (*long arrow*). The tip of the epiglottis is commonly displaced dorsal to the soft palate. (*D*) Releasing the displaced epiglottis with a blunt stylet. (*E*) The tip of the epiglottis is visible after it is released using a blunt stylet. (*F*) After visualization of the glottis assisted by a laryngoscope, endotracheal tube is inserted.

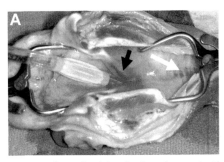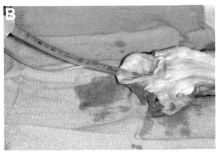

Fig. 7. Endotracheal intubation demonstration in a porcine cadaveric specimen. (*A*) If the endotracheal tube is inserted with the tip directed downward, it will most likely face the laryngeal diverticulum (*black arrow*) and will not enter the trachea (*white arrow*) as desired. (*B*) Inserting the endotracheal tube into the larynx while the tube curvature faces downward and the tip of the tube faces upward results in a successful endotracheal intubation.

Halothane is not commonly used, primarily because of the association with its use and development of malignant hypothermia in production pigs, although other inhalational anesthetics also have the potential for triggering malignant hyperthermia (MH) if the animal has the genetic predisposition.

Injectable protocols for TIVA are reported for MCPs, but these are typically recommended for minor procedures up to 20 minutes in length. Routine procedures in MCPs, such as castration, can take longer compared with other veterinary species (44 minutes in one study).[35] When planning anesthetic protocols in MCPs, one should weigh the benefits of intubation with the relative ease of an injectable protocol, because the use of injectable protocols without airway support and monitoring of the patient could be problematic for longer procedures or in compromised patients. The authors occasionally use TIVA protocols in intubated animals that may not tolerate the adverse effects of inhalational anesthetics, even at low doses (eg, animals with sepsis). With an appropriate combination of drugs, endotracheal intubation, and proper anesthetic monitoring, TIVA protocols are also used for longer procedures (60–90 minutes). PIVA protocols usually provide better homeostatic stability without significant delay in anesthetic recovery and are applied to most MCPs undergoing general anesthesia.

PERIANESTHETIC MONITORING

Anesthetic monitoring for MCPs should include electrocardiogram, pulse oximetry, temperature, capnography, and blood pressure where possible. Hypoventilation has been reported in MCPs undergoing anesthesia.[6] Using mechanical or intermittent manual ventilation resolves hypoventilation and hypoxemia (oxygen saturation by pulse oximetry of <95%). Hypotension with mean arterial pressures of less than 65 mm Hg or systolic arterial pressures of less than or equal to 85 mm Hg can also occur frequently in MCPs and may require intervention with dopamine or dobutamine (1–10 μg/kg/min continuous rate IV infusion for either), colloids, or fluid support.[6,36,37] In addition, the authors frequently use ephedrine (0.05–0.1 mg/kg, preferably IV) to improve blood pressure. Ephedrine's blood pressure boosting effect usually lasts for 10 to 20 minutes. Monitoring of circulatory function is critical for cases undergoing anesthesia for different underlying conditions, such as gastrointestinal disturbances, because the stoic nature of MCPs frequently leads to clients presenting their animals to veterinary hospitals after some degree of circulatory compromise has occurred.[38] Hypothermia is a frequent complication from anesthesia in MCPs.[6] Normal rectal temperatures of some MCP breeds, such as Vietnamese pot-bellied pigs (37.6 ± 0.8°C, 99.7 ± 1.5°F), may be lower than those reported for other pigs, and the temperature could be different based on diurnal variations.[39] Heat support can usually be performed using different methods, such as electrical heating mats (HotDog, Augustine Surgical Inc, Eden Prairie, MN), forced warm air heating devices (Bair Hugger, 3M, Maplewood, MN), or recirculating warm water blankets.[25,36]

OTHER PERIANESTHETIC COMPLICATIONS
Malignant Hyperthermia

In addition to the previously mentioned common adverse effects of general anesthesia (hypothermia, hypotension, and hypoventilation), MH is a genetic condition caused by an altered ryanodine receptor gene and may be seen in pigs undergoing general anesthesia. Predominant clinical signs of MH include a significant and rapid rise in the body temperature and hypercapnia because of a surge in muscle activity. This condition is predominantly described in domestic pig breeds, such as the Landrace, Piétrain, and Yorkshire.[40] MH is not thought to occur commonly in MCPs, although a suspected case has been reported.[41] This case involved a 7-week-old pig anesthetized with isoflurane that was successfully treated with whole-body cooling and administration of dantrolene sodium.[41] This pig was never tested for the presence of the MH gene, so it is not confirmed if this was truly MH. One should recognize the importance of temperature monitoring while under inhalational anesthesia in these cases, because MH may occur.

Pneumothorax

Pneumothorax has been reported in a pair of Vietnamese pot-bellied pigs as a result of high airway pressures during mechanical ventilation.[42] The rupture of pulmonary bullae has also been associated with pneumothorax in MCPs.[43] Pneumothorax is managed by the application of indwelling chest tubes and suction.[43]

Concerns with Fentanyl Transdermal Patches

Fentanyl transdermal patches are used as a sustained-release analgesic formulation for pigs, potentially maintaining concentrations for as long as 72 hours after application. However, clinicians should be aware that patches can become dislodged in pigs and can present a risk to the patient if swallowed.[25,44] The authors have found that covering the patch with dynamic pressure tape, such as Elastikon, and stapling the tape to the skin can be necessary to prevent dislodgement. Even with these additional security measures, pigs have been able to remove fentanyl patches.[25,44] In one case report, a fentanyl patch was ingested by a production pig and presented with dysphoria, panting, and vocalization. This progressed to depression and recumbency.[44] In that case, the pig was successfully treated with an injection of naloxone (0.012 mg/kg).[44] Clinicians should also keep in mind that the potential for release from a fentanyl transdermal patch may be longer than the short half-life of naloxone, so multiple injections could be necessary if fentanyl absorption is ongoing from the patch. Another consideration is that if a fentanyl patch is to be used in conjunction with the procedure, vigilance is warranted to ensure that the patch is not in direct contact with a heating device because this increases the release of the drug, which may result in an overdose.

Other Considerations

Obesity is common in MCPs and can complicate anesthetic events. Drugs may be administered in adipose tissue instead of IM and may take longer to reach full effect or may last longer than desired. One should consider this when deciding whether to administer additional doses of injectable sedative or anesthetic drugs, because it may result in an overdose. These pigs can also have difficulty thermoregulating during recovery from anesthesia, and lipid embolism has been identified as a cause of peri-surgical mortality in obese pet pigs.[45] Obese pigs have also been reported to have increased resistance to airflow, and inspiratory flow limitation,[46] so respiratory monitoring is crucial in these cases. Use of the American Society for Anesthesia scoring system should be considered for planning procedures for MCPs, but in a recent study, American Society for Anesthesia scores were not correlated with the likelihood of complications during MCP anesthesia.[37] This may have been caused by a small number of pigs used in that review.

Additional considerations for pet pigs undergoing general anesthesia include complications associated with surgery. Excessive hemorrhage has been reported in uterine and ovarian surgeries,[47] and identifying and collecting donor blood from pigs is challenging.

RECOVERY

During recovery, MCPs should be placed in sternal recumbency to allow for appropriate oxygenation. Oxygen supplementation during recovery via a face mask may be necessary if there is any risk for hypoxemia. Temperature should be monitored frequently, and external heat sources are frequently needed. Cold animals tend to shiver, which in turn increases their oxygen demand significantly. Because of the variability in drug absorption, delayed or prolonged absorption and action of injectable agents can occur. Pigs are obligate nasal breathers and should be monitored postextubation for any signs of upper airway obstruction. MCPs should be recovered in padded, temperature-controlled areas for comfort and to assist with any potential lingering hypothermia from anesthesia. Caution should be used when recovering pigs on straw, shavings, or blankets because of the risk of swallowing the material. Ingested blankets have been reported as gastrointestinal foreign objects that resulted in obstruction in MCPs.[36,48]

AUTHORS' RECOMMENDATIONS

In the authors' practice, the most common combination of sedative/anesthetic drugs used for MCPs include IM administration of ketamine (5–10 mg/kg), xylazine (0.5–1 mg/kg), and midazolam (0.1–0.2 mg/kg). The lower doses are usually used for sedation purposes and the higher are intended for anesthetic premedication/induction. In the latter scenarios, usually within 10 minutes after IM administration of the combination into the cervical muscles (caudoventral area to the auricle), animals demonstrate profound sedation and endotracheal intubation is possible. Alternative combinations may include a mixture of alfaxalone (1–2 mg/kg) with xylazine (same doses as previously mentioned) or dexmedetomidine (5–10 μg/kg), and midazolam (at same doses as previously mentioned). After heavy sedation is achieved with either combination, an attempt at intubation is performed. However, if the jaws are not fully relaxed or if swallowing is observed, inhalational anesthetics (isoflurane or sevoflurane) at low doses (2%–3% and 3%–4%, respectively) are administered via a tight-fitting face-mask for about 5 minutes before intubation is attempted again.

For maintenance of anesthesia, the authors' preferred method is using PIVA with low concentrations of isoflurane or sevoflurane (1%–1.5% or 1.5%–2%, respectively) in combination with IV infusion of injectable anesthetics or analgesics. Examples of the latter group include ketamine (1–3 mg/kg/h) and lidocaine (3–6 mg/kg/h). PIVA techniques usually provide better cardiovascular stability compared with the use of inhalational anesthetics alone, particularly in animals with systemic comorbidities.

Drug Regulatory Considerations

When administering drugs to MCPs, it is important to keep in mind that even though they are pets, from a regulatory perspective, there is no difference between them and a commercial pig intended for food production, because this designation is based on species. Although not common, there are documented instances of MCPs entering the food chain in the United States.[49] Because of this, clinicians should provide language advising for drug withdrawal periods. Regulatory agencies, such as the Food Animal Residue Avoidance Databank (United States: www.farad.org; Canada: www.cgfarad.usask.ca), are consulted in such cases. With the role of the MCPs as pets, the authors have found that the following statement can be used to convey this message to the client, without concerns of implying their pet will be used for food production.[25,36]

> While we understand that your MCP is a pet, we are legally obligated to inform you that there is a withdrawal period for the medications administered. Please contact us if you need this information.

FUTURE DIRECTIONS FOR SEDATION AND ANESTHESIA

There are several considerations for sedation and anesthesia of MCPs that could be focused on given the increasing popularity of these animals as companions. For instance, trazodone is a serotonin antagonist and reuptake inhibitor that is used for anxiety and sedation in multiple species.[50] Trazadone anecdotally has been used for sedation in MCPs,[51] but investigation of clinically efficacious dosages and safety is lacking. If safe for MCPs, trazodone could be used as a sedative agent, but more investigation is necessary, because the drug is hepatotoxic in dogs and cardiotoxic in other species.[52–54] Similarly, gabapentin is anecdotally mentioned as a sedative in MCPs, but currently there are no studies evaluating its efficacy.

SUMMARY

Because of the increasing popularity of MCPs in North America, there will continue to be a demand for veterinary services to support their medical needs. Therefore, a thorough understanding of sedation and anesthesia of these patients is critical to respond to the increasing demand for these animals' veterinary care and health. Practitioners should be familiar with the agents used for sedation and anesthesia and the importance of anesthetic monitoring and recovery in MCPs.

REFERENCES

1. Braun WF Jr, Casteel SW. Potbellied pigs. Miniature porcine pets. Vet Clin North Am Small Anim Pract 1993;23:1149–77.

2. Tynes VV. Miniature pet pig behavioral medicine. Vet Clin North Am Exot Anim Pract 2021;24:63–86.

3. Meier JE. Exotic companion mammal ambulatory practice, including potbellied pigs and llamas. Vet Clin North Am Exot Anim Pract 2018;21:651–67.
4. Boldrick L. Veterinary care of pot-bellied pet pigs. Orange, CA: All Pub. Co.; 1993.
5. Johnson L. Physical and chemical restraint of miniature pet pigs. Care and management of miniature pet pigs. Santa Barbara (CA): Veterinary Practice Publishing Company; 1993. p. 59–66.
6. Trim CM, Braun C. Anesthetic agents and complications in Vietnamese potbellied pigs: 27 cases (1999-2006). J Am Vet Med Assoc 2011;239(1):114–21.
7. Snook CS. Use of the subcutaneous abdominal vein for blood sampling and intravenous catheterization in potbellied pigs. J Am Vet Med Assoc 2001;219: 809–10, 764.
8. Boorman S, Douglas H, Driessen B, et al. Fatal ovarian hemorrhage associated with anticoagulation therapy in a Yucatan mini-pig following venous stent implantation. Front Vet Sci 2020;7:18.
9. Van Metre DC, Angelos SM. Miniature pigs. Vet Clin North Am Exot Anim Pract 1999;2:519–37.
10. Bollen PJ, Hansen AK, Alstrup AKO. The laboratory swine. New York, NY: CRC Press; 2010.
11. Tonge M, Robson K. Hypoxaemia following suspected intubation of the tracheal bronchus of a pig. Veterinary Record Case Reports;n/a:e19.
12. Østevik L, Elmas C, Rubio-Martinez LM. Castration of the Vietnamese pot-bellied boar: 8 cases. Can Vet J 2012;53(9):943 8.
13. Rubio-Martinez LM, Rioja E, Shakespeare AS. Surgical stabilization of shoulder luxation in a pot-bellied pig. J Am Vet Med Assoc 2013;242:807–11.
14. Rosanova N, Singh A, Cribb N. Laparoscopic-assisted cryptorchidectomy in 2 Vietnamese pot-bellied pigs (Sus scrofa). Can Vet J 2015;56:153–6.
15. Io T, Saunders R, Pesic M, et al. A miniature pig model of pharmacological tolerance to long-term sedation with the intravenous benzodiazepines; midazolam and remimazolam. Eur J Pharmacol 2021;896:173886.
16. Anderson DE, Mulon PY. Anesthesia and surgical procedures in swine. Dis Swine 2019;171–96.
17. Wallace CK, Bell SE, LaTourette PC 2nd, et al. Suspected anaphylactic reaction to ketamine in 3 Yucatan swine (Sus scrofa). Comp Med 2019;69:419–24.
18. Carpenter JW. Exotic animal formulary. 5th edition. St. Louis (MO): Elsevier Health Sciences; 2018.
19. Booth N. Drugs acting on the central nervous system. Veterinary Pharmacology and Therapeutics; 1988. p. 5.
20. Swindle MM, Smith AC. Best practices for performing experimental surgery in swine. J Invest Surg 2013;26:63–71.
21. Mitek A. Pot-bellied pig sedation. Fast facts and drug protocols 2017 2020. Available at: https://vetmed.illinois.edu/pot-bellied-pig-sedation-fast-facts-drug-protocols/. Accessed December 22, 2020.
22. Hampton CE, Takawira C, Ross JM, et al. Sedation characteristics of intranasal alfaxalone in adult Yucatan swine. J Am Assoc Lab Anim Sci 2021;60(2):184–7.
23. Poirier NC, Smith JS, Breuer RM, et al. Management of hematometra in a Boer doe. Clin Theriogenology 2020;12:39–45.
24. Ekstrand C, Sterning M, Bohman L, et al. Lumbo-sacral epidural anaesthesia as a complement to dissociative anaesthesia during scrotal herniorrhaphy of livestock pigs in the field. Acta Vet Scand 2015;57:33.

25. Høy-Petersen J, Smith JS, Merkatoris PT, et al. Case report: trochlear wedge sulcoplasty, tibial tuberosity transposition, and lateral imbrication for correction of a traumatic patellar luxation in a miniature companion pig: a case report and visual description. Front Vet Sci 2021;7:567886.

26. Smith JS, Chigerwe M, Kanipe C, et al. Femoral head ostectomy for the treatment of acetabular fracture and coxofemoral joint luxation in a potbelly pig. Vet Surg 2017;46:316–21.

27. Tendillo FJ, Pera AM, Mascias A, et al. Cardiopulmonary and analgesic effects of epidural lidocaine, alfentanil, and xylazine in pigs anesthetized with isoflurane. Vet Surg 1995;24:73–7.

28. Smith JS, Schleining J, Plummer P. Pain management in small ruminants and camelids: applications and strategies. Vet Clin North Am Food Anim Pract 2021;37:17–31.

29. Wheeler EP, Abelson AL, Wetmore LA, et al. Anesthesia case of the month. J Am Vet Med Assoc 2020;257:809–12.

30. Chum H, Pacharinsak C. Endotracheal intubation in swine. Lab Anim (Ny) 2012; 41:309–11.

31. Malavasi LM. Swine. Veterinary Anesthesia and Analgesia; Hoboken, NJ, 2015. p. 928–940.

32. Moon PF, Smith LJ. General anesthetic techniques in swine. Vet Clin North Am Food Anim Pract 1996;12:663–91.

33. Tranquilli WJ. Techniques of inhalation anesthesia in ruminants and swine. Vet Clin North Am Food Anim Pract 1986;2:593–619.

34. Murison PJ. Delayed dyspnoea in pigs possibly associated with endotracheal intubation. Vet Anaesth Analg 2001;28:226.

35. Salcedo-Jiménez R, Brounts SH, Mulon PY, et al. Multicenter retrospective study of complications and risk factors associated with castration in 106 pet pigs. Can Vet J 2020;61:173–7.

36. Cain A, Kirkpatrick J, Breuer R. A case of a linear foreign body removal in a miniature companion pig. J Dairy Vet Anim Res 2020;9:6–9.

37. Portier K, Ida KK. The ASA Physical Status Classification: what is the evidence for recommending its use in veterinary anesthesia?—A systematic review. Front Vet Sci 2018;5:204.

38. Sipos W, Schmoll F, Stumpf I. Minipigs and potbellied pigs as pets in the veterinary practice: a retrospective study. J Vet Med A, Physiol Pathol Clin Med 2007; 54:504–11.

39. Lord LK, Wittum TE, Anderson DE, et al. Resting rectal temperature of Vietnamese potbellied pigs. J Am Vet Med Assoc 1999;215:342–4.

40. Swindel MM. Swine in the laboratory: surgery, anesthesia, imaging, and experimental techniques. 2nd edition. Boca Raton (FL): CRC Press; 2007.

41. Claxton-Gill MS, Cornick-Seahorn JL, Gamboa JC, et al. Suspected malignant hyperthermia syndrome in a miniature pot-bellied pig anesthetized with isoflurane. J Am Vet Med Assoc 1993;203:1434–6.

42. Lukasik VM, Moon PF. Two cases of pneumothorax during mechanical ventilation in Vietnamese potbellied pigs. Vet Surg 1996;25:356–60.

43. Smith J, Cuneo M, Walton R, et al. Spontaneous pneumothorax in a companion Kunekune pig due to pulmonary bullae rupture. J Exot Pet Med 2020;34:6–9.

44. Jerneja Sredenšek MB, Urša Lampreht T, Kosjek T, et al. Case report: intoxication in a pig (Sus scrofa domesticus) after transdermal fentanyl patch ingestion. Front Vet Sci 2020;7:611097.

45. Newkirk KM, Fineschi V, Kiefer VR, et al. Lipid emboli in a Vietnamese potbellied pig (Sus scrofa). J Vet Diagn Invest 2012;24:625–9.
46. Tuck SA, Dort JC, Olson ME, et al. Monitoring respiratory function and sleep in the obese Vietnamese pot-bellied pig. J Appl Physiol (1985) 1999;87:444–51.
47. Cypher E, Videla R, Pierce R, et al. Clinical prevalence and associated intraoperative surgical complications of reproductive tract lesions in pot-bellied pigs undergoing ovariohysterectomy: 298 cases (2006-2016). Vet Rec 2017;181:685.
48. Ludwig EK, Byron CR. Evaluation of the reasons for and outcomes of gastrointestinal tract surgery in pet pigs: 11 cases (2004-2015). J Am Vet Med Assoc 2017; 251:714–21.
49. Lord LK, Wittum TE. Survey of humane organizations and slaughter plants regarding experiences with Vietnamese potbellied pigs. J Am Vet Med Assoc 1997;211:562–5.
50. Gruen ME, Sherman BL. Use of trazodone as an adjunctive agent in the treatment of canine anxiety disorders: 56 cases (1995-2007). J Am Vet Med Assoc 2008; 233:1902–7.
51. Mozzachio K. Routine veterinary care of the miniature pig. Mammal Medicine 2019. 2021. Available at: https://lafeber.com/vet/routine-care-mini-pig/. Accessed February 25, 2021.
52. Arnold A, Davis A, Wismer T, et al. Suspected hepatotoxicity secondary to trazodone therapy in a dog. J Vet Emerg Crit Care (San Antonio) 2021;31:112–6.
53. Soe KK, Lee MY. Arrhythmias in severe trazodone overdose. Am J Case Rep 2019;20;1949–55.
54. Atli O, Kilic V, Baysal M, et al. Assessment of trazodone-induced cardiotoxicity after repeated doses in rats. Hum Exp Toxicol 2019;38:45–55.
55. Amstel SV. Medical, surgical, and lameness conditions of pet pigs. Orlando: North American Veterinary Conference; 2011.
56. Mitek A. Pot-bellied pig sedation. Urbana, IL: University of Illinois; 2017. Available at: https://vetmed.illinois.edu/pot-bellied-pig-sedation-fast-facts-drug-protocols/.
57. Swindle M, Sistino J. Anesthesia, analgesia, and perioperative care. Swine Lab 2007;3:39–88.
58. Bigby SE, Carter JE, Bauquier S, et al. The use of alfaxalone for premedication, induction and maintenance of anaesthesia in pigs: a pilot study. Vet Anaesth Analg 2017;44(4):905–9.
59. Dubois M-S. Surgical arthrodesis for treatment of chronic shoulder joint luxation in a Vietnamese potbellied pig. J Am Vet Med Assoc 2020;257(7):750–4.
60. Lagerkranser M, Stånge K, Sollevi A. Effects of propofol on cerebral blood flow, metabolism, and cerebral autoregulation in the anesthetized pig. J Neurosurg Anesthesiol 1997;9(2):188–93.
61. Coutant T, Dunn M, Montasell X, et al. Use of percutaneous cystolithotomy for removal of urethral uroliths in a pot-bellied pig. Can Vet J 2018;59(2):159–64.
62. Needleman A, Videla R. Urolithiasis in a female miniature potbellied pig. Vet Rec Case Rep 2019;7(3):e000809.
63. Calle P, Morris P. Anesthesia for nondomestic suids. Zoo Wild Anim Med Curr Ther 1999;4:639–46.
64. Papich MG. Saunders handbook of veterinary drugs-e-book: small and large animal. Raleigh, NC: Elsevier Health Sciences; 2015.
65. Kim M-J, Park C-S, Jun M-H, et al. Antagonistic effects of yohimbine in pigs anaesthetised with tiletamine/zolazepam and xylazine. Vet Rec 2007;161(18): 620–4.

Local and Regional Anesthesia in Zoological Companion Animal Practice

Peter M. DiGeronimo, VMD, MSc, DACZM[a,b,]*,
Anderson F. da Cunha, DVM, MS, DACVAA[c]

KEYWORDS

- Benzocaine • Bupivacaine • Epidural • Lidocaine • Nerve block • Analgesia • Pain

KEY POINTS

- Diluting lidocaine or bupivacaine with sodium bicarbonate solution may potentiate their effects, but there is no clinical advantage of mixing lidocaine and bupivacaine together before administration.
- Administered as a bath, lidocaine at low concentrations may provide systemic analgesia to teleost fishes.
- In amphibians, rapid systemic absorption may limit the clinical efficacy of lidocaine and bupivacaine for local or regional anesthesia.
- Regional anesthesia of the tail, pelvic limbs, and cloaca of chelonians and some lizards may be achieved by spinal (intrathecal) administration of preservative-free lidocaine or bupivacaine.
- Ultrasound guidance may facilitate the safe administration of local anesthetics in species for which the anatomy is not well described.

INTRODUCTION

Local anesthesia is indicated as part of a multimodal approach to anesthesia by treating and preventing acute and chronic pain caused by surgery and disease, and also by helping to prevent central pain sensitization. The most commonly used local anesthetics, including lidocaine, ropivacaine, and bupivacaine, are amides that stop the conduction of action potentials that mediate nociception by blocking voltage-dependent sodium channels. The various commercially available local anesthetics differ in their duration of action and potential toxicity, with those agents having a longer duration of effect also being more toxic because of greater lipophilicity and protein-binding

[a] Adventure Aquarium, 1 Riverside Drive, Camden, NJ 08103, USA; [b] Animal & Bird Health Care Center, 1785 Springdale Road, Cherry Hill, NJ 08003, USA; [c] College of Veterinary Medicine, Midwestern University, 5715 W Utopia Road, Glendale, AZ 85308, USA
* Corresponding author. Adventure Aquarium, 1 Riverside Drive, Camden, NJ 08103, USA.
E-mail address: pmdigeronimo@gmail.com

Vet Clin Exot Anim 25 (2022) 321–336
https://doi.org/10.1016/j.cvex.2021.08.015
1094-9194/22/© 2021 Elsevier Inc. All rights reserved.

capacity.[1,2] Note that when dose recommendations of lidocaine and bupivacaine are the same for a given species, the clinician should suspect that there is a lack of research in this area. This is because for species in which these drugs have been well-studied, the dose of lidocaine is usually 4 to 5 times higher than that of bupivacaine.

The major adverse effect of systemic absorption of amide anesthetics is cardiotoxicity characterized by depression of cardiac conductivity and contractility, increased heart rate and arterial pressure, and cardiac arrest[3,4]; although in humans, hypotension and bradycardia are more commonly reported.[5] Other adverse effects include injection site reaction, seizures, needle-induced nerve injury, systemic allergic reactions, and methemoglobinemia. Ropivacaine is associated with less cardiotoxicity in comparison with bupivacaine[6,7] and may be useful to provide surgical local analgesia without cardiovascular toxicity. Species-specific adverse effects to various local anesthetics have been reported and clinicians should be aware of this possibility. Benzocaine, an ester-type local anesthetic, can cause methemoglobinemia in domestic cats. In the case reported, the cat went into acute respiratory distress after vomiting and collapsing about 15 to 20 minutes after topical application of the benzocaine.[8] In nondomestic mammals, methemoglobinemia following topical benzocaine application to the glottis was reported in a meerkat (Suricata suricatta) under human care.[9] The animal was treated successfully with intravenous methylene blue. It is questionable if benzocaine can cause the same effect in other species of felids and herpestids or in other feloid carnivores. Exposure to benzocaine by immersion has been shown to cause methemoglobinemia in some freshwater salmonids, the severity of which was found to be species-specific.[10] To be safe, this drug should be avoided in any feline species and used with caution in other taxa.

In veterinary medicine, local anesthetics may be included in multimodal analgesia and anesthetic protocols. Clinical applications include topical, subcutaneous, and intramuscular infiltration for local blocks, perineural or spinal administration for regional blocks, and systemic administration for analgesia and anesthesia. Although intra-articular administration of bupivacaine has been described for clinical use, this practice should be avoided because chondrotoxicity has been observed in vitro using canine chondrocytes,[11] in horses[12] and humans. An analysis of 43 published articles in this area provides enough evidence for the authors to conclude that intra-articular administration of large doses of anesthetics should be avoided in clinical practice, and that further studies are required to assess the possible chondrolysis associated with single-dose intra-articular injections of local anesthetics.[13] The current literature reviews do not provide information regarding the intra-articular use of local anesthetics in zoologic species and zoologic companion animals. It is possible that bupivacaine is chondrotoxic for all species; however, further research in this area is warranted.

Commercial formulations of lidocaine and bupivacaine often include preservatives or epinephrine. Preservatives extend the shelf-life of the product and are included in vials intended for multiple uses. These products should not be used for intrathecal or epidural spinal anesthesia, as preservative-free products should be used when performing these procedures. The addition of epinephrine achieves local vasoconstriction to limit rapid systemic uptake of the local anesthetic and thereby prolongs its action at the site where it is administered. Lidocaine and bupivacaine are acidic, and therefore are often buffered with sodium bicarbonate to achieve a neutral pH to reduce pain during initial injection. Conflicting reports exist, but buffering local anesthetics with sodium bicarbonate to achieve a neutral pH may decrease time to onset of action, prolong duration of effect, and increase analgesic quality.[14] It has been proposed that buffering/alkalinization is of benefit only when using formulations that include epinephrine, as the vasoconstricting activity of epinephrine is inactivated at a low pH.[14]

Although touted anecdotally, administration of mixtures of lidocaine and bupivacaine do not offer a clinical advantage over administration of either agent alone. The intention of mixing the 2 drugs is to achieve the short onset of action of lidocaine and the long duration of effect of bupivacaine. However, mixing lidocaine and bupivacaine does not produce analgesia any quicker than using either agent[15,16] and there is no difference in discomfort when injected.[15] The duration of action of bupivacaine administered as a sole local anesthetic is longer than that of lidocaine alone.[16] In humans, lidocaine and bupivacaine administered as a 1:1 mixture had no difference in onset of action than either agent alone, and no difference in duration of effect than lidocaine alone.[16]

FISH

In teleost fishes, lidocaine has been investigated for both local and systemic clinical applications. Tricaine methanesulfonate (MS-222) is a benzocaine derivative that is administered by immersion to achieve general anesthesia in fish. It has similar modes of action as local anesthetics on the conduction of action potentials along neurons and therefore it is questionable whether local anesthetics can have any therapeutic effect while a fish is under general anesthesia with MS-222. Local anesthetics may provide analgesia for some period after the patient recovers from anesthesia, and therefore their use may be clinically beneficial.

In an experimental study, lidocaine injected at the same time as the initiation of a noxious stimulus (acetic acid injection) reduced signs of pain in rainbow trout (*Oncorhynchus mykiss*) for up to 3 hours compared to controls with no adverse effects observed.[17] A subsequent review of fish analgesia calculated the dose administered to be 4.5 to 18 mg/kg lidocaine.[18] In a separate study, 20 mg/kg lidocaine injected on either side of the dorsal fin of rainbow trout anesthetized with MS-222 did not affect their recovery time from general anesthesia.[19] Trout that received lidocaine had lower opercular rates than untreated controls, but this finding was not considered clinically significant.[19] No adverse effects on food consumption, movement, or behavior were observed even though the dose administered was much higher than recommended for terrestrial vertebrates.[19] Lidocaine (2 mg/kg) diluted 1:1 with sterile saline was injected locally as part of the anesthetic protocol for a koi (*Cyprinus carpio koi*) undergoing surgical excision of a leiomyoma under general anesthesia with MS-222 with no clinically apparent adverse effects reported.[20]

Administered by immersion, lidocaine has systemic effects and may be used for analgesia, anesthesia, or euthanasia, in a dose-dependent manner. Lidocaine administered by immersion at a concentration of 1 to 5 mg/L has been reported to provide systemic analgesia to zebrafish (*Danio rerio*).[18,21] Clinical efficacy of lidocaine immersion may vary according to species and water parameters (temperature, pH, and salinity), and caution should be exercised when trying to extrapolate therapeutic concentrations across taxa. Higher lidocaine concentrations (300–800 mg/L) have been reported to anesthetize marine medaka (*Oryzias dancena*), with shorter induction times at higher concentrations and water temperatures.[22] However, similar concentrations euthanized zebrafish.[23] A surgical plane of anesthesia can be induced by 325 mg/L lidocaine, but at 350 mg/L, lidocaine immersion was associated with ~30% mortality rate.[24] Adult zebrafish were successfully euthanized with 400 to 1000 mg/L lidocaine.[23] After cessation of opercular breathing rate and heartbeat, these fish did not recover when immersed in anesthetic-free water.[23] No signs of toxicity were observed on postmortem examination and the fish exhibited less of an excitement phase than those exposed to MS-222, suggesting high-dose lidocaine baths may be used for humane euthanasia of teleost fishes.[23] Lower concentrations of lidocaine (50–150 mg/L) successfully induced anesthesia in zebrafish when combined with 2.5 mg/L propofol, but propofol alone did not.[25] This protocol had a faster onset of action, but longer recovery, than MS-222[25] and may be useful in practice if MS-222 is unavailable.

It should be pointed out that larval zebrafish were not affected by lidocaine baths even at high concentrations. Because larval fish rely more on transcutaneous, rather than branchial, respiration, they seem to be more resistant to the systemic effects of agents administered by immersion that presumably rely on uptake via the gills rather than the skin.[23] Clinicians should be aware that the opposite is true of amphibians, with larval forms (tadpoles) relying more heavily on branchial respiration than adults. Thus, therapeutic baths typically require much lower concentrations for larval amphibians than for adults.

AMPHIBIANS

According to a recently published literature review, doses of local anesthetics used for amphibians are mostly anecdotal and likely extrapolated from recommendations for mammals, with doses of up to 5 mg/kg lidocaine or bupivacaine diluted 3:1 with sodium bicarbonate solution reported.[26] Local administration of 1 mg/kg lidocaine has been recommended for amphibian surgery[27] and has been used as a ring block diluted 1:1 with sodium bicarbonate for digit amputation in an American bullfrog (*Lithobates catesbeianus*) sedated with 7 mg/kg alfaxalone administered intramuscularly.[28] Toe-clipping is a commonly used marking technique to identify amphibians. Lidocaine has been topically applied by a cotton-tipped applicator to the digit of Northern dusky salamanders (*Desmognathus fuscus*) and seal salamanders (*Desmognathus monticola*) until the animals did not withdrawal in response to touch, suggesting local analgesia before toe-clipping.[29]

Therapeutic effects of local anesthesia in amphibians are questionable because even topically administered drugs are likely to be rapidly systemically absorbed.[26] In an experimental study using bullfrogs, 5 mg/kg lidocaine SC did not cause loss of reflexes or change in heart rate but did reduce gular respiratory rate.[30] Bradypnea, progressive loss of righting, palpebral, and withdrawal reflexes occurred at higher doses (50 mg/kg lidocaine SC) with effects lasting up to 4 hours.[30] The authors of that study noted that systemic sedative effects were not associated with analgesia at the site of injection and that frogs responded to noxious stimuli at the injection site even when systemic effects were most profound.[30]

Benzocaine is a local anesthetic available over-the-counter for the treatment of oral pain in humans (10% benzocaine, Regular Strength Orajel, Church & Dwight Co., Inc. Ewing, NJ, USA). A small drop (estimated to weight ~9 mg) was applied to the shoulder or pelvic regions of red-spotted newts (*Notophthalmus viridescens dorsalis*) weighing 0.14 to 1.08 g induced immediate local limb paralysis followed by decreased activity within 3 minutes and surgical anesthesia by 15 minutes.[31] All animals recovered with 15 minutes after rinsing and soaking in anesthetic-free water.[31] Although no adverse effects were reported, clinicians should be aware of the risk of methemoglobinemia secondary to benzocaine exposure, the treatment of choice for which, in amphibians, is methylene blue administered by immersion.

REPTILES

Several local anesthetics including lidocaine, ropivacaine, bupivacaine, tetracaine, mepivacaine, EMLA cream (2.5% lidocaine and 2.5% prilocaine), and Cetacaine spray

(14% benzocaine, 2% butamben, and 2% tetracaine) have been reported for local and topical use in reptiles, and the use of lidocaine (3–5 mg/kg) and, to a lesser extent, bupivacaine to achieve spinal anesthesia has been well documented.[26]

The potential systemic effects of lidocaine administration have been investigated in central bearded dragons (*Pogona vitticeps*) sedated with 10 mg/kg alfaxalone SC.[32] Lidocaine (4 mg/kg) administered into the muscles of a forelimb had no effect on duration or depth of sedation, or on respiratory rate, but the heart rate increased by 28% to 37% for less than 10 minutes following administration.[32] Interestingly, bearded dragons anesthetized with 15 mg/kg alfaxalone SC exhibited an increased depth and duration of sedation and transient increase in heart rate following spinal (intrathecal) administration of 2 mg/kg lidocaine compared to saline controls.[33]

Although local anesthesia may be included as part of a multimodal protocol, 1 mg/kg lidocaine injected at the incision site alone was not sufficient for coelioscopy of juvenile Chinese box turtles (*Cuora flavomarginata*).[34] A drop of lidocaine infused into the facial pits of rattlesnakes (*Crotalus viridis*) apparently blocked the trigeminal nerve and stopped the animals from responding to temperature extremes, both hot and cold, for 25 minutes[35] although the clinical application of this technique is yet to be reported.

Mandibular nerve blocks can be achieved in crocodilians by infiltration of a local anesthetic into the mandibular foramen.[36,37] The technique has been described to achieve a mandibular block for dental surgery in American alligators (*Alligator mississippiensis*), Yacare caiman (*Caiman yacare*), and dwarf crocodiles (*Osteolaemus tetraspis*) using mepivacaine by both external and intraoral approaches,[36] and in juvenile Nile crocodile (*Crocodylus niloticus*) cadavers by the external approach.[37] The external mandibular foramen can be identified by palpation, whereas intraorally a needle should be advanced ventrocaudally along the lingual aspect of the ramus of the mandible.[36] In both cases, the jaw should be secured before manipulation and an appropriate speculum (eg, PVC pipe) used with the intraoral approach.[36]

Spinal administration of local anesthetics for regional anesthesia of the tail, cloaca, and pelvic limbs has been well described in chelonians.[38] The most proximal intervertebral space of the coccygeal vertebrae is identified by palpating the dorsal midline of the tail. The site should be prepared using aseptic technique and the needle advanced maintaining slight negative pressure on the syringe. Aspiration of cerebrospinal fluid confirms accurate placement of the needle. Blood should not be aspirated if the needle is correctly placed. Only preservative-free formulations of lidocaine or bupivacaine should be used when performing this procedure.[38] Examples of dosing regimens reported for chelonians have been summarized in **Table 1**. Similar techniques have been described for central bearded dragons.[33] The dorsal midline between the border of the ilia where the mobile coccygeal vertebrae meet the immobile sacrum should be prepared aseptically.[33] Intrathecal infusion of 2 mg/kg lidocaine resulted in motor and sensory block within 5 minutes of administration and lasted on average 48 minutes (range, 25–100 minutes).[33] Unlike chelonians, accurate placement of the needle cannot be confirmed by aspiration of cerebrospinal fluid in this species.[33]

BIRDS

Published reports of clinical use of local anesthetics in birds vary in dose (2–20 mg/kg lidocaine; 1.5–5 mg/kg bupivacaine) and routes of administration (topical, perineural, subcutaneous, intramuscular, and intervertebral).

In experimental studies, the cardiovascular effects of lidocaine and bupivacaine administered intravenously to chickens (*Gallus gallus domesticus*) under general

Table 1
Published dosing regimens for spinal (intrathecal) anesthesia of chelonians

Dose	Species	Notes
4 mg/kg lidocaine[38] 1 mg/kg bupivacaine[38]	Chelonians	Regional anesthesia of tail, cloaca & pelvic limbs; ~1-h duration for lidocaine and ~2-h duration for bupivacaine
0.1 mL 0.5% bupivacaine/ 10 cm straight carapace length[72]	Green turtle (*Chelonia mydas*)	Surgical excision of cutaneous fibropapillomas
3 mg/kg 2% lidocaine[73]	D'Orbigny's slider (*Trachemys dorbignyi*)	Lasted 82 min with no adverse side effects or change in heart rate
0.2 mL 2% lidocaine/10 cm straights carapace length[74]	Green turtle (*Chelonia mydas*)	Onset of action ≤3 min; full recovery by 90 min; did not affect cranial spine; sufficient for surgical excision of cutaneous fibropapillomas
0.8 mg/kg lidocaine[75]	Galapagos tortoise (*Geochelone nigra*)	Allowed for exteriorization of phallus for phallectomy; EMLA cream also applied topically; all animals were walking within 30–60 min

anesthesia with isoflurane were described. Lidocaine administered intravenously at 6 mg/kg did not induce any cardiovascular side effects, including significant changes in heart rate or mean arterial pressure (MAP),[39] suggesting that peripheral use of lidocaine at this dose is unlikely to cause systemic effects. However, 2 mg/kg bupivacaine caused a significant change in MAP (≥30% from baseline), but no change in heart rate when administered IV.[40] Intra-articular administration of approximately 2 mg/kg bupivacaine relieved signs of pain in chickens with experimentally induced arthritis, but higher doses (≥3 mg/kg) were associated with decreased activity and grooming assumed to be adverse side effects due to systemic absorption of bupivacaine, although this was not further substantiated.[41] That study concluded that the optimum intra-articular dose of bupivacaine to treat musculoskeletal pain in chickens was 3 mg bupivacaine dissolved in 0.3 mL sterile saline.[41] Other potential adverse effects were not evaluated in this study and clinicians should be cautious of intra-articular infusions of local anesthetics as they have been shown to induce chondrolysis.[12,13]

Locally infiltrated lidocaine (2 mg/kg) and bupivacaine (2 mg/kg) have been used in sedated birds for minor surgical procedures as an alternative to general anesthesia.[42] These were used to remove a cutaneous mass at the commissure of the beak of a blue-crowned conure (*Thectocercus acuticaudatus*) and amputate a digit of cockatiel (*Nymphicus hollandicus*).[42] The same doses were used as a splash and incisional block to treat a large skin wound on a chicken.[42] Adverse events were not reported in any case. Topical application of bupivacaine to chickens following beak amputation has been shown to have analgesic effects.[43]

Local anesthetics infused subcutaneously and intramuscularly at incision sites can be used as part of a multimodal anesthetic protocol for intracoelomic surgery.

Bupivacaine was used at incision sites during the surgical placement of intracoelomic radiotransmitters in eiders (*Somateria fischeri*, *Somateria spectabilis*, and *Somateria mollissima*) under general anesthesia with intravenous propofol administered to effect (mean total dose 26.2–45.6 mg/kg).[44] Although doses used were relatively high (2–10 mg/kg), adverse effects from bupivacaine administration were not observed.[44] Mortalities associated with the procedure were attributed to the use of ketoprofen in individuals that may have been dehydrated or otherwise compromised because of histologic renal lesions observed postmortem.[44] A 2:1 mixture of bupivacaine and lidocaine was used at a total dose of 1.5 to 2.0 mg/kg for similar procedures in free-ranging bar-tailed godwit (*Limosa lapponica*) and bristle-thighed curlew (*Numenius tahitiensis*) with no adverse effects attributable to their use observed.[45]

Brachial plexus blockade has been described in mallards (*Anas platyrhynchos*), chickens, and Hispaniolan amazon parrots (*Amazona ventralis*) in 3 experimental studies. Blockade was attempted in mallards using anatomic landmarks from dorsal and axillary approaches[46] and in chickens using nerve locator guidance[47] with either lidocaine or bupivacaine in both studies. In Hispaniolan amazons, blockade was attempted with lidocaine using palpation and ultrasound guidance.[48] Palpable landmarks included the space between the pectoral, triceps, and supracoracoideus aticimus muscles and the insertion of the tendons of the caudal coracobrachial and scapulohumeral muscles (**Fig. 1**).[48] Regardless of the technique used, in each study, the effects were found to be inconsistent and no mortality was associated with the use of amide anesthetics.

A nerve stimulator-guided sciatic-femoral nerve block was described in raptors undergoing surgical treatment of pododermatitis.[49] The authors of the case report considered the technique feasible and effective as no rescue analgesia was necessary during surgery and no complications were observed. A similar technique has been reported to successfully provide regional analgesia to a duck undergoing surgical fixation of a fractured tibiotarsus under general anesthesia.[50] A technique for spinal anesthesia has been developed for chickens. Administration of 0.5 to 2 mg/kg

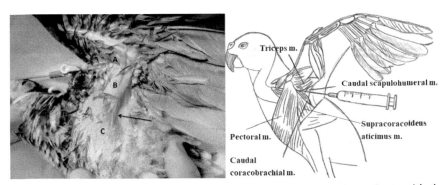

Fig. 1. Hispaniolan amazon parrot (*Amazona ventralis*) under general anesthesia with the wing extended (*left*). Feathers from the axilla have been plucked to show the radius (A), humerus (B), pectoral muscles (C), and site of injection for brachial plexus blockade (*arrow*). Diagram of a Hispaniolan amazon parrot with the wing extended (*right*). The injection site is identified by the pectoral, triceps, and supracoracoideus aticimus muscles, and the insertion of the tendons of the caudal coracobrachial and caudal scapulohumeral muscles. (*Figure adapted from* da Cunha AF, Strain GM, Rademacher N, Schnellbacher R, Tully TN. Palpation- and ultrasound-guided brachial plexus blockade in Hispaniolan Amazon parrots (*Amazona ventralis*). Vet Anaesth Analg. 2013;40: p. 98.)

lidocaine into the subarachnoid space is possible by inserting a 75 mm, 23-gauge needle directed 10° to 20° cranially between the synsacrum and first free coccygeal vertebra.[51] Onset of action was within 1.5 minutes at all doses of lidocaine administered, but the duration was dose-dependent, with the highest dose (2 mg/kg) providing regional anesthesia for approximately 20 minutes.[51] No adverse systemic effects were observed and all birds retained motor function of the pelvic limbs throughout the procedure. Cloacal temperature decreased with time but was not considered clinically significant.[51] This technique may be useful for cloacal procedures in chickens and other Galliformes. Further study is indicated for its application in Psittaciformes and other avian orders.

MAMMALS

Local anesthetics are widely used in mammals. Many techniques have been described in the literature for the prevention and treatment of pain through topical application, or via infiltration into a small area or a major anatomic region such as the brachial plexus, epidural canal, subarachnoid space, and others. The rabbit is considered a good model for epidural technique research[52] and therefore this technique is well described for the species and should be applied into the clinical management of painful conditions of rabbits. The lumbosacral space is usually identified by palpation of landmarks and needle placement in the epidural space verified by lack of resistance or the "hanging drop" technique,[53] although the use of an electrical stimulator can improve the success rate of the epidural injection.[54] This technique has been described for use in small animal practice and has been proven to be effective; it is demonstrated in a video that can be viewed by following the link provided by the QR code in **Fig. 2**. Nerve stimulation may improve the accuracy and safety of local anesthesia techniques, particularly in species for which these techniques have not been well described.

The transversus abdominis plane (TAP) block is often indicated for local anesthesia of the abdominal wall and is used in small animals for any surgery of the abdomen (eg, ovariohysterectomy, abdominal exploratory, splenectomy). As the area for the needle insertion is quite small, this technique is performed with ultrasound guidance and is considered straightforward and effective. In the author's experience, the TAP block may seem challenging, but having observed the fourth-year veterinary students successfully learn the technique, the authors believe that the learning curve for the TAP block is not as steep as for other local anesthetic techniques such as the epidural or the brachial plexus block. The TAP block has been demonstrated in a Canadian lynx (*Lynx canadensis*)[55] and in chinchillas (*Chinchilla lanigera*)[56] with good success.

Equipment needed to perform a TAP block includes an ultrasound with a linear probe, a 2″ 26g needle, and an extension set in addition to the local anesthetic. First, connect the needle to the extension set and prime the line with a local anesthetic. The procedure is performed with the patient in dorsal recumbency after the abdominal area has been clipped and aseptically prepared for surgery. Place the ultrasound probe on the area immediately caudal to the posterior margin of the last rib and lateral to the first thoracic nipple. Identify the peritoneum, internal and external fasciae of the transverse abdominal muscle, and the fasciae of the internal and external oblique muscles. Note that fasciae and peritoneum are hyperechoic to the muscle tissues. Introduce the needle within the ultrasonographic field of view at a 45° angle aiming for the area between the internal fascia of the internal oblique muscle and the external fascia of the transversus abdominalis muscle. This area will be an anechoic line between 2 hyperechoic lines (the fasciae). Maintain the needle in the ultrasonographic

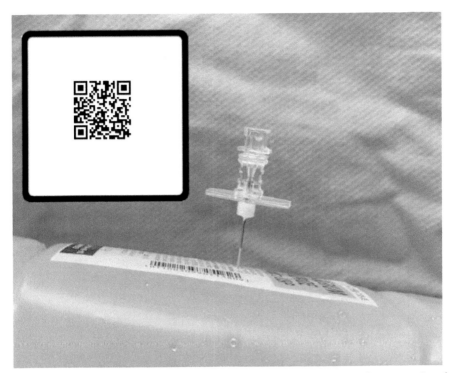

Fig. 2. QR code with YouTube link describing how to perform the "loss of resistance" and "hanging drop" techniques in a model. Please scan this code with your smartphone or copy and paste the following link: https://www.youtube.com/watch?v=vn9LM_iE3VA.

field of view throughout the procedure to avoid entering the abdomen. Once the needle is correctly placed, administer 0.2 mL of local anesthetic. The fascial plane will open and an anechoic oval will be formed as the liquid is injected. If the injection is not administered in the TAP, rather than a well-defined oval appearing, an irregular "explosion" will appear masking the area and preventing a clear view of the fascial planes. If this happens, identify another area and restart the procedure. A tutorial video of a TAP block can be viewed by following the link provided by the QR code in **Fig. 3**.

Alternatively, an incisional infiltration of local anesthetics (line block) could be prescribed to control postoperative pain of abdominal procedures. Line blocks are straightforward to perform and can be done in any species as no precise knowledge of anatomy is necessary. A large volume of local anesthetic drug is injected intramuscularly, about 1 cm away from the incision line.[57]

Clinicians should be aware that line blocks and topical local anesthetics may prolong the healing time of surgical incisions and corneal ulcers, respectively.[58] This may be mediated by the anti-inflammatory effects of local anesthetics or by localized muscle necrosis at the injection site of the line blocks.[58] In a study of dogs undergoing ovariohysterectomy, the effects of bupivacaine line blocks administered preoperatively at the incision site did not have clearly clinically relevant adverse effect on postoperative healing.[57]

Retrobulbar and auriculopalpebral blocks have been well described in domestic animals and in some cases can be transferred to other mammals with minimal adjustments based on species-specific anatomic variances.[59] Retrobulbar blocks are

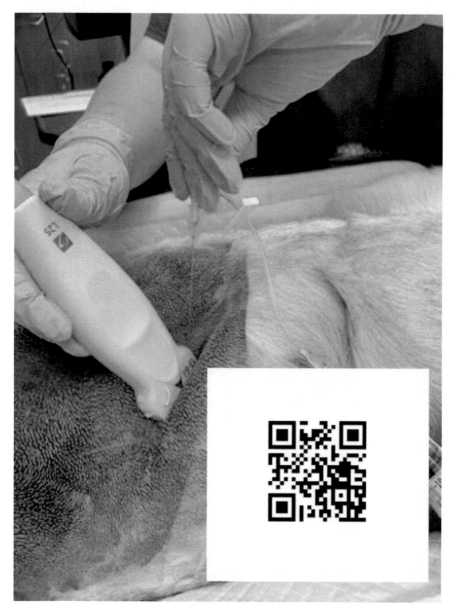

Fig. 3. QR code with YouTube link to a tutorial video on how to perform a transverse abdominal plane block using a dog model. Please scan this code with your smartphone or copy and paste the following link: https://youtube/8I892RRVJ-s.

indicated for enucleation, blepharorrhaphy, and to centralize a ventrally rotated globe for eye examinations during general anesthesia. Auriculopalpebral blocks anesthetize the palpebra and prevent blepharospasm. Gutierrez and colleagues[59] described both techniques for use in California sea lions (*Zalophus californianus*). A retrobulbar block was achieved by administering 4 mg/kg of lidocaine by transpalpebral injection at 2 points, ventrolateral and ventromedial, with 50% of the volume in each site, using a 20-ga, 1 ½ inch needle.[59] The auriculopalpebral nerve block was performed by injecting 2 to 3 mL of lidocaine subcutaneously lateral to the orbital rim, where the auriculopalpebral nerve branch courses over the zygomatic arch.[59] Although not investigated in sea lions, in domestic dogs, a peribulbar block was as effective as a retrobulbar block for analgesia of the eye during enucleation procedures and is safer, more reliable, requires less training to be performed, and has been described in detail.[60] The retrobulbar technique is considered superior to, and more effective than, common splash blocks for postoperative analgesia for enucleations.[61] Splash blocks are simple installations of a local anesthetic into a lesion and, although used often in practice, their effectiveness is questionable. It is possible that the peribulbar block is also more effective than splash blocks, but a study comparing the 3 techniques is needed.

Femoral and sciatic nerve blocks are considered ideal techniques for analgesia and anesthesia of the pelvic limb in many species.[62,63] The sciatic nerve can be located by palpation alone or with the aid of a nerve stimulator, by ultrasound guidance, or a combination of the 2. The sciatic nerve block is performed by palpating the ischiatic tuberosity and greater trochanter with the animal in sternal recumbency and then introducing a needle at the midpoint between the ischiatic tuberosity and the greater trochanter and injecting bupivacaine or ropivacaine at the site. The femoral nerve block is performed with the animal in lateral recumbency. After identifying the femoral artery by palpation, the needle is inserted between the sartorius muscle (cranially) and the femoral artery (caudally). As the femoral artery and vein are very close to the site of injection, always apply negative pressure to the syringe before injection to identify possible intravascular needle placement. The advantage of the ultrasound-guided nerve block is that one can avoid inadvertent intravascular and/or intraneural injections.

Intravenous lidocaine has been investigated in many species to treat neuropathic pain, as an anti-inflammatory and as a gastrointestinal prokinetic. The analgesic effects of intravenous lidocaine have been assessed in Sprague-Dawley rats, dogs,[64] and humans, and seem to effectively reverse the development of neuropathic pain[65] and to treat allodynia in rats.[66] In rabbits, lidocaine administered intravenously as a constant rate infusion (CRI) at 100 µg/kg/min was used for 48 hours postovariohysterectomy. The authors reported better postoperative outcomes with respect to fecal output, food intake, and glucose concentrations in rabbits receiving lidocaine compared with rabbits receiving buprenorphine (0.06 mg/kg IV q 8 h for 2 days).[67] Intravenous lidocaine CRIs have clinical application for the auxiliary treatment of functional ileus and for pain management, including postoperatively. Note that only preservative-free lidocaine without epinephrine should be used intravenously. In dogs[68] and rabbits,[69] lidocaine CRIs are often used to reduce the minimum alveolar concentration (MAC) of inhalant volatile anesthetics and to provide analgesia with no cardiovascular side effects. In cats, however, lidocaine CRIs are contraindicated as they can significantly decrease cardiac output.[70] Therefore, clinicians should be cautious of using lidocaine CRIs in species for which no studies are available as some cardiovascular side effects are likely species-specific.

SUMMARY

Locoregional anesthesia has broad applications as part of a multimodal approach to veterinary anesthesia and analgesia. Its use can reduce the MAC of inhalant anesthetics and mitigate the indication for general anesthesia. Because voltage-gated ion channels are widely conserved across vertebrate taxa,[71] local anesthetics are likely to be effective even in species in which they have not been studied. The same is not true for systemic analgesics, such as opioids for which receptor type, distribution, and affinity can vary widely by species, especially among birds and reptiles. Locoregional anesthesia should continue to be explored to improve anesthetic and analgesic options for species for which limited pharmacologic data are understood.

DISCLOSURE

The authors have nothing to disclose.

REFERENCES

1. Mather LE, Chang DH. Cardiotoxicity with modern local anaesthetics: is there a safer choice? Drugs 2001;61:333–42.
2. Heavner JE. Cardiac toxicity of local anesthetics in the intact isolated heart model: a review. Reg Anesth Pain Med 2002;27:545–55.
3. Scott DB, Lee A, Fagan A, et al. Acute toxicity of ropivacaine compared with that of bupivacaine. Anesth Analg 1989;69:563–9.
4. Groban L, Butterworth J. Local anesthetic systemic toxicity. In: Neal JM, Rathmell JP, editors. Complications in regional anesthesia and pain medicine. Philadelphia, PA: WB Saunders; 2007. p. 55–66.
5. Gristwood RW. Cardiac and CNS toxicity of levobupivacaine: strength of evidence for advantage over bupivacaine. Drug Saf 2007;25:153–63.
6. Catterall WA, Mackie K. Local anesthetics. In: Brunton LL, Lazo JS, Parker KL, editors. Goodman & Gilman's the pharmacological basis of therapeutics. 11th edition. New York, NY: McGraw-Hill Medical; 2006. p. 565–82.
7. Knudsen K, Beckman Suurkula M, Blomberg S, et al. Central nervous and cardiovascular effects of i.v. infusions of ropivacaine, bupivacaine and placebo in volunteers. Br J Anaesth 1997;78:507–14.
8. Wilkie DA, Kirby R. Methemoglobinemia associated with dermal application of benzocaine cream in a cat. J Am Vet Med Assoc 1988;192:85–6.
9. Gyimesi ZS, Burns RB. Presumptive benzocaine-induced methemoglobinemia in a slender-tailed meerkat (Suricata suricatta). J Zoo Wildl Med 2009;40:389–92.
10. Saunders J, Speare DJ, McConkey S. Methemoglobin concnetrations in three salmonid species following exposure to benzocaine or tricaine methanesulfonate. Fish Physiol Biochem 2020;46:2257–63.
11. Hennig GS, Hosgood G, Bubenik-Angapen LJ, et al. Evaluation of chondrocyte death in canine osteochondral explants exposed to a 0.5% solution of bupivacaine. Am J Vet Res 2010;71:875–83.
12. Park J, Sutradhar BC, Hong G, et al. Comparison of the cytotoxic effects of bupivacaine, lidocaine, and mepivacaine in equine articular chondrocytes. Vet Anaesth Analg 2011;38:127–33.
13. Gulihar A, Robati S, Twaij H, et al. Articular cartilage and local anaesthetic: a systematic review of the current literature. J Orthop 2015;31:S200–10.
14. Candido KD, Winnie AP, Covino BG, et al. Addition of bicarbonate to plain bupivacaine does not significantly alter the onset or duration of plexus anesthesia. Reg Anesth 1995;20:133–8.
15. Valvano MN, Leffler S. Comparison of bupivacaine and lidocaine/bupivacaine for local anesthesia/digital nerve block. Ann Emerg Med 1996;27:490–2.
16. Ribotsky BM, Berkowitz KD, Montague JR. Local anesthetics: is there an advantage to mixing solutions? J Am Podiatr Med Assoc 1996;86:487–91.

17. Mettam JJ, Oulton LJ, McCrohan CR, et al. The efficacy of three types of analgesic drugs in reducing pain in the rainbow trout, *Oncorhynchus mykiss*. Appl Anim Behav Sci 2011;133:265–74.
18. Chatigny F, Creighton CM, Stevens ED. Updated review of fish analgesia. J Am Assoc Lab Anim Sci 2018;57:5–12.
19. Chatigny F, Creighton CM, Stevens ED. Intramuscular infiltration of a local anesthetic, lidocaine, does not results in adverse behavioural side effects in rainbow trout. Sci Rep 2018;8:10250.
20. Vergneau-Grosset C, Summa N, Rodriguez CO Jr, et al. Excision and subsequent treatment of a leiomyoma from the periventiduct of a koi (*Cyprinus carpio koi*). J Exot Pet Med 2016;25:194–202.
21. Schroeder PG, LU Sneddon. Exploring the efficacy of immersion analgesics in zebrafish using an integrative approach. Appl Anim Behav Sci 2017;187:93–102.
22. Park I, Park SJ, Gil HW, et al. Anesthetic effects of clove oil and lidocaine-HCl on marine medaka (*Oryzias dancena*). Lab Anim 2011;40:45–51.
23. Collymore C, Banks EK, Turner PV. Lidocaine hydrochloride compared with MS222 for the euthanasia of zebrafish (*Danio rerio*). J Am Assoc Lab Anim Sci 2016;55:816–20.
24. Collymore C, Tolwani A, Lieggi C, et al. Efficacy and safety of 5 anesthetics in adult zebrafish (*Danio rerio*). J Am Assoc Lab Anim Sci 2014;53:198–203.
25. Valentim AM, Félix LM, Carvalho L, et al. A new anaesthetic protocol for adult zebrafish (*Danio rerio*): propofol combined with lidocaine. PLoS ONE 2016;11:e0147747.
26. Chatigny F, Kamunde C, Creighton CM, et al. Uses and doses of local anesthetics in fish, amphibians, and reptiles. J Am Assoc Lab Anim Sci 2017;56:244–53.
27. Gentz EJ. Medicine and surgery of amphibians. ILAR J 2007;48:255–9.
28. Latney LV, Miller E, Pessier AP. Nuptial pad amputation in an American bullfrog (*Lithobates catesbeianus*) with squamous cell carcinoma. J Zoo Wildl Med 2015;46:941–4.
29. Kinkead KE, Lanham JD, Montanucci RR. Comparison of anesthesia and marking techniques on stress and behavioral responses in two *Desmognathus* salamanders. J Herpetol 2006;40:323–8.
30. Williams CJA, Alstrup AKO, Bertelsen MF, et al. When local anesthesia becomes universal: pronounced systemic effects of subcutaneous lidocaine in bullfrogs (*Lithobates catesbeianus*). Comp Biochem Physiol 2017;209:41–6.
31. Brown HHK, Tyler HK, Mousseau TA. Orajel as an amphibian anesthetic: refining the technique. Herpetol Rev 2004;35:252.
32. Ferreira TH, Mans C, Di Girolamo N. Evaluation of the sedative and physiological effects of intramuscular lidocaine in bearded dragons (*Pogona vitticeps*) sedated with alfaxalone. Vet Anaesth Analg 2019;46:496–500.
33. Ferreira TH, Mans C. Evaluation of neuraxial anesthesia in bearded dragons (*Pogona vitticeps*). Vet Anaesth Analg 2019;46:126–34.
34. Hernandez-Divers SJ, Stahl SJ, Farrell R. An endoscopic method for identifying sex of hatchling Chinese box turtles and comparison of general versus local anesthesia for coelioscopy. J Am Vet Med Assoc 2009;234:800–4.
35. Chiszar D, Dickman D, Colton J. Sensitivity to thermal stimulation in prairie rattlesnakes (*Crotalus viridis*) after bilateral anesthetization of the facial pits. Behav Neural Biol 1986;45:143–9.
36. Wellehan JFX, Gunkel CI, Kledzik D, et al. Use of a nerve locator to facilitate administration of mandibular nerve blocks in crocodilians. J Zoo Wildl Med 2006;37:405–8.

37. Bianchi C, Adami C, Dirrig H, et al. Mandibular nerve block in juvenile Nile crocodile: a cadaveric study. Vet Anaesth Analg 2020;47:835–42.
38. Mans C. Clinical technique: intrathecal drug administration in turtles and tortoises. J Exot Pet Med 2014;23:67–70.
39. Brandão J, da Cunha AF, Pypendop B, et al. Cardiovascular tolerance of intravenous lidocaine in broiler chickens (*Gallus gallus domesticus*) anesthetized with isoflurane. Vet Anaesth Analg 2015;42:442–8.
40. DiGeronimo PM, da Cunha AF, Pypendop B, et al. Cardiovascular tolerance of intravenous bupivacaine in broiler chickens (*Gallus gallus domesticus*) anesthetized with isoflurane. Vet Anaesth Analg 2017;44:287–94.
41. Hocking PM, Gentle MJ, Bernard R, et al. Evaluation of a protocol for determining the effectiveness of pretreatment with local analgesic for reducing experimentally induced articular pain in domestic fowl. Res Vet Sci 1997;63:263–7.
42. Lee A, Lennox A. Sedation and local anesthesia as an alternative to general anesthesia in 3 birds. J Exot Pet Med 2016;25:100–5.
43. Glatz PC, Murphy LB, Preston AP. Analgesic therapy of beak-trimmed chickens. Aust Vet J 1992;68:18.
44. Mulcahy DM, Tuomi P, Larsen RS. Differential mortality of male spectacled eiders (*Somateria fischeri*) and king eiders (*Somateria spectabilis*) subsequent to anesthesia with propofol, bupivacaine, and ketoprofen. J Avian Med Surg 2003;17:117–23.
45. Mulcahy DM, Gartrell B, Gill RE, et al. Coelomic implantation of satellite transmitters in the bar-tailed godwit (*Limosa lapponica*) and the bristle-thighed curlew (*Numenius tahitiensis*) using propofol, bupivacaine, and lidocaine. J Zoo Wildl Med 2011;42:54–64.
46. Brenner DJ, Larsen S, Dickinson PJ, et al. Development of an avian brachial plexus nerve block technique for perioperative analgesia in mallard ducks (*Anas platyrhynchos*). J Avian Med Surg 2010;24:24–34.
47. Figueiredo JP, Cruz ML, Mendes GM, et al. Assessment of brachial plexus blockade in chickens by an axillary approach. Vet Anaesth Analg 2008;35:511–8.
48. da Cunha AF, Strain GM, Rademacher N, et al. Palpation- and ultrasound-guided brachial plexus blockade in Hispaniolan Amazon parrots (*Amazona ventralis*). Vet Anaesth Analg 2013;40:96–102.
49. d'Ovidio D, Noviello E, Adami C. Nerve stimulator-guided sciatic-femoral nerve block in raptors undergoing surgical treatment of pododermatitis. Vet Anaesth Analg 2015;42:449–53.
50. Trujanovic R, Otero PE, Larenza-Menzies MP. Ultrasound- and nerve stimulation-guided femoral and sciatic nerve block in a duck (*Anas platyrhynchos*) undergoing surgical fixation of a tibiotarsal fracture. Vet Anaesth Analg 2021;48(2):277–8.
51. Kazemi-Darabadi S, Akbari G, Shokrollahi S. Development and evaluation of a technique for spinal anesthesia in broiler chickens. N Zealand Vet J 2019;67:241–8.
52. Hughes PJ, Doherty MM, Charman WN. A rabbit model for the evaluation of epidurally administered local anaesthetic agents. Anaesth Intensive Care 1993;21:298–303.
53. Greenaway JB, Partlow GD, Gonsholt NL, et al. Anatomy of the lumbosacral spinal cord in rabbits. J Am Anim Hosp Assoc 2001;37:27–34.
54. Otero PE, Portela DA, Brinkyer JA, et al. Use of electrical stimulation to monitor lumbosacral epidural and intrathecal needle placement in rabbits. Am J Vet Res 2012;73:1137–41.

55. Schroeder CA, Schroeder KM, Johnson RA. Transversus abdominis plane block for exploratory laparotomy in a Canadian lynx (*Lynx canadensis*). J Zoo Wildl Med 2010;41:338–41.

56. Saldanha A, Martini R, Basseto JE, et al. Use of transversus abdominis plane block in chinchillas (*Chinchilla lanigera*). J Exot Pet Med 2019;31:21–2.

57. Fitzpatrick CL, Weir HL, Monnet E. Effects of infiltration of the incision site with bupivacaine on postoperative pain and incisional healing in dogs undergoing ovariohysterectomy. J Am Vet Med Assoc 2010;237:395–401.

58. Brower M, Johnson ME. Adverse effects of local anesthetic infiltration on wound healing. Reg Anesth Pain Med 2003;28:233–40.

59. Gutiérrez J, Simeone C, Gulland F, et al. Development of retrobulbar and auriculopalpebral nerve blocks in California sea lions (*Zalophus californianus*). J Zoo Wildl Med 2016;47:236–43.

60. Shilo-Benjamini Y, Pascoe PJ, Maggs DJ, et al. Retrobulbar vs. peribulbar regional anesthesia techniques using bupivacaine in dogs. Vet Ophthalmol 2019;22:183–91.

61. Zibura AE, Posner LP, Ru H, et al. A preoperative bupivacaine retrobulbar block offers superior antinociception compared with an intraoperative splash block in dogs undergoing enucleation. Vet Ophthalmol 2020;23:2225–33.

62. Aguiar J, Mogridge G, Hall J. Femoral fracture repair and sciatic and femoral nerve blocks in a guinea pig. J Small Anim Pract 2014;55:639.

63. Campoy L, Martin-Flores M, Ludders JW, et al. Comparison of bupivacaine femoral and sciatic nerve block versus bupivacaine and morphine epidural for stifle surgery in dogs. Vet Anaesth Analg 2012;39:91–8.

64. MacDougall LM, Hethey JA, Livingston A, et al. Antinociceptive, cardiopulmonary, and sedative effects of five intravenous infusion rates of lidocaine in conscious dogs. Vet Anaesth Analg 2009;36:512–22.

65. Smith LJ, Shih A, Miletic G, et al. Continual systemic infusion of lidocaine provides analgesia in an animal model of neuropathic pain. Pain 2002;97:267–73.

66. Sinnott CJ, Garfield JM, Strichartz GR. Differential efficacy of intravenous lidocaine in alleviating ipsilateral versus contralateral neuropathic pain in the rat. Pain 1999;80:521–31.

67. Schnellbacher RW, Divers SJ, Comolli JR, et al. Effects of intravenous administration of lidocaine and buprenorphine on gastrointestinal tract motility and signs of lidocaine and buprenorphine on gastrointestinal tract motility and signs of pain in New Zealand White rabbits after ovariohysterectomy. Am J Vet Res 2017;78: 1359–71.

68. Ortega M, Cruz I. Evaluation of a constant rate infusion of lidocaine for balanced anesthesia in dogs undergoing surgery. Can Vet J 2011;52:856–60.

69. Marques AEGW, Marques MG, Silveira BCR, et al. Lidocaine administered at a continuous rate infusion does not impair left ventricular systolic and diastolic function of healthy rabbits sedated with midazolam. Vet Anim Sci 2020;10: 100151.

70. Pypendop BH, Ilkiw JE. Assessment of the hemodynamic effects of lidocaine administered IV in isoflurane-anesthetized cats. Am J Vet Res 2005;66:661–8.

71. Zakon HH. Adaptive evolution of voltage-gated sodium channels: the first 800 million years. Proc Nat Acad Sci 2012;109:10619–25.

72. da Silva LCBA, Sellera FP, Nascimento CL, et al. Spinal anesthesia in a green turtle (*Chelonia mydas*) for surgical removal of cutaneous fibropapillomatosis. IOSR J Agric Vet Sci 2016;9:83–6.

73. Hirano LQL, Santos ALQ, Silva JMM, et al. Anestesia espinhal com lidocaína 2% em tigres d'água brasileiros (*Trachemys dorbignyi*). Ciência Anim brasileira 2012; 22:53–8.

74. Futema F, de Carvalho FM, Werneck MR. Spinal anesthesia in green sea turtles undergoing surgical removal of cutaneous fibropapillomas. J Zoo Wildl Med 2020;51:357–62.

75. Rivera S, Divers SJ, Knafo SE, et al. Sterilisation of hybrid Galapagos tortoises (*Geochelone nigra*) for island restoration. Part 2: phallectomy of males under intrathecal anaesthesia with lidocaine. Vet Rec 2011;168:78.

Moving?

Make sure your subscription moves with you!

To notify us of your new address, find your **Clinics Account Number** (located on your mailing label above your name), and contact customer service at:

Email: **journalscustomerservice-usa@elsevier.com**

800-654-2452 (subscribers in the U.S. & Canada)
314-447-8871 (subscribers outside of the U.S. & Canada)

Fax number: **314-447-8029**

Elsevier Health Sciences Division
Subscription Customer Service
3251 Riverport Lane
Maryland Heights, MO 63043

*To ensure uninterrupted delivery of your subscription, please notify us at least 4 weeks in advance of move.

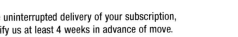

9780323896764